HANDBOOK OF PHARMACEUTICAL TECHNOLOGY

HANDBOOK OF PHARMACEUTICAL TECHNOLOGY

Dr. L.K. Ghosh
B.Pharm. (All India Topper), M.Pharm. (All India Topper), Ph.D.
Reader, Department of Pharmaceutical Technology,
Jadavpur University, Kolkata - 700032
Phone: (033) 413-1433

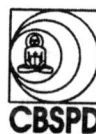

CBSPD

CBS Publishers & Distributors Pvt Ltd

New Delhi • Bengaluru Chennai Kochi Kolkata Mumbai
Hyderabad Jharkhand Nagpur Patna Pune Uttarakhand

**Handbook of
Pharmaceutical
Technology**

ISBN: 978-81-239-0850-2

First Edition: 2002
Reprint: 2003, 2006, 2008, 2010, 2013, 2018, 2019, **2025**

Published by **Satish Kumar Jain** and produced by **Varun Jain** for

CBS Publishers & Distributors Pvt Ltd
4819/XI Prahlad Street, 24 Ansari Road, Daryaganj, New Delhi 110 002, India.
Ph: 011-23266838, 23289259   Website: www.cbspd.com
                                e-mail: delhi@cbspd.com

Corporate Office: 204 FIE, Industrial Area, Patparganj, Delhi 110 092
Ph: 011-4934 4934   Fax: 011-4934 4935
                                e-mail: publishing@cbspd.com; publicity@cbspd.com

Branches

Bengaluru: Seema House 2975, 17th Cross, KR Road, Banasankari 2nd Stage, Bengaluru 560 070, Karnataka, India
Ph: +91-80-26771678/79   Fax: +91-80-26771680   e-mail: bangalore@cbspd.com
Chennai: 18/8B, Subbarayan Street, Shenoy Nagar, Chennai 600 030, Tamil Nadu, India
Ph: +91-44-42032115, 26681266   e-mail: chennai@cbspd.com
Kochi: 42/1325, 1326, Power House Road, Opp KSEB, Power House, Ernakulum Kochi 682 018, Kerala, India
Ph: +91-484-4059061-65,67   Fax: +91-484-4059065   e-mail: kochi@cbspd.com
Kolkata: 147, Hind Ceramics Cornpound, 1st Floor, Nilgunj Road, Belghoria, Kolkata-700056, West Bengal, India
Ph: +033-25633055, 033-25633056   e-mail: kolkata@cbspd.com
Lucknow: Basement, Khushnuma Complex, 7 Meerabai Marg (Behind Jawahar Bhawan), Lucknow-226001, UP, India
Ph: +0522-4000032   e-mail: tiwari.lucknow@cbspd.com
Mumbai: PWD Shed, Gala no 25/26, Ramchandra Bhatt Marg, Next to JJ Hospital Gate no. 2, Opp. Union Bank of India, Noorbaug, Mumbai-400009, Maharashtra, India
Ph: 022-66661880/89   e-mail: mumbai@cbspd.com

Representatives

| Hyderabad | 0-9885175004 | Jharkhand | 0-9811541605 | Nagpur | 0-8692091830 |
| Patna | 0-9334159340 | Pune | 0-9664372571 | Uttar akhand | 0-9716462459 |

Printed at Chaman Enterprises, Daryaganj, Delhi, India

Dedicated

to

My Mentor
Prof. B.K. Gupta

Preface

The personnel practising the noble profession of pharmacy are responsible for producing life-saving medicines, delivering the same to the patients in an effective condition and monitoring the dosage regimen during the entire course of therapy. The pharmaceutical science and technology has undergone revolutionary changes during the last few decades. A student of pharmacy, during the course of study, has to cover a huge syllabi. Before appearing in any competitive examination it is very difficult for them to have a quick look through these fast-changing syllabi. Keeping in view this problem, emphasis has been given to author this book in a most concise and exhaustive manner according to the syllabus approved by the Pharmacy Council of India.

This book encompasses four subjects, viz. Pharmaceutics I, Pharmaceutics II, Pharmacognosy and Pharmaceutical Jurisprudence (Forensic Pharmacy). Model questions are incorporated topic-wise, chapterwise or subjectwise in such a manner that in many cases informations provided through these are not included in the text to reduce the size of this book. It may be used as a textbook by both diploma and degree students and at the same time it will provide valuable and necessary information to all concerned appearing for any competitive examination in pharmacy including GATE.

I am grateful to my friend, philosopher and guide Prof. B.K. Gupta for his continuous guidance and encouragement; and to my students for their assistance during preparation of the manuscript.

I am also thankful to the authority of Jadavpur University, particularly our Vice-Chancellor, Prof. A.N. Basu, and Finance Officer, Mr. G.K. Pattanayak for their moral support.

I am also grateful to all authors whose books I have consulted.

My thanks are also due to the CBS Publishers & Distributors for their keen interest in publishing this book. I would greatly appreciate if readers bring suggestions, criticisms, omissions and errors to my attention for further improvement of this book.

L.K. Ghosh

Contents

SECTION III
Pharmacognosy 199-264

SECTION IV
Forensic Pharmacy/Pharmaceutical Jurisprudence 265-283

CHAPTER 1

Familiarization With
New Drug Delivery Systems

• New Drug Delivery Systems

The main objective of sustained/controlled/prolonged release formulation

The formulation is designed in such a way that minimum effective plasma concentration (MEC) level of drug should attain quickly and thereafter the rate of entry of drug to the body should equal with the rate of total elimination or inactivation of drug from the body. As a result the plasma drug concentration curve will run parallel to the time axis just above the MEC level. Following are the examples of some of the advantages associated with sustained released formulations :

   (i) Patient will get uninterrupted therapeutic response for a prolonged period.

   (ii) Toxicity associated with peak plasma concentrations and chances of drug resistance associated with 'deep' ineffective plasma drug concentrations would be diminished.

  (iii) Frequency of drug administration is reduced, therefore, compliance to the patient as well as nursing staffs.

  (iv) Much lesser amount of drug is essential for the entire course of therapy. On the other hand multidose conventional delivery systems are wasteful.

Few Latest Delivery Systems

   (i) Microencapsulation : In this technique the drug along with a suitable polymer(s) are transformed to numerous micro-capsules. Few hundreds of such solid microcapsules containing a definite amount of drug is then taken in a hard gelatin capsule shell or compressed into a quickly disintegrating tablet for administration to the patient. This formulation now-a-days is widely used as sustained release formulation as the entrapped drug releases slowly from the microcapsule.

(ii) Nano-particles : In this case also the entrapped or adsorbed drug is released slowly giving sustained action and the sizes of the particles permit i.v. administration.

(iii) Transdermal drug delivery system : Our skin can absorb a considerable amount of drug to initiate and continue physiological responses. The drug with moderate lipid-water partition co-efficient (not too hydrophilic or too lipophilic) can be delivered as transdermal patch alongwith pressure sensitive adhesive. The patient is directed to fix up the patch onto the particular area of skin and also remove the patch when the drug action is not required. Examples include :
   a. Transdermal scopolamine to control motion sickness.
   b. Transdermal testosterone.
   c. Transdermal oestrogen to female during post menopausal period.
   d. Transdermal antianginal preparation.

(iv) Liposomal drug delivery system.

(v) Multiple emulsions.

(vi) Monoclonal antibody tagged drug delivery system.

(vii) Drug loaded erythrocytes.

(viii) Iontophoretic techniques.

(ix) Controlled release suppository.

(x) Prodrug for sustained drug action.

MODEL QUESTIONS

1. In general, the various oral dosage forms can be ranked in which of the following expected order of availability (fastest to slowest)
   A. aqueous solution > capsule > tablet > powder > coated tablet > suspension
   B. capsule > tablet > coated tablet > powder > suspension > aqueous solution
   C. aqueous solution > suspension > powder > capsule > tablet > coated tablet
   D. suspension > aqueous solution > powder > capsule > coated tablet > tablet
   E. aqueous solution > suspension > capsule > powder > coated tablet > tablet

2. Whenever a drug is more rapidly and /or more completely absorbed from a solution than from a solid dosage form,
   A. it is due to the fact that the solid dosage form did not disintegrate
   B. it indicates that the solid dosage form is poorly formulated
   C. a solution is the only practical oral formulation
   D. it is likely that absorption is rate limited by the dissolution process
   E. none of the above.

3. The term "Prodrug" refers to a
   A. drug that is classified as being "probably effective"
   B. chemical substance that is part of the synthesis procedure in preparing a drug.

C. drug that has only prophylactic activity in the body

D. compound which may be therapeutically active but is still under clinical trials.

E. compound that liberates an active drug in the body.

4. Transdermal applications are popular for the administration of

A. antidiabetic drugs

B. cardiac stimulants

C. tranquilisers

D. coronary vasodilators.

5. Liposomes are

A. uni or multilayered vesicles of phospholipids

B. type of enzymes

C. fibrinopeptides

D. red blood cells

E. none of the above.

6. The term bioavailability refers to the

A. relationship between the physical & chemical properties of a drug and the systemic absorption of the drug.

B. measurement of the rate and amount of therapeutically active drug that reaches the systemic circulation

C. movement of drug into the body tissues over time.

D. dissolution of a drug in the G.I. tract.

E. all the above.

7. Match the following dosage forms with a primary advantage of each

(i)	Sublingual tablets	A.	Sustained action
(ii)	Kapseals	B.	Rapid solubility
(iii)	Repetabs	C.	Tamper proof
(iv)	Medihaler	D.	Metered dose
(v)	Effervescent salts	E.	Improved.

ANSWERS

1. C; 2. D; 3. E [Sometimes biologically active drugs are chemically modified in order to improve the pharmacodynamic or pharmaceutical qualities. These modified molecules (prodrug) are not active in *in vitro* but in *in vivo* condition. Upon biotransformation, the metabolite becomes active]; 4. D; 5. A [Liposome is defined as structure consisting of one or more concentric spheres of lipid bilayers, separated by water or aqueous buffer compartments. If other conditions (such as sterility, homogeneity, pyrogen free etc.) are fulfilled this delivery system can be directly administered intravenously. Phospholipids and other derivatives of phosphatidic acid are used to produce liposomal vesicles]; 6. B; 7. i - B; ii - C; iii - A; iv - D; v - E.

CHAPTER 2

Introduction to Pharmacopoeias With Special Reference to the Indian Pharmacopoeia

- Introduction to Pharmacopoeias

Pharmacopoeia is an official book consisting of monographs of different drugs and their formulations which are official in that pharmacopoeia. Monograph of a drug may include its name, formulas etc., category, dose, description, solubility, storage, standards, identification, pH, clarity and color of soluion, specific optical rotation, related substances, sulfated ash, loss on drying, assay etc. In case of individual dosage forms monographs may include other requirements. As for example, in case of tablet dosage form it may include disintegration test, dissolution test etc.

The first pharmacopoeia of India was published in 1868. It was prepared under the authority of the Secretary of State for India in Council by an Indian Pharmacopoeia Committee constituted in 1865. It was edited by Edward John Waring. After independence an Indian Pharmacopoeia Committee was constituted in 1948, which prepared the Pharmacopoeia of India (The Indian Pharmacopoeia) 1955. A supplement to the first edition of I.P. was published in 1960. This pharmacopoeia contained western & also traditional drugs. The second edition of I.P. was published in 1966 and its supplement in 1975. Similarly, the third edition of I.P. was published in two volumes in 1985 and its Addenda in 1989 & 1991. In this edition traditional drugs were not included as publication of pharmacopoeia of traditional system drugs was taken up separately and only those herbal drugs were included which had supporting definite quality control standards. Finally the latest i.e., 4th edition of I.P. was published in two volumes in 1996 by the Ministry of Health and Family Welfare, Govt. of India.

I.P.   = The Pharmacopoeia of India
B.P.   = The British Pharmacopoeia
B.P.C.   = British Pharmaceutical Codex
USP   = The United States Pharmacopoeia ⎤
N.F.   = National Formulary   ⎦ Combined

CHAPTER 3

Metrology and Pharmaceutical Calculations

- Systems of Weights and Measures
- Pharmaceutical Calculations including Conversion from One to Another System
- Percentage Calculations and Adjustments of Products
- Use of Alligation Method in Calculations
- Isotonic Solutions
- Proof Spirit, Denatured Alcohol and Alcohol Dilutions

Sensitivity of an analytical balance : The smallest weight to which the balance responds when loaded to capacity (the capacity is marked on the instrument).

Minimum Weighable Amounts : It is generally accepted that the error in the amount of any ingredients in a dispensed preparation should not be more than ± 5%. The percentage of error would be much more if weighable amount is very less. In order to avoid this, the minimum weighable amount should not be less than 100 mg (or 2 gr.). In some country like Sweden, the minimum weighable amount is 300 mg. In the USA a minimum of 200 mg is recommended in the National Formulary (N.F) for prescription balances with a sensitivity ratio of 10 mg. This is a wise precaution in case of weighing potent drugs (i.e., one with a maximum dose of 50 mg or less).

Percentage Calculations

Problem 1

Calculate the quantity of sodium chloride required for 500 ml of a 0.9% solution.

Ans.   100 ml solution contains 0.9 g sodium chloride.

500 ml solution contains (0.9 × 500/100) = 4.5 g of NaCl.

Problem 2

Send 100 ml of a solution of potassium permanganate of which 1 part diluted with seven parts of water makes a 1 in 8000 solution.

Ans.   8000 ml dilute solution contains 1 g of $KMnO_4$

∴ 1 ml dilute solution contains 1/8000 g of $KMnO_4$

∴ (1 + 7 = 8) ml dilute solution contains 1 × 8/8000 g of $KMnO_4$

This 8 ml dilute solution is actually produced by diluting 1 ml stock solution.

∴ 1 ml of stock solution contains 0.001 g of $KMnO_4$

∴ 100 ml of stock solution contains 0.001 × 100 g = 0.1 g of $KMnO_4$

Therefore, the strength of the stock solution/concentrate

= 0.1% (w/v).

Problem 3

Supply 10 capsules each containing 600 µg of hyoscine hydrobromide.

Ans.   Total amount of hyosine hydrobromide in 10 capsules is 6000 µg = 6 mg.

But the minimum weighable amount should be at least 100 mg. This 100 mg of hyoscine hydrobromide to be mixed up with sufficient amount of an inert diluent such as lactose by way of geometric dilution process. The weighable amount of this final mixture also should not be less than 100 mg containing 600 µg of hyoscine hydrobromide, to be encapsulated in hard gelatin capsule.

Parts Per Million (ppm)

1 ppm = 1 part solute per 1 million parts of solution.

similarly, 5 ppm = 5 parts solute per 1 million parts of solution.

i.e., 10,00000 parts solution contain 5 parts solute

100 parts solution contain 5 × 100/10,00000 parts solute

= 0.0005% (w/v)

i.e., 5 ppm solution = 0.0005% (w/v) solution.

Mixing Different Strengths

What is the percent of alcohol in a mixture made by mixing 5 lit of 25% (v/v), 1 lit of 50% (v/v) and 1 lit of 95% (v/v) alcohol?

Ans.   Determine the total amount of alcohol in the 3 solutions and the total amount of solution (1 lit = 1000 ml).

Assume additivity of volumes on mixing.

25% × 5000 ml = 1250 ml 100% alcohol

50% × 1000 ml = 500 ml 100% alcohol

95% × 1000 ml = 950 ml 100% alcohol

Total volume = 7000 ml ≡ 2700 ml 100% alcohol

i.e., 7000 ml mixture contains 2700 ml pure alcohol

100 ml mixture contains 2700 × 100/7000 = 38.57 ml pure alcohol.

Therefore, the strength of the final solution be 38.57% (v/v)

Alligation Alternate :

How much ml of 80% alcohol to be mixed with 200 ml of 30% alcohol to produce 70% alcohol.

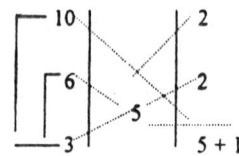

i.e., 4 parts of 80% alcohol and 1 part of 30% alcohol if mixed up then the final strength would be 70%.

Now 1 part of 30% alcohol to be mixed up with 4 parts of 80% alcohol

∴ 200 parts of 30% alcohol to be mixed up with 4 × 200 parts of 80% alcohol

= 800 ml

Calculation by Alligation Alternate or by The Method of Rectangles

Example 1 : In what proportion 10%, 6% and 3% alcohol be mixed to get 5% alcohol?

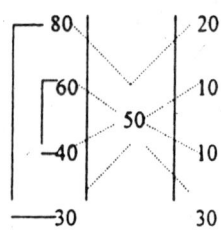

∴ Thus, the proportion for mixing would be 2 : 2 : 6 to get 5% alcohol.

Example 2 : How many parts of 80%, 60%, 40% and 30% alcohol be mixed together to get 50% alcohol?

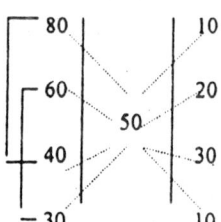

Thus, the proportion for mixing of 80%, 60%, 40% and 30% alcohol would be

(i)   20 : 10 : 10 : 30   or   2 : 1 : 1 : 3

(ii) 10 : 20 : 30 : 10   or   1 : 2 : 3 : 1

(iii) 30 : 30 : 40 : 40   or   3 : 3 : 4 : 4

Relationships of Weights and of Measures

1 fluidounce	=	30 ml (29.57 ml)
1 pint	=	473 ml
1 gallon	=	8 pint = 3785 ml
1 kilogram	=	2.2 lb.

1 pound	=	453.59 g.
1 gram	=	15.4 gr. (15.432 gr.)
1 grain	=	65 mg (64.8 mg)
1 apothecary dram	=	60 gr.
1 tumblerful	=	240 ml
1 teacupful	=	120 ml
1 wine glassful	=	60 ml
1 tablespoonful	=	15 ml
1 dessertspoon full	=	8 ml
1 teaspoonful	=	5 ml
1 fluid dram	=	4 ml = 4 × 15 = 60 minims.
1 ml	=	16.23 minims ≈ 15 minims
1 drop	=	0.062 ml = 1 minim

Proof Spirit : For tax purposes, the US government calculates the strength of pure or absolute alcohol by means of proof degrees. 100° proof spirit contains 50% (by volume) or 42.49% (by weight). Thus, 2 proof degrees equals 1% (by volume) of ethyl alcohol.

'Above Proof' and 'Below Proof' : The term 10 degrees under proof (10 UP) signifies that 100 volumes of the spirit contains 90 volumes of proof spirit plus 10 volumes of water i.e., 45% (by volume). On the other hand 30 degrees over proof (30° OP) indicates that 100 volumes diluted with water yields 130 volumes of proof spirit i.e., 65% (by volume).

Alcohol Dilutions : Measure the alcohol (say 500 ml) and the purified water (say 500 ml) separately at the same temperature, and mix. If the water and the alcohol and the resulting mixture are measured at 25°, the volume of the mixture will be about 970 ml.

During dilution of absolute alcohol with purified water there would be evolution of heat and also there is a considerable shrinkage of the volume due to **hydrogen bonding**. To prepare proof spirit, 50 volumes of C_2H_5OH are mixed with 53.71 volumes of water to allow for the contraction which occurs to yield 100 volumes of product.

Denatured Alcohol : Denatured alcohol is ethyl alcohol to which have been added such denaturing materials as to render the alcohol unfit for use as an intoxicating beverage. This may be of two types, a. Completely Denatured Alcohol and b. Specially Denatured Alcohol.

For the purpose of denaturation the materials used are, methyl alcohol, pyridine, gasoline, kerosene, methyl isobutyl ketone etc.

70% (v/v) alcohol has the **highest germicidal activity**.

Milliequivalents

1 equivalent = 1000 milliequivalents (mEq)

i.e., 1 mEq = 1 Eq. Wt / 1000

e.g., one mEq of K^+ (ion) combines with 1 mEq of Cl^- to give 1 mEq of KCl

The Eq. Wt of KCl ≅ 74.5 g of KCl ≅ 74500 mg of KCl

∴ 1 mEq of KCl ≅ 74.5 mg of KCl (1 mEq K^+ is 39 mg + 1 mEq Cl^- is 35.5 mg).

Problem 1

A solution that contains 409.5 mg of NaCl/100 ml has how many mEq of Na^+ and Cl^-?

Ans.   1 mEq wt of NaCl = 58.5 mg
i.e., 58.5 mg = 1 mEq wt of NaCl
1 mg = 1/58.5 mEq wt of NaCl
∴ 409.5 mg = 409.5/58.5 mEq wt of NaCl
= 7
∴ 7 mEq wt. of NaCl dissociates to 7 mEq of Na^+ and 7 mEq of Cl^-.

Problem 2

A prescription requires 500 ml of sodium chloride to be made so that it will contain 500 mEq of Na^+. How many grams of NaCl (MW = 58.5) are required?

Ans.   1 equivalent wt. NaCl = 1 molecular wt. NaCl = 1000 mEq of Na^+Cl^- = 1000 mEq of Na^+ as well as 1000 mEq of Cl^-
Therefore, 1000 mEq of Na^+ ≡ 58.5 g of NaCl
∴ 500 „ „ „ ≡ 29.25 g of NaCl.
Therefore, 29.25 g of NaCl is to be dissolved to make 500 ml solution containing 500 mEq of Na^+.

Osmotic Pressure

Blood plasma and lachrymal secretion (tear) have the same osmotic pressure. Taking blood plasma for comparison, a solution with lower osmotic pressure is-said to be **hypotonic** and one with a **higher** osmotic pressure **hypertonic**. Both these are **paratonic** i.e., not isotonic. 0.9% w/v sodium chloride solution is considered isotonic (same tonicity) with blood plasma. Hypertonic and hypotonic solutions are responsible for **crenation** and **hemolysis** respectively.

General Principles for Adjustment to Isotonicity

   (i) Solutions for I.V. Injection : Isotonicity is always desirable.

   (ii) Solutions for Subcutaneous Injection (less than 1 ml) : Desirable and almost essential.

   (iii) Solutions for I.M. Injection (2 ml) : Aqueous solution should be slightly hypertonic to promote rapid absorption. Aqueous depot formulation should be isotonic, a hypertonic vehicle might hasten absorption.

   (iv) Solutions for Intracutaneous Injection (0.2 ml) : Diagnostic preparations should be isotonic since a paratonic solution might cause a false reaction.

   (v) Solutions for Intrathecal Injection (within 10 ml) : These must be isotonic. The volume of the cerebrospinal fluid is only 60-80 ml, hence a small volume of paratonic solution will disturb the osmotic pressure and may cause vomiting and other effects.

   (vi) Isotonic Solutions for Topical Application : Aqueous solutions applied within the nostrils and also to areas of broken skin may prove irritant if paratonic and, therefore, it is desirable to make them isotonic with blood plasma.

   (vii) Isotonic Solutions for Ophthalmic Use : Adjustment of ophthalmic solutions depends on their volume. It is not essential for eye-drops because they are of small volume and quickly diluted by the lachrymal secretion. With eye-lotions, however, much larger volumes, are brought into contact with the eye, and isotonicity is advisable to avoid irritation of the delicate conjunctiva.

Reverse Osmosis

In case of osmosis the solvent moves from a region of lower concentration to a region of higher concentration through semipermeable membrane. Now by increasing the external pressure over concentrated solution it is possible to move the solvent from higher concentration region to lower concentration region through semipermeable membrane. This phenomenon is known as reverse osmosis.

Calculation for Solution's Iso-osmotic with Blood and Tears

1. Based on Freezing-point Data :

Determination of the depression of freezing-point is simpler and more accurate than direct measurement of osmotic pressure, and is therefore used to compare osmotic pressures.

The temperature at which blood plasma and tear freeze is –0.52°C, i.e., the dissolved substances which they contain depress the freezing point 0.52° below that of pure water and any other solution which freezes at –0.52°C will have the same osmotic pressure as blood plasma and tears.

All hypotonic solutions have a freezing point higher than these two fluids; for instance, a 1% (w/v) solution of procaine hydrochloride freezes at –0.122°C. In order to render this solution iso-osmotic an adjusting substance must be added to reduce the freezing point upto –0.52°C. The proportion of adjusting substance required is that which will produce a solution with a freezing point –0.398°C, i.e., the difference between –0.52 and –0.122°C.

Therefore, % (w/v) of adjusting substance needed = (0.52 – a)/b

where, 'a' = figure representing the freezing point of the unadjusted solution

and 'b' = figure representing the freezing point of a 1% (w/v) solution of the adjusting substance.

Problem 1

Find the concentration of sodium chloride required to render a 1.5% solution of procaine hydrochloride iso-osmotic with blood plasma. [The freezing point of a 1% (w/v) solution of procaine hydrochloride is –0.122°C, and that of a 1% (w/v) solution of NaCl is –0.576°C].

Ans. $\dfrac{0.52 - (0.122 \times 1.5)}{0.576} = 0.585\%$ w/v

[N.B. : The freezing point depression is proportionate with the concentration of the dissolved solute.]

Problem 2

Find the amount of sodium chloride to be included in 100 ml of a 0.3% solution of zinc sulphate so that, on dilution with an equal quantity of water it will be iso-osmotic with tissue fluids [The freezing point of a 1% solution of zinc sulphate is –0.086°C and that of a 1% (w/v) solution of sodium chloride is –0.576°C].

Ans.   In this particular case the general formula should be modified as

$$\frac{(2 \times 0.52) - a}{b} = \frac{1.04 - (0.3 \times 0.086)}{0.576} = 1.76$$

Therefore, in 100 ml there will be 1.76 g of NaCl.

2. Based on Molecular Concentration :

The osmotic pressure of blood plasma and lachrymal secretion is approximately 6.7 atmosphere; hence, the molarity of these fluids is $6.7/22.4 = 0.3$ M approximately. Consequently, a 0.3M solution of any non-ionizing solute will be iso-osmotic with plasma and tears.

Problem 1

Find the concentration of anhydrous dextrose needed to produce a solution iso-osmotic with blood -plasma.

Ans.   The molecular wt. of dextrose is 180 and it is non-ionising.

∴ $0.3 \times 180 = 54$ g per lit is required (The B.P. uses 5%).

If the solute ionises in solution this is assumed to be complete and the following formula is used

$$W = \frac{0.3M}{N}$$

where, W = Amount required in g per liter.

M = Molecular wt. of the solute

N = No. of ions produced from each molecule of the solute

assuming that dissociation is complete.

Solutions that are not iso-osmotic are adjusted by adding a suitable substance, such as sodium chloride or dextrose, to produce a total concentration of solutes equivalent to a 0.3M concentration of a non-ionising solute. The calculation involves three steps :

  (i) The effective molar concentration (EMC) of the medicament is found, including due allowance for ionization if necessary.

 (ii) This is subtracted from 0.3 to obtain the effective molar concentration of the adjusting substance.

(iii) The latter is converted to g per liter, again allowing for ionisation, if necessary.

If the original solution contains two or more medicaments the EMC for each is determined and the sum of these is subtracted from 0.3 to obtain the EMC of the adjusting substance.

Problem 1

Find the concentration of sodium chloride required to produce a solution iso-osmotic with blood plasma.

Solution : The molecular weight of sodium chloride is 58.5 and it dissociates into 2 ions.

∴ $W = \frac{0.3M}{N} = \frac{0.3 \times 58.5}{2} = 8.8$ g per litre (0.88% w/v)

(The B.P. uses 0.90%)

Problem 2

Find the concentration of dextrose required to make a 0.12% solution of sodium chloride iso-osmotic with blood plasma.

Solution : As sod. chloride ionises, the formula $W = 0.3M/N$ is used, substituting 'c' [representing the effective molar concentration (EMC) of medicament] for 0.3.

$$1.2 = \frac{C \times 58.5}{2}$$

$\therefore$ $C = 0.041$

Therefore, effective molar concentration of adjusting substance (dextrose) $= 0.3 - 0.041 = 0.259$.

$\therefore$ Required concentration of dextrose $= 0.259 \times M = 0.259 \times 180$

$= 46.62$ g per liter i.e., 4.662% w/v

3. Based on Sodium chloride Equivalents :

The sodium chloride equivalent or "E" value may be defined as the amount of sodium chloride that will produce the same osmotic effect as 1g of the specified chemicals.

$$\text{Sodium chloride equivalent of 'A'} = \frac{\text{Freezing point depression produced by a solution of A}}{\text{Freezing point depression produced by a sodium chloride solution of the same strength}}$$

e.g., the freezing point depression produced by 1% w/v ascorbic acid solution = 0.105°C

and the   ,,   ,,   ,,   ,,   ,, 1% w/v NaCl solution = 0.576°C

$\therefore$ Sodium chloride equivalent of 1% ascorbic acid = 0.105/0.576 = 0.18

Now the % of sodium chloride for adjustment to isotonic

$= 0.9 -$ (percentage strength of medicament solution $\times$ sodium chloride equivalent of medicament)

When adjustment is to be made with a substance other than sodium chloride first calculate the required % of sodium chloride and then divide this by the sodium chloride equivalent of the chosen adjusting substance (e.g., problem 2).

Problem 1

Calculate the % of sodium chloride required to render a 0.5% solution of potassium chloride iso-osmotic with blood plasma. Sodium chloride equivalent of 0.5% KCl = 0.76.

Solution :

$\therefore$ Percentage of NaCl for adjustment $= 0.9 - (0.5 \times 0.76) = 0.9 - 0.38 = 0.52$

Problem 2

Calculate the % of anhydrous dextrose require to render a 1% solution of ephedrine hydrochloride iso-osmotic with body fluids.

Sodium chloride equivalent of 1% ephedrine hydrochloride = 0.30; sodium chloride equivalent of anhydrous dextrose = 0.18

Solution :

$\therefore$ % of NaCl for adjustment $= 0.9 - (1 \times 0.3) = 0.6$

$\therefore$ Equivalent % of anhydrous dextrose $= 0.6/0.18 = 3.3$

MODEL QUESTIONS

1. A solution contains 3 gr. of a drug per fluidounce. What is the % w/v of the solution?

   A. 0.59%
   B. 0.66%
   C. 1.0%
   D. 6.5%
   E. 10.0%

2. In preparing a pint of a 1 : 5000 solution of $HgCl_2$, a pharmacist should use

   A. 190 mg
   B. 95 mg
   C. 19 mg
   D. 9.5 mg
   E. none of the above.

3. How many grams of aspirin must be dissolved in 484 c.c. of alcohol to make a 12% solution?

   A. 76
   B. 66
   C. 112
   D. 48
   E. 58

4. How many milliliters of concentrated HCl (37% w/w) with a specific gravity of 1.35 should be used to make 4 fluidounces of a 5% (w/v) solution?

   A. 0.12 ml
   B. 120 ml
   C. 1.2 ml
   D. 9 ml
   E. 12 ml

5. The boiling point of alcohol is 78°C. The corresponding temperature in degrees Fahrenheit is

   A. 46
   B. 10
   C. 172
   D. 156
   E. 140

6. Glycerin has a specific gravity of 1.25. One gallon weighs

   A. 128 g
   B. 473 g
   C. 591.25 g
   D. 4730 g
   E. 4800 g

7. −12°C is equivalent to

   A. 36°F
   B. 12°F
   C. 10.4°F
   D. 5°F
   E. −2°F

8. Based upon relative sensitivity requirements, the class A prescription balance is how many times more sensitive than the class B balance?

   A. 2
   B. 5
   C. 10
   D. 20
   E. 100

9. A pharmacist adds 30 ml of 6% Dilute Acetic Acid USP to a 1 liter bottle of Sodium Chloride Irrigation USP. What is the percent w/v concentration of acetic acid in the final dilution?

   A. 0.15%
   B. 0.175%
   C. 0.18%
   D. 0.19%
   E. 0.52%

10. How much Keri Lotion must be mixed with 45 g of triamcinolone cream (0.1% w/w) to obtain a final triamcinolone concentration of 0.015%?

   A. 38.3 g
   B. 45 g
   C. 210 g
   D. 255 g
   E. 300 g

11. How many ml of 17% Zephiran chloride concentrate are needed to prepare 2 quarts of a 1 : 1000 solution?

    A. 11.2   B. 17.0   C. 22.4

    D. 44.8   E. None of the above.

12. What is the minimum volume that should be measured in a 100 ml conical graduate that is calibrated in 5 ml intervals from 5 to 100 ml?

    A. 5 ml   B. 10 ml   C. 15 ml

    D. 20 ml   E. 30 ml

13. How many mg of sodium chloride should be present in the following formula to obtain an isotonic solution? (E value of cocaine hydrochloride is 0.16)

    Cocaine hydrochloride   2%
    Sodium chloride   q.s.
    Purified water q.s.   30 ml

    A. 48 mg   B. 96 mg   C. 174 mg

    D. 222 mg   E. None of these.

14. Determine the number of grains of silver nitrate needed to prepare three fluidounces of a 0.5% silver nitrate solution.

    A. 2.9 gr.   B. 6.8 gr.   C. 7.2 gr.

    D. 22.5 gr.   E. 45 gr.

15. How many grams of 2% aluminum paste must be mixed with a 10% aluminum paste to prepare exactly 120 g of 5% strength?

    A. 6 g   B. 24 g   C. 45 g

    D. 48 g   E. 75 g

16. A hospital pharmacy needs 1 gallon of Dilute Hydrochloric Acid USP (10% w/v). How many ml of Hydrochloric Acid USP (36% w/w; specific gravity = 1.18) will be needed?

    A. 320   B. 378   C. 891

    D. 1051   E. 1240

17. The injection form of Calcium gluconate $Ca(C_7H_{13}O_8)_2$, contains 1 g of drug in 10 ml of solution. How many milliequivalents of calcium are present? (atomic wt Ca = 40; mol. wt. Calcium gluconate = 430),

    A. 0.78   B. 2.30   C. 4.7

    D. 50.0   E. 430

18. Lanoxin Pediatric Elixir contains 0.05 mg of digoxin per ml. How many micrograms (μg) are there in 3 ml of the elixir?

    A. 0.0015   B. 0.015   C. 0.15

    D. 1.5   E. None of the above

19. According to USP specifications, which one of the following equivalents should be used to convert a grain measurement to milligrams when compounding prescriptions?

    A. 15.4 mg   B. 60 mg   C. 62.5 mg

    D. 64.8 mg   E. 65 mg

20. How many ml of a 0.5% gentian violet stock solution are needed to prepare one gallon of a 1 :2000 solution?

    A. 47   B. 94.5   C. 200

    D. 378   E. None of the above.

21. Dopamine 200 mg in 500 ml of normal saline at 5 µg/kg/min is ordered for a 155 lb. patient. What is the final concentration of solution in µg/ml?

    A. 0.4   B. 2.5   C. 40

    D. 400   E. 25

22. Referring to the previous question, at what rate should the solution be infused to deliver the desired dose of 5 µg/kg/min?

    A. 0.35 ml/min   B. 0.40 ml/min   C. 0.88 ml/min

    D. 2.0 ml/min   E. 5.0 ml/min

23. A physician requests one pound of bacitracin ointment containing 200 units of bacitracin per gram. How many grams of bacitracin ointment (500 units/gram) must be used to make this ointment?

    A. 182 g   B. 200 g   C. 227 g

    D. 362 g   E. None of the above.

24. A 250 ml infusion bottle contains 5.86 g of potassium chloride. How many milliequivalents of potassium chloride are present? (molecular weight of KCl = 74.6)

    A. 12.7   B. 20   C. 78.5

    D. 150   E. None of the above

25. Calcium chloride ($CaCl_2$. $2H_2O$) has a formula weight of 147. What weight of the chemical is needed to obtain 40 mEq of calcium (Ca = 40.1; Cl = 35.5; H_2O = 18)?

    A. 0.80 g   B. 1.47 g   C. 2.22 g

    D. 2.94 g   E. 5.88 g

26. The official potassium iodide solution contains 100 g of KI in a total volume of 100 ml (dl) of solution. The density of this saturated solution is approximately 1.7 g/ml. Express this concentration of the solution in terms of % (w/w).

    A. 17%   B. 59%   C. 70%

    D. 100%   E. 170%

27. For a class A prescription balance rating, a balance must have a sensitivity requirement equal to or less than

    A. 2 mg   B. 6 mg   C. 10 mg

    D. 30 mg   E. 120 mg

28. The minimum quantity that can be weighed on a balance with a sensitivity requirement of 6 mg if an error of 5% is permissible would be

    A. 6 mg   B. 24 mg   C. 60 mg

    D. 120 mg   E. 180 mg

29. How much additional sodium chloride should be added to the following prescription to maintain isotonicity? Zincfrin is an isotonic solution

    R$_x$

    Zincfrin   15 ml
    Sodium chloride   q.s.
    Sterile Water for Injection q.s. 60 ml

    A. 0.135 g   B. 0.4 g   C! 0.54 g
    D. 0.98 g   E. none (since sterile water for injection is already isotonic)

30. A physician places a patient on a daily dose of 48 units of U-80 insulin. How many ml should the patient inject each day?

    A. 0.48   B. 0.60   C. 0.80
    D. 1.0   E. 4.8

31. A patient normally uses 60 units of NPH U-100 insulin. However, only U-80 syringes are available. To what calibration mark on the U-80 syringe should the U-100 insulin be drawn to obtain the correct dose?

    A. 40 units   B. 48 units   C. 60 units
    D. 75 units   E. Impossible to measure in the U-80 syringe.

32. The freezing point depression ("D" value) for a 1% solution of pilocarpine hydrochloride is 0.14. The concentration of pilocarpine hydrochloride that would be iso-osmotic with the blood is

    A. 0.14%   B. 0.76%   C. 1.0%
    D. 2.7%   E. 3.7%

33. How much elemental iron is present in every 300 mg of ferrous sulfate ($FeSO_4 . 7H_2O$)? Atomic weights are, iron = 55.9; sulfur = 32.1; oxygen = 16.0 and hydrogen = 1.0. Iron has valances of +2 and +3.

    A. 30.2 mg   B. 60.3 mg   C. 110.3 mg
    D. 120.6 mg   E. 164 mg

34. How many 4-fluid-ounce bottle can be packaged from a 1 gallon bottle of cough syrup?

    A. 16   B. 32   C. 64
    D. 100   E. 120

35. Strong Iodine Solution USP contains 5% w/v iodine. How many mg of iodine are consumed daily if the usual dose is 0.3 ml t.i.d?

    A. 7.5 mg   B. 15 mg   C. 22.5 mg
    D. 45 mg   E. 90 mg

36. Sufficient water is added to 800 ml of a liquid chemical (density = 0.8 g/ml) to make a final volume of 4000 ml. What is the % w/v concentration of the liquid chemical in the final preparation?

    A. 12.5%   B. 16%   C. 20%
    D. 25%   E. 40%

37. The NF describes several tests for evaluating prescription balances. These tests include all of the following except

    A. arm ratio   B. rest point   C. rider & graduated beam
    D. sensitivity requirement   E. shift

38. Weights are classified by an alphabetical system for prescription work, the pharmacist should use what class (or better) weights?

    A. A   B. C   C. P   D. Q   E. T

39. According to the National Bureau of Standards (NBS), the initial calibration mark on a 100 ml graduate should be

    A. 5 ml   B. 10 ml   C. 15 ml
    D. 20 ml   E. 30 ml

40. The shrinkage that occurs when alcohol and purified water are mixed is primarily due to

    A. attractive Van der Waals forces.
    B. covalent bonding
    C. hydrogen bonding
    D. temperature changes
    E. ionic bonding.

41. Parenteral solutions that are isotonic with human red blood cells have an osmolality of approximately how many m Osm/l?

    A. 20   B. 40   C. 50
    D. 150   E. 300

42. An isotonic solution is one which

    A. does not cause hemolysis
    B. has same salt composition of plasma
    C. does not cause crenulation
    D. causes crenulation
    E. has a freezing point less than that of plasma

43. Although isotonicity is desirable for almost all parenterals it is particularly critical for which injections?

    A. intravenous   B. intramuscular   C. subcutaneous
    D. intraarterial   E. intradermal

44. The osmotic pressure of a 0.1 molar dextrose solution will be approximately how many times that of a 0.1 molar sodium chloride solution?

    A. 0.5   B. 1   C. 2   D. 3   E. 4

45. An isotonic solution has the same

    A. pH as blood
    B. fluid pressure as blood
    C. specific gravity as blood
    D. salt content as blood
    E. osmotic pressure as blood

46. All of the following substances readily permeate the red blood cell, causing hemolysis EXCEPT

    A. glucose   B. boric acid   C. propylene glycol
    D. urea   E. glycerin

47. Mixing a hypertonic solution with red blood cells will cause '............' of the red blood cells.

    A. chelation   B. bursting   C. crenation
    D. hemolysis   E. hydrolysis

48. A method for adjusting solution to isotonicity is based upon
    A. blood coagulation times
    B. boiling point elevations
    C. refractive indexes
    D. freezing point depressions
    E. milliequivalent calculations

49. All aqueous solutions that freezes at –0.52°C are isotonic with red blood cells. They are also iso-osmotic with each other. Which of the following apply?
    A. Both statements are true.
    B. Both statements are false.
    C. The first statement is false but the second is true.
    D. The first statement is true but the second is false.
    E. There is no correlation between freezing points and osmotic pressure of solutions.

50. One disadvantage in calculating isotonicity adjustment using either the sodium chloride equivalent or freezing point depression methods is
    A. E values are not accurate
    B. D values are not accurate
    C. only sodium chloride can be used for tonicity adjustments
    D. it is difficult to locate the values in the literature
    E. the adjusted solution will be iso-osmotic but may not be isotonic

51. A pharmacy has 20 g of a 5% hydrocortisone cream. How many grams of a 1% hydrocortisone cream must be added to obtain a 2% strength cream?

    A. 5 g   B. 20 g   C. 26.7 g
    D. 60 g   E. None of the above.

52. Convert the blood level of 0.2 mg/l to µg/dl.

    A. 0.0002 µg/dl   B. 20 µg/dl   C. 200 µg/dl
    D. 2000 µg/dl   E. None of the above.

53. The concentration of sodium fluoride in a community's drinking water is 0.6 ppm. Express this concentration as a percentage.

    A. 0.00006%   B. 0.0006%   C. 0.006%
    D. 0.06%   E. 0.6%

54. A 20 ml vial of a biological solution is labeled "2.0 mega units". How many units of drug are present in every ml of solution?

   A. 100   B. 1000   C. 2000

   D. 10000   E. 100000

55. A pharmacist has 50 ml of 0.5% gention violet solution. What will be the final ratio strength if the pharmacist dilutes this solution to 1250 ml with purified water?

   A. 1 : 8   B. 1 : 500   C. 1 : 1000

   D. 1 : 2500   E. 1 : 5000

56. How many grams of ammonia water (10% w/w) can be prepared from 1 lb of 28% w/w strong ammonia solutions?

   A. 84   B. 162   C. 280   D. 1270   E. 1453

57. The USP states that 1 g of a chemical is soluble in 10 ml of alcohol. What is the percentage strength of saturated solution of this chemical? (Sp. gr. of alcohol is 0.80)

   A. 10.0% (w/v)   B. 10.0% (w/w)   C. 11.1% (w/w)

   D. 12.6% (w/v)   E. 12.6% (w/w)

58. A prescription order requires 500 ml of D30W. How many ml of D40W should be used in the event of non-availability of D30W.

   A. 100 ml   B. 300 ml   C. 375 ml

   D. 400 ml   E. 500 ml

59. If a 120 lb. patient has a creatinine clearance rate of 40 ml/min, what maintenance dose will you recommend if the normal maintenance dose is 2 mg/lb of body weight.

   A. 50 mg   B. 96 mg   C. 130 mg   D. 150 mg   E. 206 mg

60. A vial of a lyophilized (i.e., freeze dried) drug is labeled "10,000 units, to reconstitute add 17 ml of sterile water for injection (SWFI) to obtain 500 units per ml." How many ml of SWFI must a pharmacist add if a 1000 unit/ml concentration is needed?

   A. 7   B. 8.5   C. 10   D. 15   E. 20

61. Cryoscopic method is familiar in the calculation of isotonic solutions. This method is based on

   A. freezing point depression of the drug
   B. molecular concentration of the drug
   C. pH of the drug
   D. sodium chloride equivalent of the drug
   E. none of the above.

62. Osmolality measures the total number of particles dissolved in a '.........' of water and depends on the electrolytic nature of the solute.

   A. kilogram   B. kiloliter   C. litre

   D. specified quantity   E. milliliter.

63. Rectified spirit contains

   A. 100% (v/v) of ethanol   B. 90% (v/v) of ethanol   C. 85% (v/v) of ethanol

   D. 70% (v/v) of ethanol   E. 50% (v/v) of ethanol

64. The amount of NaCl in 10 µl of a 1 M solution is

   A. 0.585 mg   B. 68.5 µg   C. 58.5 mg

   D. 68.5 mg   E. 5.85 mg.

65. The internal osmotic pressure of bacteria is between 5 and 20 atmosphere. The substance that is responsible for the strength of bacterial cell wall is a

   A. lipoprotein   B. mucopeptide   C. lipopolysaccharide

   D. polysaccharide

ANSWERS

1. B.   1 g = 15.432 grain (gr.)

     1 fluid ounce = 30 ml

     $\therefore$ 30 ml contain 3/15.432 g

     $\therefore$ 100 ml contain $\dfrac{3 \times 100}{15.432 \times 30} = 0.66$ g (approx.)

2. B.   1 pint = 473 ml

     Now, 5000 ml contain 1 g = 1000 mg

     $\therefore$ 473 ml contain $\dfrac{1000 \times 473}{5000} = 94.6$ mg $\approx$ 95 mg

3. E.   12% solution i.e., 100 ml solution contains 12 g of aspirin

     $\therefore$ 484 ml solutions contains 12 × 484/100 g of aspirin = 58.08 g

4. E.   4 fluidounces = 120 ml of 5% (w/v) solution contains 5 × 120/100 = 6 g of 100% HCl. Strength of conc. HCl is 37% (w/w)

     Therefore, required amount of HCl = $\dfrac{100 \times 6\,g}{37}$

     Now, 1.35 g HCl $\equiv$ 1 ml HCl

     $\therefore$ 1 g HCl $\equiv$ 1/1.35 ml HCl

     $\therefore$ 600/37 g HCl $\equiv \dfrac{1 \times 600}{1.35 \times 37} = 12$ ml

5. C.   C/5 = (F – 32)/9 $\therefore$ 78/5 = (F – 32)/9 $\therefore$ F = 172.4°F

6. D.   1 gallon = 8 pint = 8 × 473 ml = 8 × 473 × 1.25 = 4730 g

7. C.   C/5 = (F – 32)/9; $\therefore$ (–12/5) = (F – 32)/9 $\therefore$ F = 10.4°F

8. B.

9. B.   100 ml contain 6 units

     $\therefore$ 30 ml contain 6 × 30/100 units

     Now, 1030 ml contain $\dfrac{6 \times 30}{100}$ units

$$\therefore \ 100 \text{ ml contain } \frac{6 \times 30 \times 100}{100 \times 1030} = 0.1748\%$$

10. D.   100 g cream contains 0.1 g drug

$\therefore$ 45 g cream contains $0.1 \times 45/100$ g drug

Finally, 0.015 g drug is present in 100 g diluted product.

$$\therefore \ \frac{0.1 \times 45}{100} \text{ g drug is present in } \frac{100 \times 0.1 \times 45}{0.015 \times 100} = 300 \text{ g diluted product}$$

$\therefore$ Amount of Keri lotion required is $(300 - 45) = 255$ g.

11. A.   1 quart is approximately 1000 ml

Now, 1 g is present in 1000 ml

$\therefore$ 2 g is present in 2000 ml

Now, 17 g drug is present in 100 ml stock solution

$\therefore$ 2 g drug is present in $100 \times 2/17$ ml stock solution = 11.7 ml.

12. D.

13. C.   Sodium chloride equivalent of 2% Cocaine HCl = $0.16 \times 2 = 0.32$

$\therefore$ Amount of NaCl required for 100 ml = $(0.9 - 0.32) = 0.58$

$\therefore$ Amount of NaCl required for 30 ml = $0.58 \times 30/100 = 0.174$ g = 174 mg.

14. B.   Three fluid ounces = $29.57 \times 3 = 88.71$ ml contains

$$\frac{0.5 \times 88.71}{100} = 0.44355 \text{ g silver nitrate}$$

Now, 1 g = 15.4 grain

$\therefore \quad 0.44355$ g = $15.4 \times 0.44355 = 6.83$ gr.

15. E.

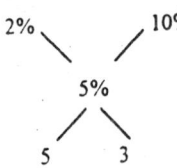

$\therefore \quad$ ratio of 2% and 10% paste would be 5 : 3

Out of 8 g 2% paste is 5 g.

$\therefore \quad$ In 120 g mixed paste (5%), 2% paste is $5 \times 120/8 = 75$ g.

16. C.   100 ml dil HCl contains 10 g HCl

$\therefore$ 1 gallon i.e., 3785 ml HCl contains $\dfrac{10 \times 3785}{100} = 378.5$ g

Now, 36 g pure HCl is present in 100 g supplied HCl

$\therefore$ 378.5 g pure HCl is present in $\dfrac{100 \times 378.5}{36} = 1051.39$ g

Now, 1.18 g HCl = 1 ml HCl

$\therefore$ 1051.39 g HCl = $\dfrac{1 \times 1051.39}{1.18} = 891$ ml.

17. C.   Mol. Wt. of Calcium gluconate = 430

∴ Equivalent wt of Calcium gluconate = 215

∴ 215 g of Calcium gluconate = 1000 mEq wt of Calcium gluconate

$$\equiv 1000 \text{ mEq Ca}$$

∴ 1 g of Calcium gluconate $\equiv 1000/215$ mEq Ca $\equiv 4.65$ mEq

18. E.   1 ml contains 0.05 mg

∴ 3 ml contains 0.15 mg = 0.15 × 1000 = 150 µg.

19. D.   Some sources use the value of 65 mg, which does not meet USP specifications. The value of 60 mg should not be used except for rough calculations in checking doses.

20. D.   2000 ml solution contain 1 unit

∴ 1 gallon = 3785 ml solution contain $\dfrac{1 \times 3785}{2000}$ units

Now, 0.5 unit present in 100 ml

∴ 3785/2000 unit present in $\dfrac{100 \times 3785}{0.5 \times 2000}$ ml = 378.5 ml.

21. D.   500 ml contain 200 mg = 200000 µg

∴ 1 ml contains 200000/500 = 400 µg.

22. C.   1 lb = 1/2.2 kg.

∴ 155 lb. = 155/2.2 kg

Delivery rate is 5 µg/kg/min

Therefore, for 155/2.2 kg drug = 5 × 155/2.2 µg

400 µg is present in 1 ml

∴ 5 × 155/2.2 is present in $\dfrac{1 \times 5 \times 155}{400 \times 2.2}$ = 0.88 ml/min

23. A.   1 g ointment contains 200 units of bacitracin

∴ 1 pound or 453.59 g contain 200 × 453.59 units of bacitracin

Now 500 units bacitracin is present in 1g ointment

∴ 200 × 453.59 units bacitracin is present in 200 × 453.59/500 g ointment = 181.4 g

24. C.   Equivalent wt of KCl = 74.6 g

∴ 74.6 g of KCl contains 1000 mEq of KCl

∴ 5.86 g of KCl contains 1000 × 5.86/74.6 mEq of KCl = 78.5 mEq

25. D.   Calcium chloride has equivalent wt 147/2 = 73.5 ≡ 1000 mEq of calcium chloride or 1000 mEq of calcium

∴ 1000 mEq = 73.5 g

∴ 40 mEq = 73.5 × 40/1000 g = 2.94 g.

26. B.   Wt of 1 ml solution is 1.7 g

∴ Wt of 100 ml solution is 170 g

Now, this 170 g solution contains 100 g of KI

∴ this 100 g solution contains 100 × 100/170 g of KI = 58.82% w/w.

27. B.   Thirty milligram is the maximum sensitivity requirement for the Class B prescription-balance.

28. D.   The minimum weight that may be weighed on any balance with a known sensitivity requirement (SR) with a given percent of error may be determined by the equation :

SR = (minimum amount that may be weighed) × (% permissible error)

∴ Minimum weighable amount = SR / % permissible error = 6/0.05 = 120.

29. B.   Out of 60 ml solution 15 ml is already sterile.

Therefore, for remaining 45 ml the amount of sodium chloride required is

0.9 × 45/100 = 0.405 g.

30. B.   The strengths of insulin were previously expressed as U-40, 80 and 100, These values refer to the number of USP insulin per ml of solution.

31. B.   Since the patient requires 60 units of the available U-100 insulin,

0.6 ml of solution is needed.

The volumes presents in both the U-80 and U-100 insulin syringes are identical, the unit calibrations are different.

In U-80 syringe 1 ml. volume reads 80 units.

∴ 0.6 ml volume reads 80 × 0.6 = 48 units.

32. E.   0.14°C depression is due to 1% solution

∴ 0.52°C depression is due to 1 × 0.52/0.14% = 3.7%

33. B.   Mol. Wt of $FeSO_4 . 7H_2O$ = (55.9 + 32.1 + 64 + 7 × 18) = 278

Now, 278 mg of ferrous sulfate contains 55.9 mg of elemental iron

∴ 300 mg of ferrous sulfate contains 55.9 × 300/278 = 60.3 mg.

The valence of iron has no significance in this type of problem since only one atom of iron is present in each molecule of ferrous sulfate.

34. B   4 fluidounce = 29.57 × 4 = 118.28 ml; 1 gallon = 3785 ml ∴ 3785/118.28 = 32

35. D.   0.3 ml t.i.d, i.e., 0.9 ml total

Now 100 ml contain 5 g = 5000 mg

∴ 0.9 ml contains $\dfrac{5000 \times 0.9}{100}$ = 45 mg

36. B.   4000 ml final solution actually contains 800 ml liquid chemical which is equal to 800 × 0.8 = 640 g.

∴ percentage w/w would be $\dfrac{640 \times 100}{4000}$ = 16% w/v

37. B.   The rest point is simply the point at which the balance indicator point stops. It may be easily shifted by adjusting the leveling screws of the balance.

A.   This test confirms that the two arms of the balance are equal in length.

C.   The rider test confirms the accuracy of the calibrated beam or dial at both the 500 mg and 1g position.

E.   The shift tests check the balance construction especially the arm and lever components.

38. D.   The accuracy of weights is expressed in tolerances which are + or – deviations from the stated weight. The class Q weights have tolerances smaller than the sensitivity requirement of the class A prescription balance. The class P weights are more accurate than class Q and are suggested for performance of the balance tests and to check other weights.

39. D.   The NBS specifications state that a graduate shall have an initial interval of not less than one fifth not more than one fourth of the capacity of the graduate. Therefore, the initial calibration mark on a 250 ml graduate should be 50 ml.

40. C.

41. E.   Osmolarity, expressed as mOsm/l, is included on the labels of many large-volume parenteral bottles. Those injections with a volume of approximately 300 mOsm/l will be iso-osmotic and presumably isotonic with the blood. For example, 5% dextrose injection has a value of 280 mOsm/l, whereas 0.9% sodium chloride injection has a value of 308 mOsm/l.

Osmolarity of a solution = millimoles of chemical present in one liter × Number of ions formed from one molecule.

For example, in case of 0.9% sodium chloride solution osmolarity = (9/58.4 mole) × 1000

$$= 154 \text{ millimoles} \times 2 \text{ (ions present in NaCl)} = 308.$$

42. A.

43. C.   A subcutaneous injection will come into contact with a large number of nerve endings and extreme pain will be felt if the solution is other than isotonic. The potential isotonicity effects of hypotonic or hypertonic intravenous solutions are offset by dilution in the large volume of blood into which they are injected, provided the volume of injection is less and rate of injection is slow.

44. A.   The osmotic pressure of the dextrose solution will be approximately one half that of an equivalent sodium chloride solution. The osmotic pressure of a substance in a solution is an example of a colligative property. Equimolar concentrations of non-electrolytes will have similar osmotic pressure. However, electrolytes ionize to form particles which quantitatively increase the magnitude of the colligative property. Since sodium chloride ionizes into two particles, a 0.1 molar solution has twice the osmotic pressure of 0.1 molar solution of a non electrolyte such as dextrose.

45. E.

46. A.   Even when boric acid, glycerin propylene glycol and urea solutions are iso-osmotic, hemolysis occurs when red blood cells are added.

47. C.   A hypertonic solution will draw water from within the cell until an equilibrium is reached with equal pressure on each side of the semipermeable cell membrane. The shrinkage of the cell as a result of fluid loss is known as crenation.

48. D.

49. C.   Aqueous solutions that have the same freezing or boiling point will have the same osmotic pressure, since these are all colligative properties. Both freezes at –0.52°C; other aqueous solutions that freeze at this point are considered to be isoosmotic with blood and with each other. The term isotonic further qualifies the relationship by indicating that the solutions have the same "tone" as the red blood cells in the blood and will not cause

changes in the cell size. Since some chemicals will readily pass through the RBC wall, equalized pressure on both sides of the cell wall is not possible without changes in the cell volume. Such solutions may be described as being iso-osmotic but not isotonic with R.B.C.

50. E. Although it is possible to experimentally determine whether a solution is iso-osmotic with a 0.9% sodium chloride solution or blood, one cannot assume that the solution is also isotonic.

51. D. ∴ 1 part of 5% cream to be mixed with 3 parts of 1% cream

∴ 20 parts of 5% cream to be mixed with 3 parts of
3 × 20 = 60 parts.

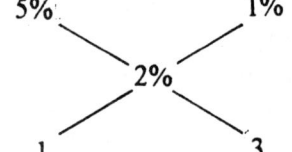

52. B. 1 lit i.e., 1000 ml contain 0.2 mg

∴ 1 ml contains 0.2/1000 mg

∴ 1 dl i.e., 100 ml contain $0.2 \times 100/1000$ mg $= \dfrac{0.2 \times 100 \times 1000}{1000}$ μg/dl $= 20$ μg/dl

53. A. 1 million i.e., 10,00000 parts contain 0.6 parts

∴ 100 parts contain $0.6 \times 100/10,00000 = 0.00006\%$ (w/v)

54. E. 1 mega units (M units) = 1000 kilo units = 1000,000 units

∴ each ml contains $2 \times 1000000/20$ units = 100,000 units.

55. E. 50 ml of 0.5% solution contains 0.25 g of gention violet

This 0.25 g gention violet actually ultimately present in 1250 ml solution.

∴ ratio becomes 0.25 : 1250 i.e., 1 : 5000.

56. D. x (g) × 10% (w/w) = 453.56 (g) × 28% (w/w)

∴ $x = 1269.96$ or 1270 grams

One can apply unitary method or alligation alternate method.

57. C. After solubilization of 1 g of chemical in 10 ml (i.e., $10 \times 0.8 = 8$ g) of alcohol, the final volume is unknown but the final weight would be $(1 + 8) = 9$ g.

∴ 9 g solution contains 1 g chemical

∴ 100 g solution contains 100/9 = 11.11 g

∴ % strength = 11.1% (w/w)

58. C. D30W i.e., 30 g dextrose is present in 100 ml solution.

∴ 500 ml such solution contains $5 \times 30 = 150$ g.

∴ D40W i.e., 40 g dextrose in 100 ml solution

∴ 1 g dextrose in 100/40 ml solution

∴ 150 g dextrose in $100 \times 150/40$ ml solution = 375 ml.

59. B. Normal maintenance dose is $2 \times 120 = 240$ mg

Normal creatinine clearance rate = 100 ml/min

Due to impaired creatinine clearance rate the maintenance dose should be $240 \times 40/100 = 96$ mg.

60. A.   After first reconstitution 500 units present in 1 ml of reconstituted preparation.

∴ 10000 units present in $1 \times 10,000/500 = 20$ ml of reconstituted preparation.

So, out of 20 ml final volume 17 ml is due to SWFI and 3 ml volume occupied by the drug.

In second case, 1000 units present in 1 ml of reconstituted preparation

∴ 10000 units present in 10 ml of reconstituted preparation

So out of 10 ml, $(10 - 3) = 7$ ml is SWFI

61. A.   Cryoscope is an instrument used to determine the freezing point depression.

62. A.   The term osmolarity is used to express the strength in milliosmol per litre and indicates the total ionic concentration of the solution.

Biochemical data often refer to osmolality of body fluids and this is the total ionic concentration per 1000 g water.

63. B.

64. A.   1000 ml = 1000000 μl contain 58.5 g = 58500 mg, therefore, 10 μl contain $58500 \times 10/1000000 = 0.585$ mg.

65. B.   In bacterial cell wall the main backbone is peptidoglycan formed by alternative linkage of N-acetyl glucosamine and N-acetyl muramic acid. The chains of peptidoglycan are cross-linked by peptide linkage which is responsible for the strength of the cell wall. Penicillin group of antibiotics actually inhibits this cell wall sythesis.

CHAPTER 4

Packing of Pharmaceuticals

- • Desirable Features of a Container
- • Type of Containers

- • Study of Glass and Plastics as Materials for Containers and Rubber as Materials for Closures, their Merits and Demerits
- • Introduction to Aerosol Packaging.

The ideal container or package should

(i) protect the contents from physical and mechanical hazards.

(ii) not interact with the products.

(iii) protect the contents from the effects of atmospheric gases.

(iv) be capable of withstanding extremes of temperature and humidity.

(v) protect the contents from both water loss and gain.

(vi) protect the contents from loss of volatile materials, light, airborne particulate contamination, animal contamination etc.

(vii) be sufficiently transparent to permit the inspection of the contents.

(viii) not shed particles into the contents.

(ix) have a "pharmaceutically elegant" appearance.

(x) be easy to label and then to identify the product.

(xi) be convenient and easy to use.

(xii) be cheap and economical.

Closures : With respect to closures, the Pharmaceutical Codex defines four types of container :

(i) Airtight container : This container protects the content from contamination with extraneous solids, liquids and vapors, from loss of volatile constituents and from changes due to efflorescence (release water), deliquescence (absorb water and liquify) and evaporation under ordinary conditions of handling, storage and transport.

(ii) Security closed container : This is an air tight container fitted with some means of preventing the unintentional displacement of the closure.

(iii) Hermetically sealed container : This container is impervious to air and other gases under ordinary conditions of handling, storage and transport. It is usually a glass ampoule sealed by fusion of the glass.

(iv) Child-resistant container : A container designed to prevent children gaining access to its content.

Glass : Main advantages among others—it is available in clear or amber (light resistant) forms and main disadvantages is, fragile, heavy and may release alkali to aqueous contents.

Ribbed or flutted bottles warns the user, even in the dark or if blind or partially sighted, that the contents are not to be taken for internal use.

There are mainly four types of glass :

(i) **Type I** glass (commonly known as neutral glass) or borosilicate glass offers a high hydrolytic resistance due to the chemical composition of the glass.

(ii) **Type II** glass has a high hydrolytic resistance due to an appropriate inner surface treatment (with SO_2 gas at very high temperature, 500°C). The surface alkali is converted into sulphate which can be washed off to expose a tough silica rich surface furnishing very little alkali to bottled products. The internal coating will be weakened by repeated sterilization or exposures to alkaline detergents. Both type I and II glasses may be used for different types of injectable preparations, depending on their physico-chemical properties.

(iii) **Type III** glass (soda glass) offer only a moderate hydrolytic resistance and should be used only for non-aqueous liquid preparations or for powder for injection or for preparations not for parenteral use.

(iv) **NP** (nonparenteral glass) is unsuitable for injection purposes.

Containers of Type II and Type III glass should be used once only. Containers for injectable preparations arc made from uncoloured glass except that coloured glass may be used for substances known to be light sensitive, in such cases, the containers should be sufficiently transparent to permit visual inspection of the contents.

Hydrolytic resistance test for glass container is done to measure the resistance to water attack of new (not previously used) glass containers at elevated temperature, the degree of attack being determined by the amount of alkali released from the glass under specified conditions.

Silicone treated glass : Glass can be coated with hydrophobic silicones and can be used on many occasions.

Plastics : They include such substances as polyvinyl chloride (PVC), low-density and high-density polyethylene and polystyrene. The main disadvantages associated with plastic containers among others, leaching of undesirable constituents to the packed materials and during partial removal of the content due to 'suck back' phenomena, may result in microbial contamination, oxidation, hydrolysis or dehydration of the contents. Specialized containers like "Rotahaler", "Spinhaler" are also made up of plastics, for administration of dry powder to the respiratory tract.

Polymethylmethacrylate (PMMA) container is clear, hard, strong, light and softens at about 100°C.

Polytetrafluoroethylene is transparent and opaque, heat resistant and remains unchanged even at 250°C. It is also resistant to solvents and chemicals and its permeability to water vapor is negligible.

Polypropylene (m.p 170°C) container can be autoclaved.

Polyamides (Nylons) container is tough, flexible and heat resistant but are sensitive to phenols, weak organic acids etc.

Plastic containers for non-injectable preparations should be tested for (a) leakage test, (b) collapsibility test, (c) clarity of aqueous extract and, (d) test for non-volatile residue. Plastic containers for injectable preparations should also comply with these tests. Besides these they also should comply with the test for water vapour permeability, transparency and extractable di (2-ethylhexyl) phthalate. Plastic containers for ophthalmic preparations should also comply with the above tests. Besides these they should also comply with the eye irritation test.

Rubber : Rubbers are generally used for construction of closures of multiple dose vials, dropping bottles and as washers. Rubber may be natural or synthetic. Natural rubber consists of latex from *Heavea braziliensis* and is an isoprene polymer. Natural rubber is compounded with addition of a number of additives to alter its physical and chemical properties, such as :

   (i) Vulcanising agent (sulphur)

  (ii) Accelerators (thiazoles)

 (iii) Activators (stearic acid, zinc oxide, zinc stearate)

 (iv) Filler (carbon black, calcium carbonate, talc, asbestos etc.)

  (v) Softeners (pine oil, mineral oil)

 (vi) Antioxidants

 (vii) Pigments (oxides and sulfides of iron, cadmium, antimony etc.)

(viii) Lubricants (zinc stearate)

 (ix) Miscellaneous substances such as paraffin wax, resin etc.

The synthetic rubbers are silicon, neoprene, nitrile or butyl rubbers.

Rubber should comply with the following test.

   (i) Test for penetrability force

  (ii) Extractive test

 (iii) Fragmentation test

 (iv) Permeability test

  (v) Compatibility test

 (vi) Sterilization test

 (vii) Self-sealability test.

Sometimes rubber closure may adsorb any formulation component from the packed material. For example, some preservatives may be adsorbed by the rubber and as a result the preservative concentration in the formulation may become insufficient to prevent microbial growth. In such cases the rubber closure before use should be kept immersed in concentrated (at least twice the concentration used in formulation) solution of that preservative so that it becomes saturated with the adsorbed preservative.

Metals : Metals includes aluminium, tin, tincoated steel and lead.

Types of metal containers include (a) collapsible tubes for semi-solid preparations (b) metal containers for tablets and capsules and (c) metal foil for suppositories, pessaries, tablets, capsules etc. The main problem associated with metal containers is that they may shed metal particles into the pharmaceutical product.

AEROSOLS

Aerosols are dosage forms containing therapeutically active ingredients that packaged under pressure in a sealed container and are released as a fine mist of spray upon activation of a suitable valve system. They are intended either for inhalation for local action in the lungs or for systemic absorption through the alveoli or for topical application to the skin or various body orifices. Inhalation aerosols are metered dose preparations which provide controlled amounts of the active ingredient(s).

The basic components of an aerosol system are the container, the propellant (which helps in the propulsion or expulsion of the materials through the microorifice by application of pressure), the concentrate containing the active ingredient(s), the valve and the actuator.

Aerosols are of two types, the two-phase system consisting of gas and liquid or the three-phase system consisting of gas, liquid and solid or liquid. The two-phase aerosol comprises a solution of active ingredient(s) in liquefied propellant and the vaporized propellant. The solvent is usually the propellant or a mixture of the propellant and co-solvents such as ethanol, propylene glycol and polyethylene glycols. The three-phase aerosol consists of a suspensions or emulsion of the active ingredient(s) and the vaporised propellants. In the suspension the ingredient(s) may be dispersed in the propellant system with the aid of suitable pharmaceutical aids such as wetting agents, solubilising agents, emulsifying agents, suspending agents and lubricating agents to prevent clogging of valves. Foam aerosols contain an emulsion of the active ingredients, surface active agents, aqueous or nonaqueous liquids and the propellants.

Propellants are liquefied or compressed gases having vapour pressure exceeding atmospheric pressure. The commonly used propellants in aerosol systems are hydrocarbons, especially the fluorochloro-derivatives of methane and ethane, the butanes and pentanes and compressed gases such as nitrogen and carbon dioxide.

The actuator or adaptor which is fitted to the aerosol valve stem is a device which on depression or other movement opens the valve and directs the spray to the desired area. The breath actuated device is controlled by the inspired air.

Aerosol containers are made of metal (stainless steel, aluminium or tin-plated steel), glass or hard plastic.

The label of the container must include among other informations : (i) the conditions under which it should be stored; (ii) a warning that the container is under pressure and that it must not be punctured, broken or incinerated even when apparently empty; (iii) the statement : "Warning, keep away from children".

In order to measure the standard of aerosol the following tests are recommended by the pharmacopoeia :

(i) Content of active ingredient delivered per spray.

(ii) Number of deliveries per container.

(iii) Pressure test.

(iv) Leak test.

MODEL QUESTIONS

1. According to the USP, a monograph's instruction "Protect from light" indicates storage in a
    A. dark place
    B. amber glass bottle
    C. light-resistant container
    D. hermatic container
    E. tight glass container

2. Glass used to make pharmaceutical containers is designated as Types I, II, III and NP. All of these glasses are composed of soda-lime except
    A. Type I
    B. Type II
    C. Type III
    D. Type NP
    E. Type II and III

3. Type II glass is prepared from Type III glass by surface treatment with

    A. lime   B. nitrogen   C. oxygen

    D. silicon   E. sulfur dioxide

4. The water resistance of glass containers is tested by measuring
    A. amount of acid released into water
    B. amount of alkali released into water
    C. changes in pH
    D. determination of silicate levels
    E. turbidity of an aqueous solution after autoclaving.

5. The containers used to package drugs may consist of several components and/or be composed of several materials. The release of an ingredient from packaging components into the actual product is best described by the term.

    A. permeation   B. leaching   C. diffusion

    D. adsorption   E. porosity

6. The term PSIG in reference to aerosols means

    A. atmospheric pressure   B. pounds per square inch gauge

    C. propellant safety in glass   D. per square inch of glass   E. none of the above

7. USP acetylsalicylic acid tablets should be packaged and stored in
   A. well-closed containers
   B. tightly-closed containers
   C. light-resistant containers
   D. tightly closed, light-resistant containers.
   E. none of the above.

8. Freons are
   A. alkanes   B. alkenes   C. alkynes
   D. fluorinated hydrocarbon   E. mixture of CO_2 and air.

9. A drug that is frequently administered by inhalation is
   A. insulin   B. isoproterenol   C. allopurinol
   D. penicillin   E. nitroglycerin

10. Which of the following is available in a metered dose aerosol?
    A. Reserpine
    B. Isoproterenol
    C. Guanethidine
    D. Dimenhydramine
    E. Diphenylhydantoin

11. Which of the following is NOT an advantage of aerosol dosage forms?
    A. Fine particle size
    B. Easy to apply
    C. Inexpensive
    D. Even application
    E. Less contamination

12. The storage temperature of aerosols should never exceed
    A. 37°C   B. 120°F   C. 95°F   D. 100°F   E. 25°C.

13. Characteristics of inhalation aerosol dosage forms include : I. avoid first pass effect of liver; II. rapid onset of action; III. can administer large amounts of drug to intended site.
    A. I only.
    B. III only.
    C. I and II only.
    D. II and III only
    E. I, II, and III.

ANSWERS

1. C (A container that reduces light transmission in the range between 290 and 450 nm to the level specified in the USP may be considered light resistant and suitable for protection from light. Many containers including amber glass bottle, plastic etc. may meet this specification); 2. A; 3. E; 4. B

(**Water attack test** is used to identify the alkalinity in type I, II, and III glass); 5. B (**Adsorption** would refer to the binding of a substance onto the surface of the container wall. **Diffusion** is the passage of a substance through a second substance. For example, volatile oil or dye may diffuse from a solution through the walls of a plastic container. **Permeation** would denote the solution of a substance in the cell wall followed by passage through the wall. Porosity indicates small holes or passages through which a substance could pass); 6. B (This indicates the intensity of pressure); 7. A (Moisture must be excluded); 8. D (These are used as propellants in aerosols); 9. B (This anti-asthmatic agent is used frequently in the form of aerosol in acute attacks of asthma); 10. B (It is anti-asthmatic drug); 11. C; 12. B (Because this dosage form contains gas under pressure); 13. C (Drug absorbed from the GI tract carried by the portal vein to the liver first which may metabolise a fraction of the drug during first passing. In case of aerosol dosage forms drugs are administered to the pulmonary tree from where the drugs are quickly absorbed through the alveolar capillary membrane to the general circulation. It is very difficult to administer large amounts of drug to intended site through this delivery system. Because a large fraction of the inhaled drug tends to come out through the expired air or during the expiratory phase of respiration).

CHAPTER 5

Size Reduction

- Objectives and Factors Affecting Size Reduction   • Study of Different Mills and Disintegrator
- Methods of Size Reduction

Size reduction or milling or comminution is the process of reducing substances to small particles of various grades.

Particle size and the related surface area of certain mass of powder has great significance in the field of pharmacy. Because some physico-chemical as well as pharmacokinetic parameters are dependent on it, such as, medicinal activity, bio-availability, solubility, stability, suspendibility, bulk-density and porosity, extractability of the active principle, onset and duration of action, viscosity and consistency of the preparations, appearance of the powder, homogeneity of the powder mixture etc.

The reduction of materials to a fine state of subdivision is an essential preliminary to the preparation of pharmaceutical capsules, insufflations (i.e., preparations inhaled directly into the lungs), suppositories, pessaries and ointments, where the requirement is that the solid constituents should be impalpable (not perceivable by touch), i.e., less than about 60 µm in diameter. Finally, for the reduction of the volume of the bulk of the crude drugs for transport facilities, e.g., evenised cascara has less volume than the hollow quills of the whole drug. In regard to the physico-chemical properties of the final product the size reduction is very important. For example, the viscosity of mucilage of tragacanth prepared from No. 60 powder will be greater than that prepared from No. 120 powder, both powders having been prepared from the same sample of gum.

Factors influencing milling

The selection of the appropriate method of size reduction depends upon material properties that may influence the process such as :

   (i) Hardness : The hardness of the material can be described by its position in a scale known as Moh's scale which is a table of materials, at the top of which is diamond with Moh's hardness > 7 which has surface so hard that it can scratch anything below it, at the bottom of the table with Moh's hardness < 3 is talc.

   (ii) Toughness : e.g., rubber, waxy substances etc. This type of material which resist milling at ambient or elevated temperature can be more easily size reduced by lowering the temperature below the glass transition point of the material, by treating the material with a liquefied gas such as liquid nitrogen. When this is carried out the material undergoes a transition from plastic to brittle behaviour and crack propagation is facilitated.

     Camphor may be effectively pulverized by addition of few drops of alcohol to camphor and then immediately trituration.

   (iii) Abrasiveness : In general, abrasiveness is a property of hard materials. The final powder may be contaminated with metal worn from the grinding mill.

   (iv) Stickiness : Complete dryness and addition of inert substances may be beneficial.

   (v) Softening temperature : In this case suitable cooling arrangement is essential.

   (vi) Material structure.

   (vii) Moisture content of the feed.

   (viii) Physiological effect : Dust of the potent drug may have an effect on the operators. Using of enclosed mill, induction of special air extraction systems and, if possible, adoption of wet grinding is desirable.

   (ix) Purity required.

   (x) Ratio of feed size to product size.

   (xi) Bulk density.

Energy requirements of the size reduction process

Only a very small amount of the energy put into a machine actually effects size reduction. This has been estimated at 2% at the most.

Mechanisms of size reduction

   (i) **Cutting :** The material is cut by means of sharp blade(s).

   (ii) **Compression :** The material is crushed by application of pressure.

   (iii) **Impact :** This may be effective in two ways such as when the material is more or less stationary and is hit by an object moving at high speed or when the moving particles strikes a stationary surface.

   (iv) **Attrition :** When the material is subjected to pressure as in compression, but the surfaces are moving relative to each other.

Mills for Dry Grinding

   a. **Cutter Mill :** Cutting is effected with rotational as well as stationary knives.

   b. **Hammer Mill :** Impact is effected with rotating hammer of different size and shape, as well as with outer stationary casing.

   c. **Ball Mill :** Here both impact and attrition is effected by the cascading action of the rotating balls contained in a cylindrical vessel rotating at optimum r.p.m. This critical angular velocity of a ball mill is very important. Because at low speed the balls slide back enmasse to the base of the drum without any relative movement between them i.e., without any size reduction. At high angular velocity the balls alongwith material to be size reduced will adhere to the inner surface of the cylinder due to centrifugal effect and again no size reduction would be effected. The cascading action may occur at about 2/3 rd of the critical angular velocity where centrifuging occurs. The main disadvantage of a ball mill is that the product may be heavily contaminated with metal.

There are some modified ball mill such as (I) Hardinge mill; (ii) Tube mill; (iii) Rod mill; and (iv) Vibration mill.

d. **Fluid Energy Mill :** Also known as jet mill or micronizer. Here fine particles are reduced to very fine particles with the help of fluid (air, superheated steam etc.) injected to feed through jet at very very high speed.

e. **Roller Mill :** In roller mill two rollers rotate along their longitudinal axes and are kept horizontally. The material is thus crushed between the two rollers due to compression. Ointments before filling in the tube are passed through roller mill to break any agglomeration or gritty particles.

f. **Disintegrator :** The disintegrator is based on impact and grinding mechanism. It is mainly used for crushing or powdering hard drugs.

g. **End Runner Mill and Edge Runner Mill :** These mills can be considered the mechanical counterparts of pestle and mortar. The end runner mill consists of a weighted pestle mounted eccentrically in a ceramic, granite or metal mortar. The pestle rotates by friction and is free to rise and fall in the morter so that its grinding action involves both impact and shear, the material being crushed and rubbed between it and the rotating morter.

The edge runner mill consists of one or two heavy steel or granite rollers mounted on a horizontal shaft and turned round a central vertical shaft on a bed of steel or granite. The stones may vary from 0.5 to 2.5 m in diameter, the larger size weighing upto about 6 tonnes. The material to be ground is kept in the path of the runners by scrapers. The reduction is partly due to crushing by the weight of the stones, but more to friction between the surfaces of contact between the runners and the bed stone. Although edge runner mills are gradually being replaced by more sophisticated machines they are still used, particularly for reducing extremely tough and fibrous materials, roots and barks—to the form of powder.

h. **Pin Mills :** These rely on the high speed rotation of a series of pins located on a plate which revolves against a similar plate leaving a small clearance for the passage of the drug being comminuted. Typical is the "Reddrop-Periflo" Mill. The upper disc is fitted to the cover while the lower disc rotated. The material is fed in through the center of the upper disc and is thrown outwards by the centrifugal force of the rotating disc and broken down to fine powder by the series of impacts as it passes outwards between the revolving and stationary pins. These mills are adopted for the fine grinding of substances with low melting points, such as resin, soap, sugar, etc.

Wet-Grinding or Levigation

This is a process of wet-grinding. The material to be ground is made into a paste with water or any other suitable non-solvent. In small scale pestle and morter and in large scale end runner mill may be used. The paste contains fine particles with a small proportion of coarse particles which have escaped or resisted grinding. The fine particles are separated from the coarse by the process of **elutriation**. In general, if the moisture content of the feed is greater than 40% then we should prefer wet-grinding process.

Size Reduction by Way of Precipitation

Precipitation is a convenient method for producing solids in a very fine state of subdivision down to 0.1 μm in diameter. Examples of pharmaceutical substances commonly prepared by precipitation are calcium and magnesium carbonates made by treating the respective chlorides with sodium carbonate solution. Hot, concentrated solutions usually produce heavy, coarse precipitates which can be fairly readily freed from contaminating salts, by washing. But the precipitates from cold dilute solutions are usually much finer and it may be difficult to free them from impurities adsorbed onto their very large surface area.

MODEL QUESTIONS

1. A roller mill is used mainly to reduce particle size in
   A. tablet granulation
   B. ointments
   C. emulsions
   D. capsules
   E. bulk powders.

2. Particle size reduction will not enhance the absorption of
   A. hydrophobic compounds
   B. hydrophilic compounds
   C. weak acids
   D. weak bases
   E. none of the above.

3. The process of grinding a substance to a very fine powder is termed
   A. levigation
   B. sublimation
   C. trituration
   D. percolation
   E. maceration.

4. The term "impalpable" refers to a substance that is
   A. not tasty
   B. not perceptible to the touch
   C. tasteless
   D. greasy
   E. nongreasy.

5. The value of particle size reduction to enhance drug absorption is limited to those situation in which the
   A. drug is very soluble
   B. drug is very potent
   C. drug is irritating to the GI mucosa
   D. absorption process is rate limited by the dissolution of drug in GI fluids
   E. absorption process occurs by active transport.

6. The various equipments are used to size reduction of materials of different nature. Match them correctly.

(i)	Rod mill	A.	Sticky material
(ii)	Fluid energy mill	B.	Abrasive material
(iii)	Cutting mill	C.	Thermolabile material
(iv)	Revolving mill	D.	Fibrous material
		E.	Thermostable material

7. In comminution, certain types of materials listed in A to E are NOT suitable for the mills mentioned below. Match them correctly.

(i)	Cutter mill	A.	Soft material
(ii)	Hammer mill	B.	Adhesive material
(iii)	Revolving mill	C.	Friable material
(iv)	Fluid energy mill	D.	Liquifiable material
		E.	Abrasive material.

ANSWERS

1. B (This mill is useful in case of semisolids); 2. B (Particle size is reduced to increase the surface area and thereby to improve the solubility according to **Noyes and Whitney** equation. But in case of hydrophilic compounds wettability and solubility is not a problem), 3. C (**Levigation** is the process of reducing the particle size of solids by the addition of a small amount of a liquid or ointment base to make a paste which is then rubbed with a spatula against a tile, camphor may be better pulverized by addition of few drops of alcohol followed by trituration. **Sublimation** is the conversion of a solid to a vapor without passing through a liquid phase. **Percolation** is the extraction process in which the desired constituents are dissolved from a granulated or powdered drug by the descent of a suitable solvent at a controlled rate through a column of the drug. **Maceration** is an extraction process in which the ground drug is soaked in the solvent until the cellular structure is penetrated and the soluble constituents have been dissolved and leached out of the drug particles.); 4. B (Usually a particle size of 50 μ or smaller is desirable); 5. D; 6. (i) - A, ii - C, iii - D, iv - B; 7. (i) - C, ii - E, iii - A, iv - B.

CHAPTER 6

Size Separation

- Size Separation by Sifting
- Official Standard for Powders
- Sedimentation Methods of Size Separation
- Working Principle of Cyclone Separator.

Sieves for pharmacopoeial testing are of wire cloth woven from brass, bronze, stainless steel or other suitable wire and are not coated or plated. The wires are of uniform circular cross-section. There must be no reaction between the material of the sieves and the substances being sifted. Sieves conform to the specifications given in the pharmacopoeia. **Sieve number** is the number of meshes in a length of 2.54 cm in each transverse direction parallel to the wires.

Numerous methods have been developed for sifting powders and determining their particle size. Of these sieving is undoubtedly the most common, being applicable to practically all powders from about 40 μm upwards. The powder under test is passed through a number of sieves of increasingly smaller mesh size and the weight remaining on each sieve is measured. The method of shaking the sieves is important. Agitation method, brushing method and centrifugal method may be adopted.

Most commercial classifiers and sifters are based on the principle of sieving.

Methods of particle size determination	Useful range
1. Sieving	Above 33 μm
2. Optical microscopy	0.2 to 100 μm
3. Electron microscopy	0.005 to 1 μm
4. Sedimentation and elutriation	2 to 50 μm
5. Gas permeability	5 to 100 μm
6. Gas adsorption	0.005 to 20 μm
7. Coulter counters	1 to 100 μm

In case of **Andreason apparatus/pipette** for measuring particle size, the basic mechanism is **sedimentation**.

"Elutriation" method is a size separation method based on sedimentation principle. It may be used to separate the coarse and fine particles present in a paste after levigation. The paste is mixed with a large volume of water or any other nonsolvent, and the mixture is allowed to stand for a short time during which the heavy coarse particles settle to the bottom of the vessel. The upper layers of liquid is poured off and the fine particles allowed to settle to the bottom which is finally separated from the vehicle.

On the large scale, elutriation tanks are used. These have stirring gear and a number of taps at regular intervals from top to bottom. On the large scale "counter-current movement" between the suspended particles and vehicle is adopted.

Sometimes the word "Light" or "Heavy" is used to express the physical character of a material. As for example, light kaolin and heavy kaolin, light magnesium carbonate and heavy magnesium carbonate etc. These light and heavy varieties are separated by elutriation technique. There is no chemical difference between these two varieties but the physical characters like bulk density etc. are different.

Official Standard for Powder : The degree of coarseness or fineness of a powder is expressed by reference to the nominal mesh aperture size of the sieves used for measuring the size of the powders.

The following terms are used in the description of powders :

I **Coarse Powder (10/44) :** A powder all the particles of which pass through a sieve with a nominal mesh aperture of 1700 μm and not more that 40% by weight through a sieve with a nominal mesh aperture of 355 μm.

II **Moderately coarse powder (22/60) :** A powder all the particles of which pass through a seive with a nominal mesh aperture of 710 μm and not more than 40% by weight through a sieve with a nominal mesh aperture of 250 μm.

III **Moderately fine powder (44/85) :** A powder all the particles of which pass through a sieve with a nominal mesh aperture of 355 μm and not more than 40% by weight through a sieve with a nominal mesh aperture of 180 μm.

IV **Fine powder (85) :** A powder all the particles of which pass through a sieve with a nominal mesh aperture of 180 μm and not more than 40% by weight through a sieve with a nominal mesh aperture of 125 μm.

V **Very fine powder :** A powder all the particles of which pass through a seive with a nominal mesh aperture of 125 μm and not more than 40% by weight through a sieve with a nominal mesh aperture of 45 μm.

VI **Microfine powder :** A powder of which not less than 90% by weight of the particles pass through a sieve with a nominal mesh aperture of 45 μm.

VII **Superfine powder :** A powder of which not less than 90% by number of the particles are less than 10 μm in size.

When the fineness of the powder is described by means of a number, it is intended that all the particles of the powder shall pass through a sieve of which the nominal mesh aperture in μm, is equal to that number.

Cyclone Separator

Cyclone separation can take the form of a centrifugal elutriation process or a centrifugal sedimentation process in which particles sediment out of a helical gas or liquid stream. Probably the most common type of cyclone used to separate particles from fluid streams is the reverse-flow cyclone. In this system particles in air or liquid suspension are often introduced tangentially into the cylindrical upper section of the cyclone where the relatively high fluid velocity produces a vortex which throws solid particles out onto the walls of the cyclone. Coarser particles separate from the fluid stream and fall out of the cyclone through the dust outlet whereas finer particles remain entrained in the fluid stream and leave the cyclone through the vortex finder. A series of cyclones having different flow rates or different dimensions could be used to separate a powder into different particle size ranges.

MODEL QUESTIONS

1. Micromeritics refers to the study of
   A. microscopes
   B. microscopic ocean life
   C. dimensions of microorganisms
   D. small particles
   E. metric systems of measurement.
2. Moderately coarse powder (a No. 40 powder) is
   A. all particles are retained on sieve no 40 but pass through 20
   B. all particles pass through no. 40 and not more than 40% through 80
   C. all particles pass through no. 40
   D. none of the above.

ANSWERS

1. D (Micromeritics is a study of all aspects of small particles including particle size, separation of particles, comminution and behavior of particles in pharmaceutical systems); 2. B.

CHAPTER 7

Mixing and Homogenisation

- Liquid Mixing and Powder Mixing
- Mixing of Semisolids
- Planetary Mixer; Agitated Powder Mixer; Triple Roller Mill; Propeller Mixer

- Colloid Mill and Hand Homogeniser
- Double Cone Mixer.

Mixing may be defined as a process where two or more components are treated so as to lie as nearly as possible in contact with a particle of each of the other components. The aim of the process is to produce one of the following :

(i) a blend of solid particles (powder mixing),

(ii) a suspension of an insoluble solid in a liquid,

(iii) a mixture of miscible liquids,

(iv) a dispersion of particles in a semisolid as in the preparation of ointments or pastes,

(v) a mixture of soluble solid ingredients in liquid,

(vi) a mixture of two or more immiscible liquids as in the case of emulsion,

(vii) a mixing stage is involved at sometime in the preparation of practically every pharmaceutical preparation.

Liquid mixing

There are four types of mixing mechanism involved in case of liquid mixing, such as i) bulk transport, ii) turbulent mixing, iii) laminar mixing and, iv) molecular diffusion. When mixing is complete, intensity and scale of segregation is zero.

Mixers for liquid and suspensions

I **Shaker mixers :** Oscillatory or a rotar movement is adopted to make the mixing effective.

II **Propeller mixers :** A propeller has angled blades which cause the circulation of the fluid in both an axial and radial direction.

III **Turbine mixers :** A turbine mixer may be used for more viscous fluids. The impeller has four flat blades surrounded by perforated inner and outer diffuser rings.

Powder mixing

Here three primary mechanisms are responsible for mixing

(i) Convective movement of relatively large portions of the bed.

(ii) Shear failure which primarily reduces the scale of segregation.

(iii) Diffusive movement of individual particles. Most efficient mixers operate to induce mixing by all three mechanisms.

Most widely used industrial powder mixers include :

I Tumbling mixers or Rotating shell mixers : Free flowing materials can be mixed in tumbling mixers which are rotating vessels of various shapes so that the charge flows with the vessel when the angle of repose is exceeded. The shapes may be double cone, 'V'-shaped, 'Y'-shaped, diamond-shaped, twin-shell-shaped and drum-shaped, together with baffles where appropriate.

II Fixed shell mixers/Agitator mixtures : These mixers depend on the motion of a blade or paddle through the charge producing a high degree of convective mixing. The 'ribbon mixer' is a common type.

The mixing of semisolids : The problems which arise during the mixing of semisolids (ointments and pastes) stem from that fact that unlike powders and liquids, semisolids will not flow easily. Material that finds its way to 'dead' space will remain there. For that reason suitable mixers must have rotating elements with narrow clearances between the mixing vessel and they must produce a high degree of shear mixing since diffusion and convective mixing cannot occur.

Mixers for Semisolids

I The planetary mixer : This mixer is also suitable for powder mixing as well as the mixing of viscous liquid. The word 'planetary' is very much appropriate. Because the paddle or impeller blades that rotates on its own axis also travels in a circular path round the mixing vessel in opposite direction.

II The sigma blade mixer : This robust mixer will deal with stiff pastes and ointments and depends for its action on the close intermeshing of the two blades which resemble the Greek letter sigma (Σ) in shape.

Triple Roller Mill : Roller mills use the principle of attrition to produce size reduction of solids in suspensions, pastes or ointments. During the manufacturing of ointment by fusion method, some portion of ointment base may solidify in the 'dead space' of the manufacturing vessel which ultimately may form agglomerate containing least/no amount of drug. This agglomerate may better be mixed with the bulk during passing through roller mill. Two or three porcelain or metal roller are mounted horizontally with an adjustable gap which can be as small as 20 μm. The rollers rotate at different speeds so that the material is sheared as it passes through the gap and is transferred from the slower to the faster roll, from which it is removed by means of a scraper.

Colloid Mills : The principle of operation of the colloid mill is the passage of the mixed phases of an emulsion formula between a stator and a high-speed rotor revolving at speeds of 2,000-18,000 rpm. The emulsion mixture, in passing between the rotor and stator, is subjected to tremendous shearing action which effects a fine dispersion.

Homogenizers and Viscolizers

In the viscolizer and the homogenizer, the mixed phases are passed between a finely ground valve seat under high pressure. This, in effect, produces an atomization which is enhanced by the impact received by the atomized mixture as it strikes the valve head. This type of apparatus operates at a pressure of 100-500 lb./sq. inch and produces, some of the finest dispersion obtainable in an emulsion.

For small-scale extemporaneous preparation of emulsions the inexpensive hand homogenizer is particularly useful. It is probably the most efficient emulsifying apparatus available to the prescription pharmacist.

MODEL QUESTIONS

1. Sigma blade mixers are commonly used in
   A. wet granulation
   B. dry granulation
   C. powder mixing
   D. crude fiber mixing
   E. all of the above.

2. Given below (A to F) are some materials. Match them properly with the mixing equipments listed below to achieve homogeneous mix.

   (i)   Double cone blender   A. Emulsions
   (ii) Ribbon mixer   B. Viscous liquid
   (iii) Turbine mixer   C. Stiff paste and ointment
   (iv) Sigma blade mixer   D. Mixing of glidant with tablet granules before punching
   (v)   Homogenizer   E. Powder
                               F. Gases.

3. Given below are the list of mixtures, match them properly with their types listed in A to D.

   (i)   Mixture of miscible liquids   A. Neutral mix
   (ii) Mixture of insoluble solid particles   B. Positive mixing with a liquid
         with a liquid
   (iii) Mixture of powder constituents   C. Racemic mixing
                                                D. Negative mixing

ANSWERS

1. A (Wet granulation has been carried out using high power sigma blade as well as heavy duty planetary mixture. The granulating time and the requirement of granulating fluid is comparatively less in this case. Sigma blade mixers are also used in powder mixing, ointment and paste mixing); 2. i - E, ii - D, iii - B, iv - C, v - A; 3. i - B, ii - D, iii - A (Miscible liquid, gases and vapours will in time completely mix spontaneously by diffusion and no energy need to be used for this to occur. This positive mixing may be contrasted with the negative mixing of insoluble solid particles with a liquid where the particles will separate out unless work is done by stirring to keep them dispersed. A mixture of powdered constituents is an example of a neutral mix. Work must be done to mix them initially but usually there is then no tendency for demixing to occur spontaneously; though demixing is possible in certain circumstances like shaking, due to difference between the components in particle size, shape and density.)

CHAPTER 8

Clarification and Filtration

- Theory of Filtration
- Filter Media

- Filter Aids and Selection of Filters
- Study of the Various Filtration Equipments

Filtration may be defined as the separation of a solid from a fluid by means of porous medium that retains the solid but allows the fluid to pass. Whereas, clarification is the removal of visible solid containing particles from the liquid to make it clear. The proportion of solids is very low, in case of liquids to be clarified.

In case of cold sterilization by filtration one term 'polishing of liquid' is used, i.e., removal of coarse contaminating particles from the liquids to be sterile by using suitable prefilter. This is done in order to increase the lifetime and efficiency of membrane filter.

The suspension of solid and liquid to be filtered is known as the "slurry". The porous medium used to retain the solids is described as the "filter medium" the accumulated solids on the filter is referred to as the 'filter cake' while the clear liquid passing through the filter is the 'filtrate'.

Mechanisms of Filtration

The following mechanisms may be involved in case of filtration process.

(i) Straining : Just like sieving, the pores of the filter media are smaller than the particles to be separated out.

(ii) Impingement : Smaller contaminating particles may impinge and accumulate on the top of the fiber materials of the filter media whose dimension is higher than the particles.

(iii) Entanglement : Smaller contaminating particles may become entangled in the mass of fibers of the filter media. Both impingement as well as bridging may be involved in this case.

(iv) Attractive forces : In this case electrostatic forces are responsible. An example of this technique is electrostatic precipitator.

Rate of Filtration

The equation correlating the rate factors is known as "Darcy's Law" and may be expressed as

$$\frac{dV}{dt} = \frac{KA\Delta P}{\mu l}$$

where,

V = volume of filtrate

t = time of filtration

K = constant for the filter medium and the filter cake

A = area of filter media

ΔP = pressure drop across the filter medium and filter cake

μ = viscosity of the filtrate and

l = thickness of cake.

According to Darcy's law, rate of filtration is directly proportional with the area of filter medium. This may be achieved by :

(i) Using larger filters.

(ii) Using a number of small units in parallel as in the case of filter press.

(iii) In the rotary filter, the filter cake is removed continuously, giving in effect, an infinite area of filtration.

In case of simple filtration, a pressure difference (ΔP) may be achieved by maintaining a head of slurry above the filter medium. The pressure drop may also be achieved by either of the following ways :

(i) Reduced pressure/negative pressure : The pressure below the filter medium may be reduced below atmospheric pressure by connecting the filtrate receiver to a vacuum pump and creating a pressure differential across the filter which may be upto one atmospheric pressure theoretically. In this case the chances of accident due to bursting is not there as the vessel may collapse but not explode. But this technique is not applicable if the desirable filtrate is highly volatile i.e., with low B.P. In laboratory scale negative pressure may be created by using 'Buchner funnel' or 'Hirch funnel' connected with a venturimeter which is again connected with a water delivery tap.

(ii) Positive pressure : This may be upto 15 bars as in the case of some industrial plant. In this case very high pressure difference is achieved but there is a chance of explosion.

Viscosity of the liquid may be reduced by increasing the temperature in case of thermostable, non-volatile materials or by diluting the liquid/slurry. Now if the volume is doubled by diluting with an equal volume of the liquid, the rate must be more than double to show any advantage.

Materials Used for Filter Media

(i) Woven materials : Felts, cloths in wool, cotton, silk, glass, metal, synthetic fibres like rayon, nylon etc.

(ii) Perforated sheet metal.

(iii) Beds of granular solids built up on a supporting medium e.g., gravel, sand, asbestos, paper pulp, kieselguhr etc.

(iv) Porous solids : Sintered glass, sintered metal, earthenware, porous plastics etc.

(v) Membrane filter, i.e., bacteriological filter prepared by using cellulose esters.

Filter Aids : Usually the resistance to flow due to the filter medium itself is very low, but will increase as a layer of solids build up blocking the pores of the medium and forming a solid, impervious cake. The object of the filter aid is to prevent the medium from becoming blocked and to form an open, porous cake, so reducing the resistance to flow of the filtrate. Thus, the filter aid must be a light, porous, inert solid and may be used in either or both of two ways.

Firstly, by forming a pre-coat over the medium by filtering a suspension of the filter aid sufficient to give a coating upto 0.5 kg/m^2.

Secondly, a small proportion of the filter aid (0.1 to 0.5%) is added to the slurry, ensuring that the filter cake has a porous structure. Example of filter aid is kieselguhr. Filter aids are limited usually to clarification processes, that is, where the solids are discarded.

Filter Press : Plate and frame press is of wide application in pharmaceutical practice. Here plates and frames are fitted with a filter cloth in between and many such units are mounted on two parallel support bars.

If it is necessary to wash the filter cake, the ordinary plate and frame press is unsatisfactory and in such case a modified design known as "Washing Plate and Frame Press" is used.

Edge Filters : Filters such as the leaf or press act by presenting a surface of the filter medium to slurry. Edge filters use a pack of the filter medium, so that filtration occurs on the edges. In the pharmaceutical industry greatest use is made of the "Metafilter", which can be used as a strainer for coarse particles, but for finer particles a bed of a suitable material such as kieselguhr is first build up. In the second case the structure is only giving support to kieselguhr which actually acts as true filter medium.

Sintered Filters : Among the sintered filters, sintered glass filters is widely used. In this case fine wool or particles or powders of borosilicate glass are molded or sintered at very high temperatures in a suitable shape such as flat or convex plates in such a way that its porosity is reduced but not choked. If manufactured properly this filter may be used to remove microorganism. But application of (+)ve or (−)ve pressure is essential here. Sintered glass filters are graded from coarse to fine by numbering 1 to 5. Grade No. 5 is used in bacterial filtration.

Candle Filters : These are made of unglazed porcelain either cylindrical or in the shape of flanged test tube, generally known as candle. Candle filters can be obtained in various grades of porosity, varying from a relatively coarse filter to fine grades. The domestic water filter consists of candle filter. The ceramic candle filters are, however, somewhat, fragile and now a days candle made of polytetrafluoroethylene (P.T.F.E) are used.

Other Industrial Filters :

(i) **Filter Leaf :** A perforated leaf-like metallic sac is used to give support of the filter cloth wrapped onto the outward surface.

(ii) **Sweetland Filter :** Here a number of leaves are connected to a common outlet, to provide a larger area of filtration.

(iii) **Rotary Filter :** Rotating perforated drum fitted with filter cloth is used to present an infinite surface area to filtration. The device is so designed that it consist of application of vacuum, arrangement for washing, drying and removal of the cake.

(iv) **Seitz Filter**

Besides these membranes made of mixed cellulose esters are most commonly used to filtered out the contaminating microorganisms to get sterile filtrate i.e., sterilization by filtration, also known as cold sterilization.

In order to remove the microorganisms from the air (microorganisms are adhere with the suspended dust particles), HEPA Filter (High Efficiency Particulate Air Filter) is used. The Laminar air flow hood used in the industry to make aseptic area is actually fitted with this HEPA filter.

MODEL QUESTIONS

1. The mechanisms involved in the filtration process are the following except
   A. straining
   B. precipitation
   C. impingement
   D. entanglement
   E. attractive forces.
2. While in operation the area of filtration in case of rotary filter becomes
   A. $2\pi rh$
   B. $2/3\ \pi rh$
   C. infinity
   E. constant
3. Fill in the blanks with appropriate word(s)

The suspension of solid and liquid to be filtered is known as the "...... (i) ......". The porous medium used to retain the solids is described as "...... (ii) ......"; the accumulated solids on the filter is referred to as the "...... (iii) ......", while the clear liquid passing through the filter is the "...... (iv) ......".

ANSWERS

1. B; 2. C; 3. (i) slurry, (ii) filter medium, (iii) filter cake, (iv) filtrate.

CHAPTER 9

Extraction and Galenicals

• Extractive Preparations and Extracts • Galenicals

There are three classes of extractive preparations such as (i) Tinctures; (ii) Fluid extracts and, (iii) Extracts.

(i) **Tinctures :** Tinctures are defined as alcoholic or hydroalcoholic solutions prepared from vegetable materials or from chemical substances, e.g., Belladonna Tincture and Iodine Tincture.

(ii) **Fluid Extracts :** Fluid extracts are liquid preparations of vegetable drugs containing alcohol as a solvent or as a preservative or both, so made that each ml contains the therapeutic constituents of 1g of the standard drug that it represents e.g., *Cascara sagrada* Fluid Extract.

(iii) **Extracts :** Extracts may be defined as concentrated preparations of vegetable or animal drugs obtained by removal of the active constituents of the respective drugs with suitable menstrua, evaporation of all or nearly all of the solvent, and adjustment of the residual masses or powders to the prescribed standard.

Three forms of extracts are recognized :

(a) Semi-liquid or liquid of syrupy consistency, e.g., Hyoscyamus Extract.

(b) Plastic masses, known as **pilular** or solid extracts, e.g., Pure Glycyrrhiza Extract

(c) Dry powders, known as powdered extracts, e.g., Belladonna Extract.

Galenicals : The crude extracts of active constituents, in the form of dry extracts, a viscous soft extract, a concentrated infusion or a tincture, obtained by the solvent extraction of the constituents contained within plant or animal tissues are known as Galenicals.

Extraction can be defined as the removal of soluble material from an insoluble residue, either liquid or solid, by treatment with a liquid solvent. The extraction of a soluble constituent from a solid by means of a solvent is commonly referred to as **Leaching**.

MODEL QUESTIONS

1. Separation of the active constituents from the crude drug is desirable due to which of the following reason?
   A. Potency is more readily controlled.
   B. Deterioration, e.g., by enzyme action is diminished.
   C. Preparations of the drug are more easily formulated, more stable, more palatable and more elegant.
   D. Smaller bulk facilitates storage and transport.
   E. Injection of the crude material may be undesirable or dangerous.
   F. Tabletting or formation of other unit dosage form may not be possible with the crude materials.
   G. All of the above.
2. In one of the extraction processes the crude drug particles are taken in a closed vessel along with solvent with occassional shaking for few days. This is known as
   A. Percolation   B. Maceration   C. Infusion
   D. Digestion   E. Decoction
3. Unorganized drugs (drugs having no cellular structure like gum exudate, latex, etc.) may be better extracted by
   A. Decoction   B. Continuous hot extraction   C. Repeated maceration
   D. Maceration   E. Percolation.
4. It is preferable to use a percolator that is slightly conical in shape because of the following reason(s) :
   A. Sloping sides allow better expansion of the bed than would cylindrical columns.
   B. The cylindrical columns have the disadvantage that solvent often fails to permeate through material near the sides at the bottom.
   C. It is not essential that a percolator be always conical shaped.
   D. A and B.
   E. None of the above.
5. An ideal process of tea preparation is
   A. Infusion   B. Decoction   C. Soxhlation
   D. Maceration   E. Digestion.
6. Raising the temperature of the solvent has the effect of hastening the leaching process during extraction. This is due to
   A. increase rate of diffusion.   B. stronger convection currents.
   C. better solubility of the active principles.

D. lowering the viscosity.   E. A and C.   F. all of the above.

7. Percolation process of extraction excludes
   A. organized drugs.   B. unorganized drugs.   C. soft drugs.
   D. woody drugs.   E. thermolabile drugs.

8. Tinctures
   A. are made by direct solution of a volatile oil.
   B. representing 100 g of drug in 100 ml of finished tincture.
   C. are aqueous solutions of active constituents of drugs.
   D. are sweetened, flavored aqueous alcoholic solutions of drugs.
   E. none of the above.

9. All of the following are reasons why aromatic waters are not commonly used except
   A. most are saturated solutions.
   B. poor solvent properties.
   C. unpleasant taste.
   D. preparation requires 12 to 24 hours.
   E. susceptibility to mold growth.

10. Iodine Solution USP contains iodine and
    A. alcohol   B. isopropanol   C. potassium iodide
    D. sodium iodide   E. PVP.

11. Iodine Tincture USP differs from Iodine Solution USP in that the tincture contains
    A. potassium iodide as the hydrotropic agent
    B. more iodine
    C. Alcohol USP as the vehicle
    D. Diluted Alcohol USP as the vehicle
    E. less iodine.

12. Decoction process of extraction is taken for
    A. soft drug   B. woody drug   C. unorganized drug.
    D. semisolid drug   E. all of the above.

13. Glycerin in tincture card co. (compound cardamom tincture) is used
    A. as viscosity enhancer   B. as preservative   C. as sweetening agent
    D. as humectant   E. to dissolve tannin.

14. The infusion process of extraction is used for
    A. hard woody drug   B. soft spongy drug   C. volatile oil
    D. unorganized drug   E. all the above.

15. Fill in the blanks.
    (i)   The extraction of soluble constituent from a solid by means of a solvent is commonly referred to as "...... (i) ......".
    (ii) The dissolution of traces of solid from the wall of the glass or polymeric packaging material to the aqueous content of the container is commonly referred to as "...... (ii) ......".
    (iii) The solvent used in the extraction process is known as "...... (iii) ......".

    (iv) The solid residue remaining after extraction is termed as "...... (iv) ......".

    (v) The solution obtained after macerating the crude drugs is also known as "...... (v) ......".

16. State True or False.

    (i) In case of "Percolation" process of extraction the marc is pressed only to avoid wastage of solvent.

    (ii) In case of "Maceration" process of extraction the liquid expressed from the marc is of equal strength with that separated by straining.

    (iii) In case of "Reserved Percolation", the first concentrated fraction of the percolate is kept aside as reserved and residual 2nd diluted fraction is subjected to evaporation to concentrate.

    (iv) "Digestion" process of extraction is a form of maceration in which gentle heat is used during the process of extraction.

    (v) "Infusion" process of extraction is a form of maceration of drugs for a short period of time (from 15 minutes to 2 hrs.) with either cold or boiling water.

    (vi) Decoctions were prepared by boiling the drug for 15 minutes with water.

    (vii) In case of thermostable drug the Soxhlation (continuous hot extraction) may be used to extract a drug for the purposes of assay.

    (viii) In case of "Soxhlation" the same solvent (menstruum) is recycled repeatedly as fresh solvent.

ANSWERS

1. G; 2. B; 3. C (Because expression of marc is not possible in case of unorganized drug. Percolation process of extraction is not at all applicable to unorganized drugs); 4. D; 5. A; 6. F; 7. B; 8. E (The first one 'A' is a process of preparing aromatic water; the second one is applicable in case of fluid extracts. Tinctures are usually 5-20% in strength); 9. D [Although there is a method of manufacture that requires 24 hours for preparation (known as simple solution method, the waters could be prepared by the alternate solution method using talc as dispersing agent. This method requires less than one hour. As most are saturated solution, chemicals particularly electrolytes often "Salting out" the volatile oil. The solutions are usually bitter and in absence of preservatives, susceptible to microbial growth]; 10. C (Iodine and KI react to form KI_3, which is readily soluble in water. There is no loss of antibacterial activity since the iodine is readily available from the complex. This phenomenon of forming a more water soluble complex without loss of activity is known as **hydrotropy**.); 11. D (Iodine Tincture also contain KI, not as hydrotropic agent because iodine is soluble in hydroalcoholic mixture. Presence of KI allow the tincture to be diluted with water without precipitation); 12. B (For soft drug infusion process and for unorganized drug repeated maceration may be suitable); 13. E (In wild cherry syrup also glycerol serves the same purpose); 14. B. 15. i) leaching, ii) leaching, iii) menstruum, iv) marc, v) miscella. 16. i) True, ii) True, iii) True, iv) True, v) True, vi) True, vii) True, viii) True.

CHAPTER 10

Heat Processes

- Evaporation and Distillation Including Simple Fractional, Steam and Vacuum Distillation
- Waters Official in I.P.

Theoretically, every substance can exist as solid, liquid and gaseous states. Usually a change from one state to another involves either addition of heat or subtraction of heat. The heat of fusion is the amount of energy required to destroy the crystal structure of solid and thus melt it. The amount of heat required to change 1 gram of liquid into the vapour state at the normal boiling temperature of the liquid is known as the heat of vaporization and is generally expressed in calories.

The transition of a solid to liquid state due to application of heat is known as 'Fusion' or 'Melting'. Similarly, the transition of liquid to gas due to application of heat is known as 'evaporation' (below the boiling temperature) or 'boiling' (occur at boiling temperature). The transition of solid to gas due to application of heat is known as 'sublimation'. The transition from gas to liquid/solid due to subtraction of heat is known as 'condensation'. Finally, the transition of liquid to solid due to subtraction of heat is known as 'solidification'.

In case of evaporation the vapor is usually formed at the surface of liquid at any temperature usually below the boiling point of liquid. Usually condensation and collection of vapor is not done in case of evaporation but evaporation is carried out when concentrated liquid residue is required.

Factors Affecting Evaporation

Evaporation is the free escape of vapor from surface of liquid at a temperature below its boiling point.

The rate of evaporation (m) is the weight of vapor produced in unit time. This rate is proportional to surface area exposed to atmosphere (S), the difference between maximum vapor pressure of the liquid at a given temperature (F) and the actual vapor pressure above the surface of the evaporating liquid at the same temperature (f); and is inversely proportional to atmospheric pressure on the surface of liquid (P).

Therefore, $m \propto \dfrac{S(F-f)}{P}$

Besides this the following pharmaceutical and technical factors may affect the rate of evaporation :

   (i) Temperature

  (ii) Temperature and time of evaporation

 (iii) Temperature and moisture content

 (iv) Type of product

  (v) Film deposits.

Various Devices Used for Evaporation

1. Evaporating pans : A "steam pan" consists of an inner pan, jacketed with an outer pan through which steam is passed.

2. Vacuum pans : These are used for the concentration of thermolabile substances.

3. Tube evaporators.

4. Lillie film evaporator.

5. Climbing film evaporators.

6. Horizontal film evaporators.

DISTILLATION

Distillation is by far the oldest method of purifying water and other solvents. A liquid will start boiling when its vapor pressure becomes equal with the atmospheric pressure. The vapor so generated is then passed through a condenser which condenses the vapor to liquid form collected in a receiver. The majority of distillation stills consist of an evaporating vessel where boiling water produces steam which is then condensed back to water. Various systems are used to prevent water droplets carrying pyrogens, foreign matters and gases over from the evaporator to the condenser in the water vapor. A classical example is baffles.

In case of a mixed solvent e.g., alcohol and water binary liquid system, the liquid will start boiling when the partial vapor pressure of alcohol plus partial vapor pressure of water becomes equal with the atmospheric pressure. The vapor so produced would be enriched with more volatile component (m.v.c.) than the mother liquor composition. Therefore, the distillate will contain much higher percentage of m.v.c than the original mother liquor. By repeating this process we can purify one liquid from another having different boiling points. This is the principle of **fractional distillation**.

In case of rectification of alcohol, its concentration can be gradually increased in fractionating column. Thereafter 95% alcohol + 5% water cannot be further purified by way of fractional distillation. Because they form an "**azeotropic mixture**". The vapor composition of an azeotropic mixture is exactly equal with the original mother liquor composition. So further purification by fractional distillation is not possible.

Steam Distillation

The volatile oil present in different parts of plant cannot be heated at high temperature or the temperature of their boiling, because they will decompose. They can be separated from the crude material by way of Steam Distillation, keeping them immersed in water in a vessel through which steam is injected. The vapor of volatile oil and water so produced is collected in a receiver through condenser. The condensate in the receiver forms two distinct layers the top of which is volatile oil and the bottom layer consists of a saturated solution of that volatile oil in water which may be returned back to the vessel containing crude drug for better yield or may be collected as aromatic water. Therefore, separation of volatile oil and preparation of aromatic water are the two main objectives of steam distillation.

Vacuum Distillation

We know that pure water boils at 100°C under one atmospheric pressure. We also know that it freezes at 0°C. The dissolved solutes have great influence in the b.p., m.p., tonicity etc. of water. According to the Raoult's law there would be elevation of b.p. and depression of freezing point of water due to the presence of dissolved solid. Now this boiling point is also dependent on the adjacent atmospheric pressure. Because a liquid will start boiling when its vapor pressure becomes equal with the adjacent atmospheric pressure. In case of pressure cooker and autoclave b.p. of water increases with in these pressure vessels on the other hand water will boil at much lower temperature in a vacuum vessel fitted with high power vacuum pump giving effect to mass transfer at much lower temperature. This principle is used in case of vacuum distillation of thermolabile materials.

   Purified Water : Purified water is prepared by distillation, reverse osmosis, by means of ion exchange (deionisation or demineralization) or by any other appropriate means from suitable potable water that implies with all relevant statutory regulations. It contains no added substances. However, the different methods of producing it present different potential for contamination. Purified water produced by distillation by using properly designed distillation still may be sterile, provided the production equipment is suitable and sterile. Water obtained by ion-exchange treatment or by reverse osmosis may contain micro-organisms and it will be necessary to monitor the bacterial quality of the water frequently, particularly with the use of the purifying systems following periods of shutdown for more than a few hours.

   Water for Injection : Water for injection is apyrogenic distilled water intended for use in the preparations of medicines for parenteral administration when water is used as a vehicle (water for injection in bulk) and for dissolving or diluting substances or preparations for injectable preparation (sterile water for injection). Water for injection is not intended to be sterile. It should be stored and distributed under condition designed to prevent production of pyrogens or endotoxins (e.g., stored at 80°C).

   Sterile Water of Injection : This article is water for injection which is sterilised within 12 hours of collection so that it remains apyrogenic and distributed in sterile containers. It is intended mainly for use as a solvent for injectable preparations such as powders for injection that are distributed dry because of limited stability of their solutions. It should be packaged only in single dose containers of not larger than 1 liter size.

MODEL QUESTIONS

1. A solution of alcohol and water is boiling at 88°C which is much higher than the boiling point of alcohol. What would be the partial pressure of alcohol at that temperature?
   A. Equal with the atmospheric pressure.
   B. Higher than the atmospheric pressure.
   C. Less than the atmospheric pressure.
   D. All of the above.
   E. None of the above.

2. The principle objective(s) of steam distillation is/are
   A. separation of volatile oil.
   B. preparation of aromatic water.
   C. to use latent heat of steam as source of heat during distillation.
   D. A and B.
   E. none of the above.

3. The process of reverse osmosis can be used to prepare
   A. Alcohol USP.　　　　B. Isopropyl Alcohol USP.　　C. Purified Water USP.
   D. Milk of Magnesia USP.　　E. all of the above.

4. Official forms of water include (I) water for injection; (II) bacteriostatic water for injection; (III) sterile water for injection.
   A. I only.　　　　B. III only.　　　　C. I and II only.
   D. II and III only.　　E. I, II, and III.

5. Water for injection differs from sterile distilled water as it is free from
   A. carbon dioxide　　　　B. pyrogens
   C. preservatives.　　　　D. antioxidant.

6. The method of preparation must be indicated on lables for
   A. Water for Injection USP.
   B. Stronger Rose Water NF.
   C. Bacteriostatic Water for Injection USP.
   D. Purified Water USP.
   E. Milk of Magnesia USP.

7. Water for Injection USP may be prepared from tap water by
   A. chemical treatment with $KMnO_4$.
   B. deionization followed by filtration through pyrogen retaining filters.
   C. reflux distillation.
   D. simple distillation.
   E. sterilization by autoclaving.

8. The form of water most commonly used as a solvent during the manufacture of parenterals is
   A. deionized water.
   B. distilled water.

C. Bacteriostatic Water for Injection USP.

D. Water for Injection USP.

E. Sterile Water for Injection USP.

9. The USP has established limits on dissolved solids in the official waters, assuming that such values should reflect the relative purity of the waters. Which of the following has the lowest permissible level of dissolved solids?

A. Bacteriostatic Water for Injection USP

B. Purified Water USP

C. Potable water

D. Sterile Water for Injection USP (in 30 ml vials)

E. Sterile Water for Injection USP (in 1 liter bottles)

10. Fill in the blanks :

(i) 95% alcohol water mixture cannot be further concentrated by fractional distillation as they form .... mixture.

(ii) The vapor composition of an azeotropic mixture becomes .... with the composition of the original azeotropic mixture.

ANSWERS

1. C; 2. D; 3. C; 4. E (Besides this purified water and sterile water for irrigation are also official); 5. B; 6. D; 7. D [Freshly prepared distilled water (produced using properly designed distillation still) is non sterile but free from pyrogens). Although pyrogen retaining filters are available, deionized water is too contaminated to be used. Sterilization will destroy microorganisms but will not destroy pyrogens]; 8. D [Water for injection is pyrogen-free water and are used as vehicle in the preparation of parenterals (including large volume). After admixture with pyrogen free drug and excipients, the product is terminally sterilized immediately after filling and sealing in the final container is done. Water for injection should be freshly prepared or stored at 80°C to prevent further contamination with pyrogen]; 9. B

	(USP Limit)	(I.P. Limit)
Freshly prepared distilled water	10 ppm	10 ppm
Sterile water for injection	40 ppm (for 30 ml vial)	40 ppm (vial capacity ≤ 10 ml)
	20 ppm (for 1 liter bottle)	30 ppm (vial capacity > 10 ml)

Autoclaving and storing the water in glass will cause leaching of soluble solids from the container walls]. 10. i. azeotropic; ii. equal.

CHAPTER 11

Introduction to Drying Processes

> • Study of Tray Dryers, Fluidised Bed Dryer,   • Desiccation.
>   Vacuum Dryer and Freeze Dryer

Drying is an important operation in pharmaceutical practice. Correct drying can prevent deterioration or can ensure that a product is readily soluble or is free flowing etc.

Tray Dryers/Compartment Dryers/Shelf Dryers

The widely used tray dryers is directed circulation form in which electrically heated air is directed mechanically from lower tray to upper tray and saturated hot air is exhausted through the outlet. The outlet air temperature must be sufficiently high to prevent recondensation of moisture vapour before leaving the drying chamber. It is a batch operation and used to dry a variety of materials including crude drugs, chemicals, tablet granules, powders etc.

A slight modification of this drying is to obtain semi-continuous operation with greater efficiency by having counter current movement of air and drying solid. A further modification of tray dryer is "tunnel dryer" where hot air entered at one end and some means of moving the material to be dried at the opposite end of the tunnel. So the outgoing material met the incoming air to ensure maximum drying and the outgoing air contacted the wettest material so that the air was as nearly saturated as possible.

In case of tray dryer and tunnel dryer the heat and subsequent mass transfer occur from the surface of the bed of the moist material. This is responsible for '**case hardening**' the main problem associated with such type of dryers which may be tackled by using a modified tunnel dryer known as 'rotary dryer' used successfully for continuous drying on a large scale of any powdered or granular solid. Total drying time in tray dryer may be 12 to 24 hrs or more.

Fluidised Bed Dryer

In fluidised bed dryer, the particulated matter to be dried is contained in a more or less conical vessel, the base of which is perforated, enabling a hot fluid (usually air) to pass through the bed of solids from below with such velocity that the particles remain suspended in hot air permitting heat and mass transfer throughout the entire outer surfaces of the individual particles. The term "boiling bed" being commonly used to describe this fluidized state, which offers a means of rapid drying (within 30 minutes to three hours per batch). Therefore, the problem of case hardening is not associated with fluidised bed dryer and total degradation due to heat is also minimized. This dryer can be used for drying any powder material particularly the tablet granules.

Another problem associated with tray dryer as well as fluidised bed dryer is solute migration during drying, which is migration of soluble solute from inner portion of the particles towards periphery along with solvent during drying and its ultimate deposition at the surface. Therefore, the fines generated, if any during drying, will contain higher percentage of drug which is responsible for variation of active constituents content in individual tablets or capsules. In case of using soluble coloring agent this may be responsible for 'mottling' of the compressed coloured tablet which is uneven distribution of colour at the surface of the tablet.

Vacuum Dryer

A classical example is vacuum tumbling dryer. In this case the application of vacuum facilitates quick evaporation and drying, comparatively at reduced temperature. Therefore, it is applicable in case of moderately heat stable materials.

Freeze Dryer

Freeze drying also known as sublimation drying or lyophilization or cold drying is applicable to dry biological products for example, antibiotics (other than penicillin), blood products, vaccines (such as BCG, yellow fever, small pox), enzyme preparations (such as hyaluronidase) and microbiological cultures etc.

In case of freeze drying the frozen materials to be dried is kept at a temperature and pressure below the **triple point** temperature and pressure of water. In that condition further addition of heat at a controlled rate is responsible for direct mass transfer from solid ice to vapour by by-passing the liquid state. The vapour so produced is quickly removed by using powerful exhaust system.

Dryers for Dilute Solutions and Suspensions

The objective of these dryers is to spread the liquid to a large surface area for heat and mass transfer and to provide an effective means of collecting the dry solid. Two main types are used, the first (Drum Dryer) spreading the liquid to a thin film and the second (Spray Dryer) dispersing the liquid to a spray of small droplets.

The drum dryer can handle a variety of materials, either as solutions or suspensions; substances that are dried by this method include milk products, starch products, ferrous salts, and suspension of kaolin or zinc oxide, aluminium hydroxide, magnesium hydroxide etc.

Spray dried substances include borax, citric acid, hexamine, sodium phosphate, gelatin, acacia, extracts, starch, milk, soap, detergents etc.

Desiccation : Desiccation is the removing of admixed water from a solid substances. In the laboratory a drying equipment called "desiccator" is used to remove admixed water. The desiccator is a tightly closed glass vessel containing a very hygroscopic substances, known as desiccants, at the bottom to absorb water vapor given out by the substances being desiccated or dried. Vacuum desiccator accelerates drying. The materials used as desiccants include :

(i) Silica gel impregnated with an indicator, cobalt chloride which gives blue color in anhydrous state but turns pink or red in moist state.

(ii) Anhydrous calcium chloride (fused).

(iii) Lithium chloride.

(iv) Concentrated sulphuric acid etc.

MODEL QUESTIONS

1. Mottling of the compressed colored tablet is
   A. uneven distribution of colour at the surface of tablet due to migration of soluble colours towards periphery during drying
   B. uneven distribution of colour during coating with colouring agent
   C. erosion of the coloured coat from the surface of the tablet
   D. all the above.

2. Mannitol may be included in lyophilized products as a
   A. preservative
   B. sweetener
   C. tonicity adjuster
   D. bulking agent
   E. buffer.

3. Fluidised bed drier is well adopted in the pharmaceutical industry for the drying of
   A. powders before filling capsules
   B. fibrous materials before passing through cutter mill
   C. granules before compression into tablets
   D. empty capsules before filling
   E. powders before mixing and granulation.

4. For drying blood plasma the following technique is used :
   A. Spray drying
   B. Freeze drying
   C. Vacuum drying
   D. Fluid bed drying
   E. Tray drying.

5. Given below (A to G) are some materials. Match them properly with the drying equipments listed below for proper and efficient drying.

(i)	Drum dryer	A.	Tablet granules
(ii)	Spray dryer	B.	Antibiotic solution
(iii)	Freeze dryer	C.	Crude drugs
(iv)	Fluidised bed dryer	D.	Suspension of kaolin
(v)	Tray dryer	E.	Gelatin
(vi)	Vacuum tumbling dryer	F.	Moderately heat stable granular materials
		G.	Human blood as such.

ANSWERS

1. A; 2. D; 3. C; 4. B; 5. i) - D; ii) - E; iii) - B; iv) - A; v) - C; vi) - F

CHAPTER 12

Sterilization

- Concept of Sterilization
- Sensitivity of Microorganisms
- Steam Sterilization including Heating with a Bactericide and Tyndallization

- Pasteurization
- Sterilization by Dry Heat, Infrared Radiation, Ionizing Radiation and U.V. Radiation
- Sterilization by Filtration and Gas

Sterilization is the process of destroying or removing all forms of living microbial organisms. A *sterile object* in the microbiological sense is free of living microorganisms. Sterility is an absolute term and should not be used in a relative sense. The product would be either sterile or non-sterile and can never be semi-sterile or almost sterile.

Sterilization can be effected in various ways which can be conveniently categorized as follows :

1. **Physical Methods :**
    A. *Heat :* (i) Dry heat (including red heat incineration, flaming, infrared radiation and hot air oven). (ii) Moist heat (including autoclave/steam sterilization, heating with bacterio-static agents, Tyndallization).
    B. *Radiation :* (i) UV. (ii) Ionization (γ)
    C. *Filtration :* Applicable to solutions and gases and involves passing the solution and gases through a filter medium to retain the microorganisms.

2. **Chemical Methods :** Formaldehyde vapor, Ethylene oxide and glutaraldehyde are normally used as chemical agents/ sterilizer.

Sensitivity of microorganisms : The vegetative forms of bacteria, fungi and yeast along with the larger viruses, are the most sensitive to heat radiation and chemicals. They are about a hundred to a thousand times more sensitive to ionization and UV radiation than are bacterial spores and they show a significant response in moist heat at 60-70 °C. The thermophilic bacteria, the smaller viruses, a few resistant forms of mold spores and some of the more sensitive bacterial spores are killed at temperatures between 70 and 90°C, while bacterial spores on the whole must be subjected to temperatures in the range 90-115°C with full hydration before significant reduction in viability occurs with a reasonable time span. However, within this general pattern, individual species of microorganisms may vary markedly in the degree of the response to moist or dry heat radiation and chemicals.

The reference organism selected for moist heat efficiency is usually *Bacillus stearothermophilus*, for dry heat spores of certain strains of *B. subtilis* or *Clostridium tetani*, for ionizing radiation spores of *B. pumilus* and for gaseous sterilization the Fort Detrick strain of *B. subtilis* is used. These choices are made on the basis of their high resistance to the particular sterilizing agents and also on account of case of recovery and propagation.

Steam Sterilization : The process involves heating in an autoclave employing saturated steam under pressure. The following combinations of temperature and time are recommended in I.P.

Holding Temperature (°C)	Minimum holding time (min)
115-118	30
121-124	15
126-129	10
134-138	3

Other combinations of time and temperature may be used provided that they can be demonstrated to be effective. The prescribed conditions are those to be maintained throughout the load, during the holding period of the sterilization cycle.

The above combinations are chosen according to the nature of the product to be sterilized and its sensitivity towards heat, e.g., when surgical dressings are sterilized by steam, the steam used should not contain more than 5% of entrained moisture. Surgical dressings are conveniently sterilized by maintaining a temperature of 134-138°C for 3 minutes but other suitable combinations of temperatures and time may be used.

Moist heat is more effective as a sterilizing agent than dry heat. This is believed to be true for two reasons :

1. Moist heat has greater penetrating power; and

2. Death is believed to result from the coagulation of the protein of the protoplasm. An increase in the water content of the protoplasm decreases the temperature required to coagulate the protein.

The principle of autoclave : Water boils at 100°C under 1 atm pressure where its vapour pressure becomes equal with 1 atm pressure. If the vapor pressure is increased, the boiling temperature will be increased. If the steam pressure is increased inside the autoclave to 15 lb. per sq. inch (2 atm. Absolute), the temperature will rise to 121°C.

The Relationship between Pressure and Temperature

Pressure (lb. per sq. inch)	Corresponding Temperature (°C)
5	109
10	115
15	121
20	126
25	130
30	135

Precautions to prevent sterilization failure by autoclave :

1. Incomplete evacuation of air from the sterilizing chamber—The temperature of a mixture of steam and air at a given pressure is less than that of pure steam alone. This means that although the autoclave is kept at the desired pressure, the temperature may not be sufficient to give complete sterilization.

2. The prescribed temperature must have to be maintained throughout the load during the entire holding period and a pressure gauge reading alone may not be sufficient to ascertain this.

3. The steam must have access to the materials to be treated. For example, suppose it is desired to sterilize some cotton contained in a bottle. If the bottle is closed with a rubber stopper, the steam cannot enter and in such a condition, the autoclave will be no more effective than a hot air sterilizer kept at 121°C for 15 min. This treatment is not sufficient to destroy microorganisms in a dry-air sterilizer. On the other hand, if the mouth of the bottle is covered with one or more thickness of muslin, permitting free access of steam, the cotton should be sterilized.

Applications of autoclave : Autoclave is used to sterilize anything, which is not injured by steam and high temperature. This includes most types of solid and liquid media with and without carbohydrate, gelatin media, distilled water, saline solution, rubber tubing and stopper, discarded cultures and contaminated media prior to washing, laboratory coats and aprons, canned foods, etc.

Sterilization by Heating with a Bactericide : This process may be used for sterilizing aqueous preparations, which are unstable at the higher temperatures attained in the steam sterilization process. However, it has lower margin of safety and should be used only when steam sterilization is not applicable.

In this process the medicament is dissolved or suspended in a suitable solution of the following bactericides so as to achieve the concentration of bactericides given below :

For Injections :

| (i) | Chlorocresol | 0.2% w/v |
| (ii) | Phenylmercuric acetate or nitrate | 0.002% w/v |

For eye drops :

(i)	Benzalkonium chloride solution sufficient to give a final concentration of 0.01% w/v of benzalkonium chloride.	
(ii)	Phenylmercuric acetate or nitrate	0.002% w/v
(iii)	Thiomersal	0.01% w/v
(iv)	Chlorhexidine acetate	0.01% w/v

The preparation is distributed in suitable container which are then sealed so as to exclude microorganisms and heated for a sufficient time to ensure that the entire contents of each container are maintained at about 100°C for thirty minutes.

The bactericide used must not interfere with the therapeutic efficiency of the product, nor be incompatible with the product, its container or its closure.

Sterilization by heating with a bactericide must not be used for

(i) Solutions of medicaments for intrathecal, intraatrium, intracisternal or any other route of injection giving access to the cerebrospinal fluid, or

(ii) Intracardiac or intraocular injections.

The use of a combination of heat and antimicrobial agent is synergistic and, provided the time of exposure is sufficient, permits the use of a lower sterilizing temperature. An interesting modification of heat/chemical synergism is found if the formulation has a high or low pH value because the synergism between the toxic effects of extremes of pH and heat on bacteria enables sterilization to be achieved at 98°-100°C without the addition of a bactericide, for e.g., Phenobarbitone Injection B.P. It is possible also that a medicament may possess intrinsic antimicrobial activity, which may permit sterilization at the lower temperatures.

Tyndallization by Using Arnold Sterilizer : Arnold sterilizer employs streaming steam at a temperature of approximately 100°C (212°F) for a period of 20 min or more on three consecutive days. The length of the exposure period will depend on the nature of the materials being treated and the size of the containers. Agar, for e.g., must be completely melted before recording the beginning of the exposure period.

A temperature of 100°C for 20 min is not sufficient to destroy spores. A much higher temperature is required to effect a complete sterilization in one operation over a relatively short exposure period. However, sterilization in the Arnold sterilizer may be realized by employing the intermittent method. The first exposure period kills all vegetative cells present. Then the materials are kept at a warm temperature for 24 hr. During this holding period, any spores present should germinate into vegetative cells. The second heating period again will destroy all vegetative cells. It sometimes happens that all spores do not germinate into vegetative cells before the second exposure period. Therefore, an additional 24 hr period is allowed to elapse to all spores to germinate to vegetative cells.

It may be seen that unless the spores germinate, the method will fail to sterilize. Failure may be due to the following :

1. The medium may be unsuitable for the germination of the spores, e.g., distilled water is not a favorable environment for the growth of bacteria and will not permit spores to germinate into vegetative cells.

2. Spores of anaerobic bacteria, if present, will not germinate in a medium in contact with atmosphere.

3. If any preservative is present in the product, it may not allow to germinate the spores.

The Arnold sterilizer is used principally for the sterilization of gelatin, milk and carbohydrate media. Higher temperatures in the autoclave, or longer single exposures in the Arnold, may hydrolyze or decompose carbohydrates and prevent gelatin from solidifying. Obviously, such media would then be unsuitable for use.

Pasteurization : Pasteur developed the procedure of gentle heating (Pasteurization) to prevent the spoilage of beer and wine by undesired contaminating microbes. This process was later used to prevent milk-borne diseases of man.

In the pasteurization of milk, the temperature employed is either 63° to 66°C for 30 minutes (the "holder" method) or 72°C for 20 seconds (the "flash" method). Pasteurization is effective because the common milk-borne pathogens (*Mycobacterium tuberculosis*, *M. bavis*, and *Brucella abortus*) do not form spores and are reliably destroyed by this procedure; in addition, the total bacterial count is generally reduced by 97%-99%.

Dry Heat Sterilization : This process of sterilization may be used for heat-stable non-aqueous products and powders. A preparation to be sterilized by dry heat is distributed in the final containers, which are then either finally sealed or temporarily closed to exclude microorganisms, is then heated so as to ensure that the entire contents of each container are maintained at 160°C for two hours, unless otherwise stated in the individual monograph, or at any other equally effective combination of temperature and time. Containers, which have been temporarily closed during the sterilization procedure, are then finally sealed using aseptic technique so as to exclude microorganisms.

Dry heat sterilization is usually carried out in a sterilizing oven designed specifically for this purpose. The oven may be heated by gas or electricity and is normally provided with a fan or blower to circulate the heated air to assure adequate heat distribution throughout the chamber and with suitable temperature recording devices. The sterilizer should be loaded in such a manner as to permit free circulation of heated air throughout the chamber. The effectiveness of any dry heat sterilization schedule should be determined under actual working conditions by means of thermocouples or other suitable devices placed in representative locations within the load and after a proper schedule has been determined, the chamber should be loaded in substantially the same manner for all subsequent cycles in which the particular material is to be treated. Suitable biological indicators may be employed to demonstrate the effectiveness of the sterilization cycle.

Applications of hot air sterilization : The hot air sterilizer is used for sterilizing all kinds of glassware such as test tubes, pipettes, petri-dishes, and flasks. In addition, it may be used to treat other laboratory materials, instruments, equipment (e.g., forceps, scalpels, scissors, throat swabs) which are not burned or injured by the high temperature of the sterilizer. Under no condition, must the sterilizer be used to sterilize rubber goods and laboratory coats, as such materials would burn. The same applies to culture media, as the liquid would boil to dryness. The hot-air oven is also used to sterilize dry materials in sealed containers, and powders, fats, oils and greases (e.g., petroleum jelly) that are impermeable to moisture. These materials are penetrated very slowly by heat and must therefore be sterilized in small lots.

Mechanism of hot-air sterilization : Irreparable degradations of essential cell constituents such as enzymes and other proteins by oxidation are the most probable mechanism of dry heat sterilization.

Infrared Radiation : This may be employed to sterilize metal instruments and glass syringes in central supply departments, but has no routine use in the microbiology laboratory. The infrared rays are directed from electrically heated element on to the objects to be sterilized, and temperatures of 180°C can be attained. Heating at or above 200°C by infrared *in vacuo* has been employed as a means of sterilizing surgical instruments. Cooling is hastened and oxidation prevented during the cooling period by admitting filtered nitrogen to the chamber.

Sterilization by Ionizing Radiation : Some materials can be sterilized by exposure of the product in its final container or package to ionizing radiation in the form of γ-radiation from a suitable radioisotope source such as Cobalt-60 or Cesium-137 or of electrons energized by a suitable electron accelerator. A dose of 2.5 M rads is generally accepted as adequate, although other doses levels may be employed. As with other sterilization processes, the effectiveness of the radiation cycle should be confirmed by a series of experiments and by determination of the sterilization microbial burden and by the use of suitable dosimeters. Suitable biological indicators may also be used.

The types of radiation available for sterilization may be categorized as either *corpuscular* or *electromagnetic*. The former consists of α-rays (He nuclei), β-rays (electrons), protons and neutrons. However, α-rays, β-rays and protons do not have sufficient penetrative power to be useful and only fast neutrons are used in practice, and only to a limited extent. The most widely used kinds of radiation are the electromagnetic radiation of very short wavelength X-rays and γ-rays. These are called *ionizing radiation* because the principle means of energy dissipation in their passage through matter is the ejection of an electron, leaving a positively charged ion. Within cells this primary event is followed by further chemical reactions including damage in DNA, some of which cause the death of the cell.

As with heat, bacterial spores are more resistant to radiation in the dry state than in the fully hydrated conditions and the resistance is also increased under anoxia. However, radiation is still more efficient than heat under dry anoxic conditions (and is probably, for those conditions, the method of choice). Radiation, like heat, can cause damage of the article to be sterilized. The amount of degradation is greatest for pharmaceuticals in aqueous solution, as the damage is mediated through radiation-induced free radicals in water. For practically all aqueous solutions of drugs, the amount of degradation is so great that it precludes the use of radiation as a method of sterilization. The amount of degradation to surgical instruments, sutures, etc., and, in the absence of water, to drugs, makes radiation an attractive and valuable alternative sterilization method to heat. The necessary apparatus is much expensive for installation in a hospital. It is employed commercially for the sterilization of large amounts of pre-packed disposable items such as plastic syringes and catheters, which are unable to withstand heat.

Ultra Violet Radiation : UV light is also a type of electromagnetic radiation, but has much less quantum energy than γ-rays so that, in general, UV is capable of producing only increased excitation, not ionization of molecules that absorb it. This process is less drastic and less lethal than ionization and so UV irradiation is not as efficient a method of sterilization as γ-irradiation.

UV sterilization is usually brought about using a wavelength of 2537 Å (253.7 nm) which is a high-emission wavelength for the mercury lamps that are used as the UV source. A tentative life-span has been assigned to the UV lamps, because of the gradual change in the crystal lattice structure of the outer glass covering, the wavelength of the emitted radiation slowly shifts and become less effective. UV, however, does not penetrate normal packaging materials such as glass or plastics and as a consequence, is not used as a method of sterilizing pharmaceutical dosage forms. It has the added disadvantage that most bacteria have active enzyme processes that under favorable environmental conditions, can repair UV-induced damage, so that recovery of UV-irradiated cells is a common phenomenon.

Its main application as a sterilizing agent is for air sterilization and also for the surface sterilization of aseptic work areas and surgical instruments, but even here its efficiency is doubtful.

Mechanism of UV sterilization : It has been found that a maximum biological efficiency exists at 253.7 nm, which is also the absorbance peak of isolated DNA. This suggests strongly, therefore, that DNA or the nucleic acid, is the target for UV-induced lethal events. The absorption and subsequent reactions are predominantly in the pyrimidines of the nucleic acid. One important alteration is the formation of a pyrimidine dimer in which two adjacent pyrimidines become bonded. Unless specific intracellular enzymes remove dimers, DNA replication can be inhibited and mutations can result.

The major Purines	The major Pyrimidines
Adenine	Cytosine
Guanine	Thymine
	Uracil (in RNA in place of Thymine)

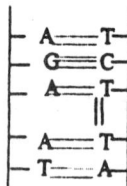

Thymine dimer (T == T) formation is the cause of damage

Photoreactivation : If a suspension of bacteria is exposed to UV light for several minutes, only a small fraction will be able to form colonies in a nutrient medium and thus appear to be viable. However, if a sample of the irradiated cells is then exposed to visible light for several minutes, the fraction of survivors in the sample will be much higher, as if, these bacteria had been exposed to UV light for a shorter time. Thus, a fraction of cells that were apparently damaged have been photoreactivated by the exposure to visible light. Photoreactivation never reaches 100% efficiency, i.e., not all the cells recover. Photoreactivation is actually due to a light dependent enzyme that recognizes thymine dimers in DNA and cleaves them so that the normal DNA structure can be restored.

Excision repair (dark reactivation) : Some microorganisms possess a second mechanism for repairing damage to DNA caused by UV irradiation. This mechanism is not light dependent and requires a sequence of enzyme reactions. Two enzymes, a dimer-specific endonuclease and a dimer-specific exonuclease, excise the dimer together with a number of neighboring nucleotides. The missing piece of the DNA strand resulting from the excision is repaired by enzymatic insertion of nucleotides complementary to the good strand. Two enzymes accomplish this : a DNA polymerase synthesizes the required segment, and a DNA ligase reestablishes its location in the strand.

Sterilization by Filtration : This process depends upon the physical removal of organisms by the mechanisms comprising of sieving, adsorption, surface tension effects in retained capillary films and trapping in the convolutions of the filter channels. This process is used for the sterilization of heat-sensitive solutions. A suitable filter medium of nominal pore size 0.22 μm or less, yields a sterile and relatively particle-free filtrate and does not alter substantially the composition of the liquid passed through it.

The solution to be sterilized is passed through the filter (usually made of cellulose derivatives, plastic, porous ceramic or of suitable sintered construction or suitable combinations of these) and collected in the sterile receiver by the application of positive pressure to the non-sterile side of the system or application of vacuum to the sterile side. Care must be taken to avoid excessive positive or negative pressure. Prolonged filtration must also be avoided to prevent the growth of a contaminant through the filter medium and entry into the sterile solution. Appropriate measures should be taken to avoid loss of solute by adsorption on to the filter. After filtration the solution is aseptically distributed in the previously sterilized final containers which are then sealed so as to exclude microorganisms.

Filter elements of porcelain or sintered material that are used repeatedly should be tested for cracks or leaks prior to each use. Fiber-shedding filters such as asbestos filters are to be avoided. If, however, the use of such filters is unavoidable, a fiber-retaining filter must be used downstream of the asbestos filter. The effective pore size of the sterilizing filters should be confirmed before use and the continued integrity of the filters confirmed after use.

The process of sterilization by filtration must be validated by monitoring the microbial load in the solution to be filtered. For filters of a sintered or fritted construction, a procedure such as the bubble-point procedure should be used and for membrane-type filters, a bubble-point procedure or diffusion rate test should be used, in accordance with the manufacturer's recommendations.

The integrity of any new or modified filtration system should be determined before it is placed in service.

Application of filtration technique : Serum, physiological salt solutions containing $NaHCO_3$ (after loosing CO_2 it will be converted to more alkaline Na_2CO_3), enzymes and bacterial toxin in solution, and heat sensitive solutions such as solutions of antibiotics.

Gas Sterilization : The process involves exposure of materials to sterilizing gases such as ethylene oxide. The process is difficult to control, the gas itself being toxic and when mixed in certain proportions with air, explosive. It must be ensured that the process is applied only to materials compatible with the sterilizing gas.

Factors affecting activity : The sterilizing efficiency of the gases (ethylene oxide and formaldehyde) is related to the following factors :

(i)   Concentration of the gas.

(ii) Time of exposure.

(iii) Temperature of exposure.

(iv) Humidity of the sterilizing atmosphere and of the microenvironment of the contaminating bacteria.

(v) Physical nature and penetrability of the load.

(vi) Atmospheric preconditioning of the load before sterilization.

Organisms treated in a dried state are several-fold more resistant than when preconditioned in an atmosphere of high relative humidity (RH) before treatment, almost regardless of the RH of the sterilizing environment.

With gases, certain minimum concentrations are necessary as otherwise exposure times become unduly prolonged. At temperatures of 40-50°C, ethylene oxide concentrations in excess of 400 mg/L are necessary. Then with a sterilizing environment humidity in the range of 30-60%, the load having been preconditioned for 24-hours, at RH in excess of 60%, inactivation factors of the order of 10^{17} for *B. subtilis* spores on non-hygroscopic surfaces can be achieved in about 2 hours. This is assuming rapid and complete penetration of the load preferably aided by the evacuation of the sterilizing chamber before treatment. Because of the uncertainties of the efficiency of the process exposure time of 3-4 hours in the above conditions are more usual to allow a wide safety margin.

With formaldehyde, concentrations of the order of 3.5 mg/L or higher are necessary, and then at a temperature of 25°C a RH in excess of 50% and with preconditioning of the load as before, inactivation factors of the order of 10^{10} for *B. subtilis* spores on test pieces can be produced with 3 hours exposure. However, formaldehyde suffers from the great disadvantage of low penetrability. It cannot penetrate polymeric packaging films as can ethylene oxide and the tendency to polymerize to the inactive forms on surfaces at low exposure temperatures can cause a fall in the active concentration. This loss can occur fairly rapidly and can only be minimized by increasing the exposure temperature and reducing the size of the load. Input concentrations as high as 2 g/L of formaldehyde, at temperatures of 90°C in sub-atmospheric conditions, with an exposure time of 3 hours have been used to sterilize dressing packs containing resistant spores. Prior evacuation of the sterilizer chamber was shown to be necessary and even then was not satisfactory for instruments with a narrow lumen such as capillary tubes. For these reasons, formaldehyde must be regarded as uncertain in its action and sterilization protocols can only be devised as a result of test on standard loads. The increase in the temperature of exposure to the maximum that the load can stand, and prolonged exposure to high concentrations are the factors essential to success.

The material to be sterilized is exposed to a mixture of ethylene oxide with a suitable inert gas such as CO_2 or fluorinated hydrocarbons to minimize the explosion risk. After sterilization adequate time should be allowed for the disposal of residual ethylene oxide and other volatile residue. Products sterilized in this manner should be monitored to assure acceptable levels of residual gas and its degradation products.

The sterilization cycle must be monitored by employing modern instrumentation for controlling the concentration of ethylene oxide, the temperature, the time and the moisture content in the sterilizing chamber. As with the other sterilization procedures, the microbial burden on the articles to be sterilized should be worked out, since this is an important factor, which influences the effectiveness of the process.

Generally only ethylene oxide and formaldehyde are used in practice. Propylene oxide is sometimes employed instead of ethylene oxide, being easier to handle. Other gases infrequently used are β-propiolactone and ozone.

MODEL QUESTIONS

1. Define the terms mentioned below :
     (a) Polishing   (b) Cold Sterilization   (c) Impaction
2. Talcum powders are most effectively sterilized by a
     A. autoclave   B. dry heat   C. gas sterilization
     D. millipore   E. freeze-drying.

3. Plastics are normally sterilized with
   A. direct flame   B. oven heat   C. ethylene oxide
   D. steam under pressure   E. steam under vacuum.

4. α-particles are very similar to
   A. X-rays   B. H atoms   C. He atoms
   D. Neutrons   E. Protons.

5. γ-rays are very similar to
   A. X-rays   B. α-radiation   C. β-radiation
   D. neutrons   E. antineutrons.

6. The ideal antiseptic concentration of ethyl alcohol is
   A. 95%   B. 70%   C. 100%
   D. 50%   E. 75%.

7. The word "sterilization" means
   A. freeing an object from life of any kind
   B. removal of organisms capable of causing infections
   C. inhibition of growth of bacteria
   D. all the above
   E. none of the above.

8. The mechanism of dry heat sterilization is primarily
   A. oxidation   B. reduction   C. coagulation
   D. denaturation   E. none of the above.

9. The preferred method of sterilization for mineral oil and oil vehicle of injection is
   A. autoclave   B. bacterial filtration C. gas sterilization
   D. dry heat   E. radiation.

10. Ethylene oxide sterilizes by a mechanism primarily involving
    A. coagulation   B. oxidation
    C. alkylation of the functional groups of nucleic acids
    D. hydrolysis   E. denaturation.

11. HEPA (High Efficiency Particulate Air) filters are widely used in
    A. autoclaves   B. laminar flow hoods   C. face masks
    D. oxygen masks   E. gas sterilizers.

12. The word "sterility"
    A. can be expressed as % basis
    B. may be used in a relative sense
    C. is an absolute term
    D. all the above.

13. Tyndallization means
    A. autoclaving with a bactericide
    B. successive heating with a bactericide
    C. successive heating at low temperature

    D. successive heating at low temperature and incubation

    E. all the above.

14. Most common bactericidal agent used for sterilizing intraocular injection is

    A. chlorocresol   B. thiomersal   C. benzalkonium chloride

    D. all the above   E. none of the above.

15. Thermal death point takes place when

    A. all bacteria of a given species are killed after 10 minutes exposure

    B. all bacteria of a given species are killed after 20 minutes exposure

    C. all bacteria are killed instantaneously

    D. half of the virulent organisms are killed

    E. lysis of bacteria begins.

16. A test used to check leakage of bacterial filters is

    A. the seep test   B. the millipore test   C. the seitz test

    D. bubble point   E. none of the above.

17. Propylene syringes are

    A. completely transparent

    B. unbreakable

    C. autoclavable

    D. lighter in weight than polyethylene syringes

    E. cheaper than polyethylene syringes.

18. Nylon is rarely used in the manufacture of syringes because it

    A. is too easily broken

    B. cannot be autoclaved

    C. may react with acidic drugs

    D. is destroyed by dilute mineral acids

    E. is not flexible.

19. The most abundant products of ultraviolet irradiation of DNA are

    A. thymine : thymine dimers

    B. adenine : adenine dimers

    C. cytosine : adenine dimers

    D. guanine : guanine dimers.

20. One of the following emissions from the decay of radionuclide is commonly used in sterilization. Identify.

    A. γ (gamma)   B. X-ray   C. α (alpha)

    D. Positron   E. All the above.

21. One of the organism mentioned below is used as a biological indicator in I.P. for ethylene oxide sterilization. Choose the correct one.

    A. *Bacillus stearothermophillus*

    B. Spores of *Bacillus subtilis*

    C. *Bacillus pumilus*

    D. Spores of *Bacillus cereus*

    E. All the above.

22. Two method of sterilization are given for the materials listed from (A) to (D). Match them correctly.

    (i) Dry heat   A. Rooms
    (ii) γ-radiations   B. Plastic syringes
                         C. Talcum powder
                         D. Intravenous admixture.

23. Given below are the reference organisms selected for measuring the efficiency of the following sterilization processes (i-v). Match them correctly.

    (i) Moist heat   A. Spores of *B. pumilus*
    (ii) Dry heat   B. Spores of *B. subtilis* or *Clostridium tetani*
    (iii) Ionizing radiation C. *B. stearothermophilus*
    (iv) Gaseous sterilization D. Fort Detrick strain of *B. subtilis*
    (v) Filtration   E. *Pseudomonas diminuta*

24. Permitted limits of ethylene oxide in various products are mentioned below. Match them.

    (i) Opthalmic preparations   A. 5 ppm
    (ii) Hard gelatin capsule shells B. 10 ppm
    (iii) Surgical materials   C. 15 ppm
    (iv) Intrauterine devices   D. 25 ppm
                                      E. 35 ppm

25. In the "Flash method" of Pasteurization the holding temperature is ...... I ...... °C and holding time is ...... II ...... seconds, whereas in the case of "Holder method" it is ...... III ...... °C and ...... IV ...... min respectively.

ANSWERS

1. A high degree of clarification is termed "Polishing" a solution. This term is applied when particulate matter down to approximately 2 μm in size is removed. A further step, removing particulate matter down to 0.2 μm in size would eliminate microorganisms and would accomplish "Cold Sterilization". Filters are thought to function by one or, usually, a combination of the following : (1) sieving or screening, (2) entrapment or impaction, and (3) electrostatic attraction. When a filter retains particles by sieving, the particles are retained on the surface of the filter. Entrapment occurs when a particle smaller than the dimensions of the passageway (pore) becomes lodged in a turn or impacted on the surface of the passageway. Electrostatic attraction causes particles of opposite charge to that of the surface of the filter pore to be held or adsorbed to the surface.

2. B; 3. C; 4. C; 5. A; 6. B; 7. A; 8. A; 9. D; 10. C; 11. B; 12. C; 13. D; 14. E, nothing is allowed; 15. A; 16. D; 17. C. Other plastics used for syringes cannot withstand autoclave temperature and must be gas sterilized; 18. C; 19.A; 20. A; 21.B; 22. i-C, ii-B; 23. i-C,ii-B, iii-A, iv-D, v-E; 24. i-B, ii-E, iii-D, iv-A. Ethylene oxide is used as a sterilant. After sterilization, the residues which may be present in the final product are ethylene oxide, ethylene chlorohydrin and ethylene

glycol. The FDA has proposed the residual limits of ethylene oxide and derivatives (parts per million) in the finished products as follows :

Drug product	Ethylene oxide (ppm)	Ethylene chlorohydrin (ppm)	Ethylene glycol (ppm)
1. Ophthalmics (for topical use)	10	20	60
2. Injectables	10	10	20
3. Intra-uterine devices	5	10	10
4. Surgicals scrub sponges	25	250	500
5. Hard gelatin capsule shells	35	10	35

25. I = 72, II = 20, III = 63-66, IV = 30.

CHAPTER 13

Processing of Tablets

- Definition
- Different Types of Compressed Tablets and Their Properties
- Processes involved in the Production of Tablets
- Tablets Excipients, Defects in Tablets
- Evaluation of Tablets
- Physical Standards including Disintegration and Dissolution
- Tablet Coating - Sugar Coating; Film Coating, Enteric Coating and Microencapsulation.

Tablets are solid dosage forms each containing a unit dose of one or more medicaments. They are intended for oral administration. Some tablets are swallowed whole or after being chewed, some are dissolved or dispersed in water before administration and some are retained in the mouth where the active ingredient is liberated. Preparations intended for administration by other routes, for example, the form of implants and pessaries, may also be presented in the form of tablets.

Tablets are obtained by compression of uniform volumes of powders or granules by applying high pressures and using punches and dies. The particles to be compressed consist of one or more medicaments, with or without auxiliary substances such as diluents, binders, disintegrating agents, lubricants, glidants and substances capable of modifying the behavior of the medicaments in the digestive tract. Such substances must be innocuous and therapeutically inert in the quantities present.

Because of their composition, method of manufacture or intended use, tablets present a variety of characteristics and consequently there are several categories of tablets, such as

  (i) Uncoated tablets

 (ii) Coated tablets like sugar coated, film coated, etc.

(iii) Enteric coated tablets.

(iv) Dispersible tablets

 (v) Modified-release tablets.

(vi) Soluble tablets.

(vii) Effervescent tablets

(viii) Tablets for use in the mouth.

Processes Involved in the Production of Tablets

Before starting formulation the individual ingredients are treated properly as required for e.g., size reduction, drying, sieving through appropriate sieve etc. Tablets may be prepared by three individual processes such as :

(i) Wet granulation process of tablet production.

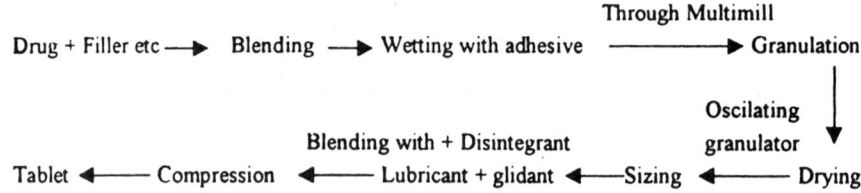

(ii) Dry granulation process of tablet production.

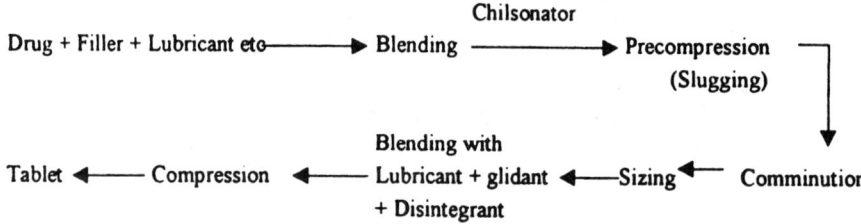

(iii) Direct compression process of tablet production.

Drug + Filler + Disintegrant + Lubricant + Glidant etc. ⟶ Blending

Tablet ◄—— Compression

Tablet Excipients/Additives/Adjuncts

(i) *Granulating fluids :* Starch paste 10%, methyl cellulose 1%, acacia mucilage, gelatin solution 5 to 10%, purified water, alcohol, sucrose solution. Acacia sometimes increases the disintegration time of the finished tablet.

(ii) *Binders :* Acacia, tragacanth, gelatine, sucrose.

(iii) *Disintegrants :* Dry starch (potato and maize), arrow root. In case of pessaries some agent like cocoa butter etc. melts at body temperature and helps in disintegration. In case of effervescent tablet, citric acid and tartaric acid in combination with NaHCO3.

(iv) *Lubricants :* During compression there is a tendency for the granules to stick to the surface of the punches. Thus, tablets, have a pitted surface and this is known as "picking". To prevent this, lubricating agents are used e.g., stearic acid, stearates like magnesium stearate, purified talc, liquid paraffin etc.

(v) *Glidants :* Finely divided grade of silica. The purpose of the glidant is to promote flow.

(vi) *Diluents :* Lactose, dextrose, dextrine, dicalcium phosphate.

Defects in Tablets

(i) *Binding in the Die :* This may be due to poor lubrication under dried granules and a dirty or blemished die.

(ii) *Picking and Sticking :* Here the problem is caused by adhesion of material to the punch faces. If localised portions of the tablet surface are seen to be missing; this is called picking. The tablet has a dull rough appearance when "Sticking" occurs due to adhesion of the tablet to the whole die walls and punch face. This may be due to under-dried granules, poorly maintained punch faces or the use of a lubricant lacking in anti-adherent properties.

(iii) *Fissured or Pitted Surface :* If this is not due to sticking or picking the most likely cause is the presence of granules which are uniform in size and lack the fines necessary to fill the voids.

(iv) *Capping, Lamination and Chipping :* In capping, the top or bottom part of the tablet separates from the main body. In lamination, the tablet breaks into two or more layers. In chipping, a small portion of the tablet may come off. These faults may be due to inadequate removal of air from the granules in the die-cavity before and during compression. Excessive fines, incorrectly prepared or overdried granules or too small a top punch/die-bore clearance, all hinder escape of air from the die cavity and may be the cause of these.

(v) *Excessive weight variation :* This problem is associated with poor granule flow and separation of granule constituents. Thus, granules which are under-dried, too large, too fine or contain a large proportion of fines, are incorrectly lubricated or comprise elements with widely differing densities or sizes, may all be suspected as possible cause of excessive weight variation.

(vi) *Variation of Medicament Content :* This may be due to inefficient mixing or due to "solute migration" during drying as discussed elsewhere.

(vii) *Soft-Tablets :* Apart from the use of too low a compaction pressure this problem usually arises when granules have been inadequately dried or the intergranule bonds have been weakened either by traces of air in the granule bed (insufficient to cause capping) or by excessive proportions of fatty lubricant such as magnesium stearate.

(viii) *Protracted Disintegration :* In this case the tablet either rapidly breaks down to form large particles that persist for a long period, or fine particles are produced, but the overall disintegration time is excessive. This fault may be due to :

a. an adhesive granulating agent which is too "strong"
b. high degree of compaction
c. hydrophobic tablet ingredients like excessive quantities of fatty lubricant or gelling of the granulating agent.
d. Insufficient or wrong type of disintegrating agent.

This problem may be tackled by incorporation of small amount of hydrophilic surfactant or incorporation of hard PEG (polyethylene glycol) or incorporation of disintegrating agent during moist granulation as well as lubrication of the granules.

(ix) *Mottled Tablets :* Already discussed elsewhere(Chapter 11).

(x) *Double Impression :* This defect may occur in those tablets on which letters are printed, practically the monogram of the lower punch is impressed upon the tablet during compression by the upper punch and a second impression (though light) may be there on the same surface of the tablet by the same lower punch during ejection of the tablet by the lower punch. This is due to the uncontrolled rotation of the lower punch.

Evaluation of Tablets

(i) Size and shape.

(ii) Hardness : The Monsanto tablet hardness tester is used.

(iii) Friabiiity : The Roche friabilator is used to find out the amount of fines erroded from the surface of the tablet.

(iv) Content of active ingredients : Unless otherwise specified in the individual monograph the average content of 20 tablets is measured and it should be within specified limits.

(v) Uniformity of weight : This test is not applicable to coated tablets other than film-coated tablets and to tablets that are required to comply with the test for uniformity of content for all active ingredients. Weigh 20 tablets selected at random and calculate the average weight. Not more than two of the individual weights deviate from the average weight by more than the percentage shown in the following table and none deviates by more than twice that percentage.

Average weight of tablet	Percentage deviation
80 mg or less	10
More than 80 mg but less than 250 mg	7.5
250 mg or more	5

(vi) Uniformity of content : This test is applicable to tablets that contains less than 10 mg or less than 10% w/w of active ingredient.

(vii) Disintegration : This test is not applicable to modified release tablets and tablets for use in the mouth.
a. Uncoated tablets : Unless otherwise directed in the individual monograph, use water as the medium and add a disc to each tube. Operate the apparatus for 15 minutes unless otherwise directed.
b. Coated tablets : Unless otherwise directed in the individual monograph, use water as the medium and add a disc to each tube. Operate the apparatus for 30 minutes for film-coated tablets and for 60 minutes for other coated tablets unless otherwise directed in the

individual monograph. For coated tablets other than film coated, if any of the tablets have not disintegrated, repeat the test on a further 6 tablets, replacing the water in the vessel with 0.1M hydrochloric acid. The tablets comply with the test if all 6 tablets have disintegrated in the acid medium.

   c. Enteric-coated tablets : If the tablet has a soluble external coating, immerse the basket in water at room temperature for 5 minutes. Suspend the assembly in the beaker containing 0.1M hydrochloric acid and operate without the discs for 120 minutes, unless otherwise stated in the individual monograph. Remove the assembly from the liquid. No tablet shows signs of cracks that would allow the escape of the contents of disintegration, apart from fragments of coating. Replace the liquid in the beaker with mixed phosphate buffer pH 6.8, add a disc to each tube and operate the apparatus for a further 60 minutes. Remove the assembly from the liquid. The tablets pass the test if all six have disintegrated.

   d. Dispersible and soluble tablets : Disintegrate within 3 minutes when examined by the disintegration test for tablets and capsules, using water at 24° to 26°C, unless otherwise stated in the individual monograph.

   e. Effervescent tablets : The tablets comply with the test if each of the 6 tablets tested disintegrates in the prescribed manner in water at 20° to 30°C within 5 minutes unless otherwise stated in the individual monograph.

The underside of the disintegration tube is fitted with a stainless steel sieve having nominal mesh apertures of 2.00 mm and 635 μm wire diameter. Temperature is maintained at 37° ± 2°C unless otherwise specified in the individual monograph.

(viii) Uniformity of dispersion : This test is applicable only to dispersible tablets. 2 tablets in 100 ml water should disperse completely and smooth dispersion should pass through a sieve with a nominal mesh aperture of 710 μm.

 (ix) Dissolution test : The disintegration test does not give any guarantee about the rate or extent of solubilisation of the active ingredient in the media. Therefore, dissolution test is performed usually at 37° ± 0.5°C temperature to get such information. The rate of dissolution must be within prescribed limits.

Coated Tablets

The most common of the various types of coated medication are sugar-coated, film-coated and enteric-coated tablets.

The sugar coat is used to mask unpleasant tastes and odors, to protect a tablet ingredient from decomposition during storage or to improve the appearance of the tablet. The sugar coating process is as complex as is the coating itself. In most instances, the first step of the process involves the application of a poorly water-soluble polymer such as shellac to protect the tablet and tablet ingredients from the aqueous fluids used in subsequent steps of the coating process. This application undoubtedly retards the release of the drug in the gastrointestinal tract. In general, it must be assumed that a sugar coating will affect the bioavailability of a drug relative to that observed with the uncoated tablet.

This dosage form should not be used when a prompt clinical response is desired. 'Pan Coating' is a popular technique of sugar coating.

The simple, nonenteric film coat is prepared by depositing a few layers of a film-forming polymer, like hydroxy-propyl methyl cellulose (HPMC) or high molecular weight polyethylene glycols (PEG), on a conventional tablet. The film coat masks objectionable tastes and protects, to some degree, tablet ingredients from moisture during storage. A well formulated product should show little difference in bioavailability compared to that of an uncoated tablet. The film coat should disrupt quickly in the fluids of gastrointestinal tract, independent of pH.

An enteric coat is usually a special film coat designed to resist gastric fluids and to disrupt or dissolve in the intestine. **The enteric coat** is used to protect a drug, for example, erythromycin, from degrading in the stomach and to minimize gastric distress caused by some drugs, for example, aspirin or ammonium chloride. Because of inter subject differences in gastric emptying, the bioavailability of drugs from enteric-coated tablets is probably more variable than with any other form of coat discussed previously.

The modern approach to enteric coating makes use of polymers like cellulose acetate phthalate or shellac and anionic copolymers of methacrylic acid and its esters, which are insoluble at pH 1 to 3 but soluble at pH 5 to 7. Most are polymeric acids with ionizable carboxyl groups. The apparent pKa of these polymers is important. If the pKa is too low, appreciable ionization takes place at low pH, and the coating does not perform its intended function in the stomach. A high pKa may prevent release of drug in the intestine. In practice, polymers with pKa values ranging from 4 to 7 have been found useful.

Microencapsulation : Wurster (according to the inventor's name) air-suspension technique is a popular method of coating individual drug particles with polymeric material to produce microcapsules (it is equally effective to coat granules or tablets by suspending them in a column of hot air and spraying with a coating solution). Differential coating is also feasible by this technique. Different fraction of differentially coated microcapsules may be blended with uncoated drug particles/granules to achieve sustained release action. Other techniques of microencapsulation include : coacervation phase separation technique, emulsion polymerization technique etc.

Press coating or compress coating

The principle of this process is that a layer of drug coating material is pressed onto a preformed tablet. By this technique two chemically incompatible ingredients may be formulated in the same tablet.

MODEL QUESTIONS

1. The Wurster process can be used to
   A. directly compress tablets
   B. automatically fill capsules
   C. coat tablet
   D. determine the disintegration time for tablets
   E gas-sterilize parenteral solutions.

2. Poorly manufactured tablets may have small pinholes on the surface. This phenomenon is known as

    A. capping   B. mottling   C. cracking

    D. impacting   E. picking.

3. Picking of tablets may be caused by all of the following EXCEPT

    A. scratch punches

    B. excessive compression pressure

    C. static charges on the powder

    D. unsatisfactory lubricant

    E. a granulation which is too damp.

4. Which of the following is NOT used primarily as a diluent in tablet formulations?

    A. Calcium stearate   B. Lactose   C. Dicalcium phosphate

    D. Starch   E. Mannitol.

5. Which of the following is not a function of the lubricant in a tablet formulation?

    A. Reducing punch and die wear.

    B. Facilitating tablet ejection from the die.

    C. Improving flow properties of granules.

    D. Improving tablet wetting in the stomach.

    E. Reducing powder adhesion onto the dies and punches.

6. All of the following ingredients have been commonly used as the coating agents for film coating EXCEPT

    A. zein

    B. carnauba wax

    C. hydroxyethyl cellulose

    D. sodium carboxymethyl cellulose

    E. hydroxy propyl methyl cellulose.

    F. cellulose acetate phthalate

    G. polyethylene glycol.

7. A sweetener that is widely employed in chewable tablet formulas is

    A. cyclamate sodium   B. glucose   C. mannitol

    D. sucrose   E. lactose.

8. An excellent choice of diluent for a compressed vaginal tablet formulation would be

    A. lactose   B. starch   C. talc

    D. sucrose   E. all are equally effective.

9. Which of the following is the first process that must occur before a drug can become available for absorption from a tablet dosage form?

    A. Solubilization of the drug in the blood.

    B. Dissolution of the drug in the GI fluids.

    C. Dissolution of the drug in the GI epithelium.

    D. Ionization of the drug.

    E. Disintegration of the tablet.

10. *In vitro* dissolution rate studies on drug products are useful in bioavailability evaluations only if they are correlated with
    A. USP disintegration limits
    B. disintegration rates
    C. *In vivo* studies in humans
    D. the chemical stability of the drug
    E. *In vivo* studies in at least three species of animals.

11. An ingredient that is added to a tablet formula to improve flow properties of granules into a die for compression is known as a (an)
    A. lubricant   B. surfactant   C. disintegrant
    D. glidant   E. emollient.

12. The disintegration time for sugar coated tablet is
    A. 15 minutes   B. 30 minutes   C. 60 minutes
    D. 75 minutes   E. 120 minutes.

13. Enteric coating is achieved by using
    A. hydroxy propyl methyl cellulose (HPMC)
    B. carboxy methyl cellulose (CMC)
    C. polyvinylpyrrolidone (PVP, povidone)
    D. cellulose acetate phthalate
    E. ethyl cellulose.

14. Subcoating is given to the tablets
    A. to increase the bulkiness
    B. to avoid deterioration due to microbial attack
    C. to prevent the solubility in acidic medium.
    D. to avoid stickiness
    E. all of the above.

15. Tablets are placed into a coating chamber and hot air is introduced through the bottom of the chamber. Coating solution is applied through an atomizing nozzle from the upper end of the chamber—This technique is called
    A. sealing before sugar coating
    B. coating by air suspension
    C. spray pan coating
    D. chamber coating
    E. compressed coating.

16. Shellac is used for the purpose of coating of tablets as
    A. polishing agent   B. film coating agent   C. enteric coating agent
    D. sub-coating agent for sugar coating   E. none of the above.

17. Lamination is
    A. separation of a tablet into two or more distinct layers
    B. partial and complete separation of the top and bottom crowns of a tablet from the main body of the tablet
    C. process of sub-coating of tablet

   D. removal of a small portion of a tablet
   E. none of the above.
18. Select the equation that gives the rate of drug dissolution from a tablet
   A. Fick's law
   B. Henderson Hasselbalch equation
   C. Noyes Whitney equation
   D. Michelis Menten equation.
19. Lactose is not used as diluent in the formulation of one of the following :
   A. Pyrazinamide   B. Ibuprofen   C. Sulphacetamide
   D. Isoniazid   E. All the above.
20. Tablet intended to be placed beneath the tongue is known as
   A. chewable tablet   B. lozenges   C. buccal tablet
   D. sublingual tablet   E. disintegrating tablet.
21. "Chilsonator" is a
   A. dry compactor machine B. chilling machine   C. sonicator
   D. homogenizer   E. none of the above.
22. The principle factor that makes enteric coated tablets unpredictable in drug therapy is
   A. pH   B. premature release of drug   C. failure to release drug
   D. state of health of patient   E. varying thickness of the coating.
23. The advantage of foamtabs is primarily
   A. improved tastes   B. improved solubility   C. faster absorption
   D. increased tablet hardness   E. better stability.
24. A substance used frequently to polish tablets is
   A. sodium chloride   B. lactose   C. air-dried talc
   D. starch   E. calcium chloride.
25. Film coatings are
   A. enteric coatings   B. sustained release   C. very brittle
   D. very flexible   E. very thick.
26. The most common disintegrator in compressed tablets is
   A. dextrose   B. lactose   C. starch
   D. potassium bitartrate   E. powdered sucrose.
27. Tablet hardness range is normally
   A. 0.2 - 0.5 kg.   B. 0.5 - 1.0 kg.   C. 1.0 - 2.0 kg.
   D. 2.0 - 3.5 kg.   E. 3.5 - 7.0 kg.
28. A substance that is often used to subcoat tablets is
   A. sugar   B. carnauba wax   C. shellac
   D. sodium stearate   E. sodium chloride.
29. Why are nitroglycerin tablets relatively unstable?
   A. They become insoluble

   B. They are hygroscopic
   C. They are deliquescent
   D. The drug migrates from the tablets
   E. They tend to crumble.

30. Splitting off of the face of a tablet is called

   A. capping   B. fissuring   C. slugging
   D. whiskering   E. picking.

31. An instrument use to measure durability of tablets to shock and abrasion is a

   A. tensiometer   B. dart penetrometer   C. chilsonator
   D. brittleometer   E. friabilator.

32. Splitting of the top of a tablet is known as capping. Reasons for capping include all of the following EXCEPT
   A. excessive lubricant
   B. insufficient binder
   C. too dry a granule
   D. excessive pressure of compression
   E. excessive fine powder.

33. Match the given ingredients from A to E with the purpose for which it is incorporated in the formulation of tablets

   (i)   Glidant   A. pre-gelatinised starch
   (ii) Diluent   B. pyramine
   (iii) Adherent   C. colloidal silica
   (iv) Disintegrant   D. calcium sulphate
                         E. sodium alginate

34. The ingredients mentioned in A to E are used in various stages of sugar coating of tablets. Match them.

   (i)   Seal coating   A. Gelatin
   (ii) Sub coating   B. Carnauba wax
   (iii) Syrup coating   C. Methanol
   (iv) Polishing   D. PEG 4000
                         E. Cane sugar

35. Listed are some tablet additives. Match them with their correct use given in A to D.

   (i)   Acacia   A. Binder
   (ii) Lactose   B. Glidant
                         C. Diluent
                         D. Lubricant

36. Tablets are evaluated by the following techniques. They are

(i)	(ii)	(iii)	(iv)	(v)	(vi)	(vii)
....	....	....	....	....	....	....

ANSWERS

1. C; 2. E; 3. B (Excessive compression would result in hard tablets that would not stick to the punches and would not be picked. However, excessively hard tablets may not disintegrate in the body-fluids); 4. A (Most stearates act as lubricant); 5. D (Lubricating agents usually imparts a hydrophobic character to the tablet. This waterproofing property might retard disintegration and dissolution); 6. B (Carnauba wax and bees wax combinations are commonly used as a polishing coat for sugar coating, but not for film coating. Cellulose acetate phthalate produces a special type of film coat known as enteric coat); 7. C (Mannitol is not as sweet as sucrose, it leaves a cool taste in the mouth and is nonhygroscopic. Mannitol is also easily compressed by wet granulation); 8. A (Lactose is readily compressible, water soluble and inert ingredient. It will also encourage the growth of *Doderlein bacilli*, a microorganism present in the healthy vagina); 9. E (Due to limited surface area the dissolution of drug from the intact tablet is negligible except for very water soluble drugs. Table disintegration is responsible for increasing the available surface area and higher drug solubility according to Noyes and Whitney equation. In this context granule disintegration is more important than tablet disintegration. Before absorption the drug must have to be solubilized); 10. C; 11. D (Dry potato and corn starch act as glidant as well as disintegrating agent); 12. C; 13. D; 14. A (In case of sugar coating, after dedusting the first step is SEALING to protect the tablet against the effects of water in subsequent coating solution. A 30 to 50% solution of shellac in alcohol or other suitable organic solvent is employed for sealing, care being taken to avoid over generous application as this leads to a prolongation of the disintegration time.

The next step of sugar coating is SUBCOATING which is built up in successive layers by wetting the tablets with an adhesive solution (usually sugar solution mixed up with acacia, gelatin or both), gradual dusting with filler (talc, precipitated calcium carbonate etc) and then thoroughly drying. This stage of the process is continued until the tablets have rounded appearance and the edge are well covered); 15. B; 16. C; 17. A; 18. C ('A' is related with diffusion of drug from a zone of higher concentration to a zone of lower concentration. 'B' is related with the calculation of pH. 'D' is related with the enzyme kinetics); 19. D; 20. D (This sublingual tablet do not disintegrate beneath the tongue, rather the content is solubilized, which due to high lipophilicity quickly absorbed and enters into general circulation by by-passing the liver); 21. A; 22. C (Many enteric coating do not reliably release the drug in the intestine and eliminated through the faces intact without disintegration); 23. A (to diminish chalky taste); 24. C; 25. D (This is because of the use of elastic film forming polymers); 26. C (Dry corn or potato starches are mainly used); 27. E; 28. C (Shellac is sometimes included in a sealing subcoat in the production of sugar-coated tablets. It will prevent the tablet from absorbing water from the subsequent coating solutions); 29. D (This is because of high vapor pressure of nitroglycerin); 30. A; 31. E; 32. A (Excessive lubricant may render the granulation too slippery, preventing cohesiveness, but will not cause capping).

33. (i) - C; (ii) - D; (iii) - E; (iv) - A

34. (i) - D; (ii) - A; (iii) - E; (iv) - B

35. (i) - A; (ii) - C

36. (i) Hardness; (ii) Friablility; (iii) Content of active ingredient(s); (iv) Uniformity of weight; (v) Uniformity of content; (vi) Disintegration; (vii) Dissolution test.

CHAPTER 14

Processing of Capsules

- Hard and Soft Gelatin Capsules
- Different Sizes of Capsules
- Filling of Capsules
- Handling and Storage of Capsules
- Special Applications of Capsules.

Capsules are solid dosage forms in which the drug or a mixture of drugs is enclosed in hard gelatin capsule shells, in soft, soluble shells of gelatin, or in hard or soft shells of any other suitable material, of various shapes and capacities. They usually contain a single dose of active ingredient(s) and are intended for oral administration. The consistency of soft shells may be adjusted by the addition of substances such as glycerin and sorbitol. Excipients such as opaque fillers i.e., opacifier (titanium dioxide), anti-microbial preservatives, sweetening agents, flavouring agents and one or more coloring agents permitted under the Drugs and Cosmetics Rules, 1945 may be added. Capsules may bear surface markings.

The contents of capsules may be of solid, liquid or paste-like consistency. They consist of the medicament(s) with or without excipients such as vehicles, solvents, diluents, lubricants, fillers, wetting agents and disintegrating agents.

The contents of capsules other than modified release (sustained-release) capsules do not contain any added coloring agent.

Hard Capsules : Hard capsules contain the medicament(s) in the solid form. Where two mutually incompatible drugs are present in the mixture, one of the drugs can be put as a tablet or pellet or in small capsule and then enclosed with the other drug in a large capsule.

Soft Capsules : Soft capsules shells are usually forms filled with medicament and sealed (FFS technology) in a combined operation on machines. In some cases, shells for extemporaneous use may be preformed. The shells which are thicker than those of hard capsules are formed to produce capsules which are spherical, oval or cylindrical with hemispherical ends. The shells may sometime contain as medicament. They may contain a preservative to prevent growth of fungi.

The contents of soft capsules usually consist of liquids or solids dissolved or dispersed in suitable excipients to give a paste-like consistency but may also consist of powders or granules. As soft gelatin shells contain appreciable amounts of water, migration of capsule contents, particularly of water soluble ingredients may occur.

Modified-Release Capsules : Modified release (sustained release) capsules are hard or soft capsules in which the contents or the shell, or both, contain auxiliary substances or are prepared by a special process designed to modify the rate at which the active ingredients are released.

Enteric Capsules : Enteric capsules are hard or soft capsules prepared in such a manner that the shell resists the action of the gastric fluid but is attacked by the intestinal fluid to release the contents.

The pharmacopoeial standards of capsules are more or less similar with that of tablet.

Disintegration : The disintegration test is not applicable to modified release capsules. For those hard capsules and soft capsules for which the dissolution test for tablets and capsules is included in the individual monograph, the test for disintegration is not required. Unless otherwise directed the D.T. of hard capsules is 30 minutes and for soft capsules it is 60 minutes. The D.T. of enteric capsules is similar to that of enteric tablets.

Sizes of Hard Gelatin Capsule Shells

The hard gelatin capsule is made in a range of eight sizes from 000, the largest, to size 5, the smallest. The most popular sizes in practice are size 0 to size 4. The sizes of capsules and their corresponding volumes are given below :

SIZE NO.	5	4	3	2	1	0	00	000
Volume in ml.	0.15	0.25	0.30	0.40	0.55	0.75	0.95	1.36

Veterinary capsule

Hard capsule shells are made by dipping moulds into a gelatin solution, the film on the mould dried, the shell cut to length and then stripped from the mould.

Type A gelatin (**pharmagel A**) is derived from an acid treated precursor and exhibits an isoelectric point in the region of pH 9, whereas type B gelatin (**pharmagel B**) is from an alkali-treated precursor and has its isoelectric zone in the region of pH 4.7. Although capsules may be made from either type of gelatin, the usual practice is to use a mixture of both types.

Blends of bone and pork skin gelatins of relatively high gel strength are normally used for hard capsule production. The bone gelatin produces a tough, firm film, but tends to be hazy and brittle. The pork skin gelatin contributes plasticity and clarity to the blend, thereby, reducing hazy or cloudiness in the finished capsule.

ROTOFIL is an automatic high speed capsule filling machine designed by Eli Lilly and Company specially to fill pellets. **ACCOFIL** is another high speed automatic capsule filling machine designed by perry industries. **ROTOWEIGH** is a high-speed capsule weighing machine sold by Eli Lilly and Co. **ROTOSORT** is a filled capsule sorting machine sold by Eli Lilly and Co. It is a mechanical sorting device that removes loose powder, unfilled joined capsules, filled or unfilled bodies and loose capsules.

Storage condition of hard gelatin capsule (filled or unfilled) is very important. If the capsule shell is stored at dry environment then water may be removed from the shell and it becomes brittle. From humid environment the shell can absorb water and becomes soft. Therefore, it should be stored at an optimum temperature in an air tight container.

Strip packaging of tablets and capsules is normally done in automatic stripping machine. Two aluminium or polymeric foils are pressed through hot roller to seal the tablets or capsules placed in proper position. A layer of nylon type polymeric material is there in the inner side of the foil which melts by the heat supplied from hot roller and perfectly sealed the strip, which may be tested as follows :

Few strips of tablets or capsules are kept immersed in a colored solution containing in a closed vessel fitted with a vacuum pump and pressure gauge. A certain degree of vacuum is created inside the vessel keeping the strips in fully immersed condition in coloured solution. Thereafter, the vacuum is removed and strips are washed and dried and defoiled to check the tablets or capsules. No tablets or capsules should be damaged by the coloured solution. But if the sealing is not proper then during application of vacuum the air present inside the cavity of strip would be released through microcapillary channel. Now after removal of vacuum i.e., when atmospheric pressure is regained over the vessel the coloured solution would be entered to the cavity of the strip through the microcapillary channel as it is then remain as vacuum. The entered coloured solution would be responsible for damaging the tablets/capsules.

MODEL QUESTIONS

1. Valproic acid capsules if chewed will cause
   A. irritation of the mouth and throat
   B. destruction of the drug
   C. staining of the teeth
   D. hyperventilation
   E. blurring of the vision.
2. The USP weight variation test for capsule dosage forms states limit for the variation of weight of individual capsules from the observed average weight of a sample of 20 capsules. None of the capsules may have net content weights varying more than '………' from the average.
   A. 5%
   B. 10%
   C. 15%
   D. 20%
   E. 25%

3. Rotosort is a machine used to sort out
   A. coated tablets
   B. sealed ampoules
   C. filled capsules
   D. sealed containers.

4. In capsules, ROTOFIL is used for filling
   A. powders   B. pellets   C. liquids
   D. corrosive liquids E. none of the above.

5. "OOO" represents
   A. dose of a tablet in a day
   B. three tablets per dose
   C. tablet size
   D. capsule size
   E. none of the above.

6. In the preparation of capsule shell the ingredients mentioned are present for specific purpose. Match them.

   (i)   Preservative   A. Mineral oil
   (ii)   Aids solubility   B. Essential oil
   (iii) Organoleptic additive   C. Titanium dioxide
   (iv)   Opacifier   D. Fumeric acid
                                    E. Propyl paraben

7. The hard gelatin capsule sizes are mentioned in their number. Their approximate capacity are listed in A to E. Match their correct volume.

   (i)   0   A. 0.10 ml
   (ii)   1   B. 0.15 ml
   (iii) 3   C. 0.30 ml
   (iv)   5   D. 0.55 ml
               E. 0.75 ml

8. Some materials used in the manufacture of pharmaceutical dosage forms are given. Match them with correct use mentioned in A-D.

   (i)   Sorbitol   A. Preservative for capsules
   (ii)   Titanium dioxide   B. Plasticizer in soft gelatin capsules.
                             C. Lubricant for tablets.
                             D. Opacifier for gelatin mass.

ANSWERS

1. A (This compound is acidic and corrosive); 2. E; 3. C; 4. B; 5. D.
6. (i) - E; (ii) - D; (iii) - B; (iv) - C.

Additional components of the gelatin mass is given below :

Purpose	Ingredients
(i) Preservative	Methyl paraben, propyl praben
(ii) Aids solubility; reduces aldehydic tanning of gelatin	Fumaric acid
(iii) Organoleptic additives (flavouring for odour and taste)	Essential oil and ethyl vanillin
(iv) Opacifier	Titanium dioxide
(v) Colorants	Approved water-soluble dyes, certified lakes, pigments and vegetable colors etc.
(vi) To produce chewable shell and taste	Sugar (sucrose)

7. (i) - E; (ii) - D; (iii) - C; (iv) - B.

8. (i) - B; (ii) - D (The plasticizers used with gelatin in soft capsule manufacture are relatively few. Mainly glycerin, sorbitol or their combinations are used. The ratio by weight of dry plasticizer to dry geletin determines the "hardness" of the gelatin shell.)

CHAPTER 15

Immunology

- Host Parasite Relationship
- Study of Immunological Products like Sera, Vaccines, Toxoids and their Preparations.

Host parasite relationship

Parasite may be defined as a microorganism or some larger species (e.g., worms) that lives in or on and obtain its nourishment from a living host and is sometimes potentially pathogenic. Parasites are not always harmful to host.

The principle types of relationship between host and parasites are as follows :

(i) **Symbiosis :** The participants are of mutual benefit to each other, for e.g., termites and their intestinal protozoa neither of which can live without the other.

(ii) **Commensalism :** The participants live in close and constant association without any evidence of injury, or of benefit to each other, e.g., members of the normal microbial flora of the respiratory tract or of the skin in man.

(iii) **Parasitism :** One participants (parasite) derives significant benefit from the other (host).

The host parasite relationship may be altered by antimicrobial drugs in several ways, such as :

a. alteration of tissue response

b. alteration of immune response

c. alteration of microbial flora.

Infection : Infection is the invasion of microorganism into the host tissue. After invasion of microorganism a competition for superiority starts between the host and the invaded organism. If the parasite is successful, disease results. If the host is successful, disease does not occur and immunity may develop.

Contamination : When bacterial or viral suspension (live cell) i.e., pathogenic organism come in contact with the host tissue without making any infection, then this phenomenon is known as contamination. Bacteria can survive for a long period but virus dies within a short period. It should be noted that contamination by pathogen may lead to produce infection under favorable condition.

Routes of infection : Bacteria enters into the body through different ways. Some enter, through broken skin (occasionally through unbroken skin), some by the way of respiratory passages, some by the way of alimentary tract. The organism of typhoid fever or cholera vibrio, if rubbed into the broken skin would not produce an infection and may or may not produce disease. Therefore, the bacteria must enter the body by the route with which they are adopted, e.g., influenza virus through nose.

Pathogenic organism is one which is capable of producing disease in the body or capable to infect a body. Thousands of bacterial species have been isolated but only a few of those are capable of producing diseases in man. Some are pathogenic for human but not for animal. Similarly reverse may also happen. The ability of an organism to invade and produce disease process depends upon the species concerned and host.

Pathogenicity : Pathogenicity denotes the ability of microorganisms to cause disease or result in the production of progressive lesions.

Virulence : Virulence is the degree of pathogenicity. This property may be subdivided into toxigenicity, i.e., ability to produce toxic substances; invasiveness i.e., ability to enter host tissue, multiply and spread. Virulence is estimated by the minimum lethal dose i.e., the smallest dose of the organism that will kill a particular species of animal.

Infectious and communicable diseases : Infectious diseases are those in which infection occurs from one person to another through air as well as by other means e.g., food, water, stool and by direct contact. Example includes typhoid, poliomyelitis, T.B. etc. Communicable diseases are those which are transported from one individual to another by air or dust particles. An infectious disease is not necessarily a communicable disease.

Immunity : The power to resist the effects of the invasion of pathogenic microorganisms is called "immunity" and the lack of ability to resist infection in called "susceptibility".

There are three kinds of immunity namely, natural immunity, naturally-acquired immunity and artificial immunity.

I. Natural Immunity : Normal body due to the constitutional makeup, possess a series of defence mechanism that is capable to resist microbial invasion to its tissues and give it a natural immunity or inherent resistance towards most organisms. It is not acquired through previous contact with infectious agent. The following are examples of natural immunity.

(i) **Racial** : e.g., Negroes can resist yellow fever but susceptible to T.B., whereas white men are very susceptible to yellow fever. Indians are also resistant to yellow fever.

(ii) **Species** : e.g., Cholera, typhoid, dysentery occur in human beings but cannot be even produced experimentally in animal. Leprosy (*M. leprae*) does not occur in any animal. It is unexplainable why differences in species susceptibility occur.

(iii) **Individual** : Resistance to infection varies with different individuals of the same species and race. Individual immunity is totally inheritant or hereditary in nature. Besides this nutritional status, exposure to ionizing radiation, hormonal balance etc., may greatly influ-ence individual susceptibility.

(iv) **Age** : e.g., between the ages of 2-5 years 75% of children are susceptible to diphtheria, but with older children the proportion is less and most adults are immune. Resistance to tuberculosis (*M. tuberculosis*) is higher at 5-15 years of age than before or after. Many age differences in specific infections can be related to physiologic factors, for e.g., *Gonococci vaginitis* occurs mainly in small girls.

(v) **Hormonal and metabolic influence** : Many known hormones influence susceptibility to infection. In diabetes mellitus there is increased susceptibility to infections of the urinary tract, vagina and pyogenic infections of tissue. The latter be due in part to altered metabo-lism, elevated glucose, reduced influx of phagocytic cells and depression of phagocytosis.

(vi) **Placental** : Mother carries immunity and transmits it towards the fetus. After child is born it can carry the immunity for some length of time. This can be termed as immunologic tolerance. If mother is affected by some disease and gain immunity the child also carries the immunity for some period against that disease. Most infants are immune to measles for the first 4-6 months of life, due to placental transfer of antibodies from mother to fetus. This is an example of a naturally acquired passive immunity.

II. Naturally-acquired Immunity : This immunity is acquired as a result of infection by the causative organisms. The infection may be due to both virulent and non-virulent organisms and in both cases an appreciable amount of antibody may be produced which will prevent subsequent infection by the same organism in the near future. This immunity may last for life (e.g., polio, smallpox etc.).

III. Artificial Immunity : Artificial immunity is also acquired immunity achieved artificially. This acquired immunity may depend on the presence and amount of specific γ-globulin molecules or antibody in the blood elicited in response to the stimulus of foreign protein or other large molecular substances which is called antigen. It is very specific in the sense that it protects against one particular pathogen or its toxic products. It has been found that not only living virulent microorganisms, but also attenuated (reduced virulency) microorganisms, dead microorganisms and in many cases substances prepared from, but quite free from, bacteria, will stimulate the body to produce antibodies. These substances are referred to as "antigens" or antigenic substances.

There are some substances which are not antigenic as such but when introduced in the body may combined with a body protein to produce a complete antigen which will subsequently produces antibody. Such substances are known as "hapten".

Acquired immunity may be of three types :

(i) Naturally acquired active immunity—already discussed.

(ii) Artificially acquired active immunity : This is the immunity which are given to the individ-ual artificially by means of giving different vaccines in the different forms. The immunity produced by artificial means, may last for life or may be of shorter duration but usually extends over many years.

(iii) Artificially acquired passive immunity : A susceptible individual when invaded by disease producing microorganisms, cannot often respond quickly to the stimulation produced by the micro-organisms and as such the formation of antibodies does not keep space with the infection and in this unequal contest, the patient may succumb. In such instances, the injection into the patient of antibodies provides an immediate means of defence and greatly increases the chances of recovery. The preparations containing the ready-made antibodies are called antiserums and the immunity obtained by their use is called passive immunity, because it is conferred. **Passive immunity lasts for a short time only,** usually less than three months. Antiserums are used for transient prophylaxis, usually for persons who have been in contact with infection, but have not yet exhibited symptoms. In such cases immediate immunization is indicated and a relatively small dose of serum may prevent or shorten an attack.

Phagocytosis : Phagocytosis is the ingestion of bacteria by certain cells of the body, whereby the bacteria are more or less altered and rendered harmless or killed and digested. Phagocytosis is effected by two different kinds of body cells, (a) the cells of the reticulo endothelial system and, (b) the white blood corpuscles.

Normal blood-serum contains a thermolabile substance called "**complement**" which destroys bacteria by lysis, i.e., solution or disintegration. Complement alone cannot effect lysis Antibodies such as cytolysins or bacteriolysins must be present.

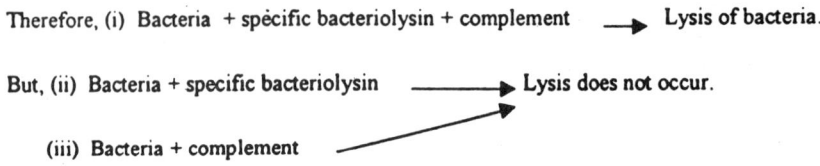

Therefore, (i) Bacteria + specific bacteriolysin + complement ⟶ Lysis of bacteria.

But, (ii) Bacteria + specific bacteriolysin ⟶ Lysis does not occur.

(iii) Bacteria + complement

Vaccines

Vaccines are preparations of antigenic substances that are administered for the purpose of inducing in the recipient a specific and active immunity against the infective agent or toxin produced by it. They are prepared form bacteria, viruses, rickettsiae or toxins.

Vaccines may contain living microorganisms suitably treated to attenuate (by drying, or using less nutrient media, or having unfavorable temperature, or continuous change of host) their virulence but retain their antigenic potency or they may consist of pathogenic organisms which have been killed or inactivated. Some vaccines consist of antigenic fractions or substances produced by the same pathogenic organisms but rendered harmless whilst retaining their antigenic efficiency. Vaccines may be prepared from one species only or from a mixture of two or more species.

Vaccines may be prepared by the method described in the individual monographs or by the general methods given below or in any other manner provided the identity of the antigens is maintained and the vaccines are free from microbial contamination and extraneous agents. Suitable adjuvants may be added during the preparation but streptomycin, penicillin or other β-lactam antibiotics may not be added at any stage of manufacture or in the final vaccine. A suitable bactericide may be added to sterile and inactivated vaccines. The final products are distributed aseptically into sterile containers which are then sealed to exclude extraneous micro-organisms. Unless otherwise indicated in the monograph, the final vaccine may be filled into single dose or multiple dose containers but vaccines in multidose containers must invariably contain a bactericide.

Vaccines may be classified as follows :

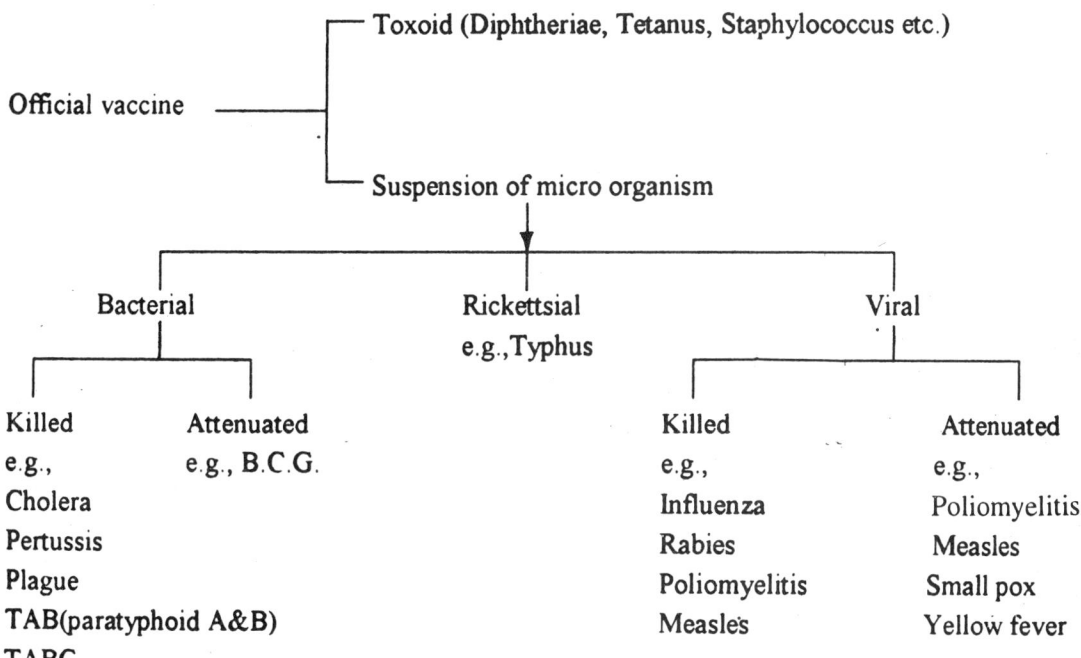

Bacterial Vaccines

Bacterial vaccines are either sterile suspensions of live or killed bacteria or sterile extracts of derivatives of bacteria. They may be simple vaccines prepared from one species or may be mixed vaccines prepared by blending two or more simple vaccines from different species or strains.

Bacterial vaccines may be prepared from cultures grown on suitable solid or liquid media. The whole culture or parts of may be used in preparing the vaccine. The identity, antigenic potency and purity of each bacterial culture must be carefully controlled.

Vaccines containing killed organisms may be prepared by killing the organisms by chemical or physical means provided the antigenic potency of the vaccine is preserved. Vaccines containing living bacteria may be prepared from strains which are avirulent for humans but which stimulate the production of antibodies active against pathogenic strains of the same species. The final vaccines must be free from any substance known to cause toxic, allergic or other undesirable immunological reactions in humans.

Bacterial vaccines are suspensions of varying degrees of opacity in colorless or slightly colored liquids or they may be freeze-dried so that the water content is not more than 2% (w/w) unless otherwise stated in the individual monograph. They may be standardized in terms of international opacity (measured by photoelectric nephelometer) units or where appropriate, by numbers of living or killed bacteria determined by direct cell count or by viable count.

Bacterial Toxoids

Bacterial toxoids are toxins or material derived therefrom, the toxicity of which has been reduced to a very low level or completely eliminated by chemical or physical means without destroying their immunising potency. The toxins are obtained from selected strains of specific micro organisms, grown in media free from ingredients known to cause toxic, allergic or other undesirable immunological reactions in humans. Toxoids treated with formaldehyde are known as formal toxoids (F.T.). There are Alum precipitated toxoid also (APT).

Bacterial toxoids may be liquid or may be prepared by adsorbing on mineral carriers such as aluminium phosphate, aluminium hydroxide or any other suitable adsorbent; the adsorbed product may be separated, washed and suspended in a saline or other appropriate solution isotonic with blood.

Bacterial toxoids are clear or slightly opalescent liquids, colorless or slightly yellow. Adsorbed toxoids may be white or greyish white suspensions or pale-yellow liquids with a sediment at the bottom of the container. Freeze-dried preparations are greyish white or yellowish white powders or pellets.

Viral and Rickettsial Vaccines

Viral and rickettsial vaccine are suspension of viruses or rickettsiae and are prepared from infected tissues or blood obtained from artificially infected animals, from cultures in fertile eggs, or from cell or tissue cultures. Viral vaccines may be live or killed and they may be freeze dried. Live vaccines are usually prepared using attenuated strains of the specific organism. Killed vaccines may be inactivated by suitable chemical or physical means.

Mixed Vaccines : Mixed vaccines are mixtures of two or more vaccines. A suitable antibacterial substance may be added to inactivated or live viral and rickettsial vaccines provided that it has no action against the specific organisms.

It is to be noted that there are several forms of vaccines such as

(i)	Simple	Consisting of only one species of organism e.g., plague.
(ii)	Mixed	Two or more species e.g., Typhoid, Paratyphoid.
(iii)	Univalent	Contains only one strain of organism.
(iv)	Polyvalent	Contains two or more strains.
(v)	Autogenous	Contains bacteria obtained from patient to whom the vaccine is to be injected.

Storage : Vaccines must be stored at a temperature between 2°C and 8°C and should not be allowed to freeze unless otherwise specified in the individual monograph. Freeze-dried preparations must be stored at a temperatures below –20°C or as specified in the individual monograph. At higher temperature vaccines deteriorate rapidly.

Labelling : The label states :

(i) for liquid vaccines, the total number of ml in the container and, for dried vaccines, the number of doses in the container;

(ii) unless otherwise indicated the minimum number of units per dose or per ml or, for viral vaccines, the minimum viral titre;

(iii) the dose and route of administration;

(iv) the name and proportion of any antibacterial preservative or other auxiliary substances added to the vaccine;

(v) the date after which the vaccine is not intended to be used;

(vi) the conditions under which it should be stored;

(vii) for dried vaccines, the liquid to be used for reconstitution and its volume;

(viii) that the vaccine should be used immediate after reconstitution;

(ix) unless otherwise directed that the vaccine should be shaken well before use;

(x) any contra-indication to the use of the vaccine.

Standards : Vaccines, reconstituted when necessary, comply with the following requirements unless otherwise stated in the individual monograph. Phenol, if present, must not be more than 0.25% (w/v). Thiomersal, if present, between 0.005% (w/v) and 0.02% (w/v), Free formaldehyde, if present, not more than 1.25 mg per dose. Unless otherwise stated all vaccines comply with tests for sterility and test for abnormal toxicity.

Some Vaccines Official in I.P.

(i) **Diptheria and Tetanus Vaccine (adsorbed) I.P. :** Prepared by mixing formal toxoids prepared from the toxin produced by the growth in suitable media of *Corynebacterium diptheriae* and *Clostridium tetani* respectively.

   Storage : As stated under vaccines.

   Category : Active immunizing agent.

(ii) **Diphtheria, Tetanus and Pertussis (Whooping cough) vaccine (adsorbed) I.P.** is a sterile suspension prepared from diphtheria formal toxoid + purified tetanus formal toxoid + a suspension of killed *Bordetella pertussis*.

   Storage : As stated under vaccines.

   Category : Active immunising agent.

(iii) **BCG Vaccine (Freeze-dried) i.e., Bacillus Calmette-Guerin Vaccine** is a preparation containing live bacteria obtained from a strain derived from bacillus of Calmette and Guerin and known to protect human beings against tuberculosis.

   Category : Active immunising agent.

   Storage : Store in light-resistant glass-container at a temperature between 2° and 8°C.

(iv) **Plague Vaccine** is a sterile suspensions of killed plague bacilli, *Yersinia pestis*, of the 195/p strain.

(v) **Typhoid Vaccine** is a sterile suspension or a freeze dried solid prepared from one or more strains of *Salmonella typhi*.

   Storage : Store at a temperature between 2°C to 8°C. The liquid vaccine must not be allowed to freeze.

(vi) **Typhus Vaccine** is a sterile suspension of killed rickettsiae of strain or strains of epidemic typhus rickettsiae (*Rickettsia prowazeki*).

(vii) **Yellow Fever Vaccine,** live, is an aqueous suspension of chick embryo tissue infected with 17D strain of yellow fever virus.

(viii) **Typhoid Paratyphoid A Vaccine** is a sterile suspension or a freeze-dried solid prepared from one or more strains of *Salmonella typhi* and *S. paratyphi A*.

(ix) a. **Rabies Vaccine, Human (cell culture)** is a freeze dried preparation which is produced on the basis of seed-lot system. It may be prepared by growing an approved strain of rabies virus in an approved cell culture.

   b. **Rabies Vaccine, Human (Neural tissue).**

(x) **Poliomyelitis Vaccine**, live (oral) is an aqueous suspension of attenuated strains of polio-virus(sabin), type 1, 2 or 3 of known history and originally obtained from the WHO or any other approved source and grown in suitable approved cell cultures. It may contain any one of the three virus types or a mixture of two or three of them. This particular species of organism produces minor infection in the intestine and lacks the capacity to produce further infection in the nervous system. As a result the body acquires an immunity which lasts for 1 to 2 years.

   Storage : Below –20°C. When thawed it should be kept at a temperature of 2° to 8°C and used within 4 months. When exposed to higher temperature it should be used within a few hours.

(xi) **Measles Vaccine**, live—is a sterile aqueous suspensions of live attenuated measles virus.

(xii) **Japanese Encephalitis Vaccine, Human (Mouse Brain)** is a sterile freeze-dried prepara-tion containing inactivated Japanese encephalitis virus. The vaccine is prepared immediately before use by reconstitution with a suitable sterile liquid.

   Storage : At a temperature below 10°C.

(xiii). **Cholera Vaccine** is a homogeneous suspension of killed cholera vibrios (*Vibrio cholerae*) of a strain or strains selected for high antigenic efficacy and purity.

Antisera (Immunosera)

Antisera are native (unconcentrated) sera or preparations from native sera containing specific immunoglobulins that have prophylactic or therapeutic action when injected into persons exposed to or suffering from a disease caused by a specific microorganism.

Antisera are prepared by injecting antigens which are preparations of cultures of the specific organisms or venoms or their products into healthy humans or animals such as horses so as to produce in them antibodies which are normally associated with the globulin fraction of serum. Antigens commonly used for this purpose are toxins, toxoids, venoms and bacterial and viral vaccines. Non-lethal amounts of the toxin or the corresponding toxoid/vaccine are injected in gradually increasing dose into animals. Specific antitoxins are formed in the serum and the animals become actively immune. During the process of immunization, the animals should not be treated with penicillin. When a satisfactory degree of the immunity is produced, larger volumes of blood are withdrawn from the animals and the plasma or serum is processed to produce specific antisera. The globulins may be obtained from the immune serum by enzyme treatment and fractional precipitation or by other physical or chemical methods. Antisera is a passive immunising agent.

Storage : Antisera should be stored at a temperature between 2° to 8°C and should not be allowed to freeze unless otherwise stated in the individual monograph.

Some Antisera Official in I.P.

(i) **Diphtheria Antitoxin** is a preparation containing the specific antitoxic globulins or their derivatives obtained by purification of hyperimmune serum or plasma of healthy horses or other suitable animals and having the specific activity of neutralizing the toxin formed by *Corynebacterium diphtheriae.*

(ii) **Gas-gangrene Antitoxin (Oedematiens)** having the specific activity of neutralising the alpha toxin formed by *Clostridium oedematiens.*

(iii) **Gas-gangrene Antitoxin (Perfringens)** having the specific activity of neutralising the alpha toxin formed by *Clostridium perfringens.*

(iv) **Gas-gangrene Antitoxin (septicum)** having the specific activity of neutralising the alpha toxin formed by *Clostridium septicum.*

(v) **Human Normal Immunoglobulin (Normal Immunoglobulin; Immune Human Serum Globulin; Human Gamma Globulin)** is a sterile solution or freeze-dried preparation containing immunoglobulins, mainly immunoglobulin G (IgG).

(vi) **Rabies Antiserum (Antirabies Serum)** is a preparation containing the specific globulin or its derivatives obtained by purification of hyperimmune serum or plasma of healthy horses or other suitable animals having the specific activity of neutralising the rabies virus.

(vii) **Scorpion Venom Antiserum** to neutralise the venom of one or more species of scorpion.

(viii) **Snake Venom Antiserum (Snake Antivenin)** have the power of specifically neutralising the venom of one or more species of snakes.

(ix) **Tetanus Antitoxin** is a preparation containing the specific antitoxic globulins or their derivatives having the specific activity of neutralising the strain formed by *Clostridium tetani.*

MODEL QUESTIONS

1. Gamma globulin fraction is separated from serum by
   A. centrifugation   B. filtration   C. dialysis
   D. salting out   E. agglutination.

2. All of the following biologicals may be administered to humans. Which one is the most dangerous in respect to body response and potential toxicity?
   A. Antiserums   B. Antitoxins   C. Toxins
   D. Toxoids   E. Vaccines.

3. Biologicals can be used to obtain either active or passive immunity. Which one of the following pairs is NOT correct?
   A. Antiserum, passive immunity
   B. Antitoxin, passive immunity
   C. Human immune serum, active immunity
   D. Toxoid, active immunity
   E. Vaccine, active immunity.

4. The Schick test is used to determine susceptibility to

A. diphtheria   B. measles   C. polio

D. T.B.   E. typhoid fever

5. All of the following biologicals are used for active immunization EXCEPT
   A. bacterial vaccines
   B. bacterial antigens
   C. multiple antigen preparations
   D. toxoids
   E. toxins
   F. human immune sera.

6. Immune serum globulin (gamma globulin) is usually administered by what type of injection?
   A. Intradermal   B. Intramuscular   C. Intravenous
   D. Subcutaneous   E. Any of the usual methods of injection.

7. The Sabin poliomyelitis vaccine is
   A. administered orally as a live attenuated vaccine
   B. available only in a monovalent form
   C. available only in a trivalent form
   D. a killed vaccine
   E. similar to the Salk vaccine.

8. The Mantoux test uses
   A. diagnostic diphtheria toxin
   B. DPT toxin
   C. Mumps skin test antigen
   D. Old tuberculin
   E. Scarlet fever streptococcus toxin.

9. The intermediate tuberculin skin test (intermediate strength PPD) contains
   A. 2 tuberculin units
   B. 5 tuberculin units
   C. 25 tuberculin units
   D. 250 tuberculin units
   E. 500 tuberculin units.

10. All of the followings are used for the prophylaxis or treatment of disease EXCEPT
    A. antitoxins   B. antivenins   C. globulins
    D. serums   E. serum albumin.

11. The usual storage condition specified for biologicals is
    A. below 2°C   B. 2 to 8°C   C. cool place
    D. 8 to 15°C   E. room temperature.

12. All of the following statements concerning toxoids are true EXCEPT
    A. toxoids are detoxified toxins
    B. toxoids are antigens
    C. toxoids produce permanent immunity
    D. toxoids are often available in a precipitated or adsorbed form
    E. toxoids produce artificial active immunity.

13. Several vaccines and toxoids are precipitated and adsorbed onto aluminium hydroxide, aluminium phosphate, or other suitable media. This process results in a dosage form that, in comparison to fluid products, is
    A. more effective orally
    B. more slowly absorbed
    C. more stable
    D. less irritating upon injection
    E. less likely to cause abscesses.

14. All of the following are viral infection EXCEPT
    A. influenza   B. measles   C. mumps
    D. poliomyelitis   E. typhoid fever   F. smallpox
    G. yellow fever   H. hepatitis.

15. All of the following are bacterial infections EXCEPT
    A. cholera   B. plague   C. rabies
    D. pertussis   E. tuberculosis   F. leprosy
    G. typhoid fever.

16. Most vaccines are administered in two or more doses separated by a time interval of several weeks. The exception to this statement is in the administration of
    A. BCG Vaccine   B. Pertussis Vaccine   C. Typhoid Vaccine
    D. Plague Vaccine   E. Cholera Vaccine.

17. The route of administration of antitoxins in the prophylactic treatment of tetanus would be
    A. I.M.   B. I.V.   C. S.C.
    D. either S.C. or I.M   E. intradermal.

18. Which of the following preparations will induce passive (rather than active) immunity?
    A. Tetanus toxoid
    B. Botulism antitoxin
    C. Typhoid vaccine (killed)
    D. Mumps virus vaccine, attenuated
    E. Cholera vaccine (killed).

19. The capacity of the syringe commonly known as the tuberculin syringe is
    A. 0.1 ml   B. 0.5 ml   C. 1.0 ml   D. 2.0 ml   E. 5.0 ml.

20. Vaccine prepared from a patient's own infection is called
    A. autogenous vaccine   B. simple vaccine   C. stock vaccine
    D. monovalent vaccine   F. polyvalent vaccine.

21. An example of immunization with attenuated living infectious agent
    A. anaphylaxis   B. vaccination   C. any antigen injection
    D. Neisser-Wechsberg phenomenon   E. anaboliser.

22. The poliomyelitis virus ordinarily enters the body through the
    A. ear   B. skin   C. mouth
    D. lungs   E. none of the above.

23. Passive immunity usually gives which of the following protection to the patient?

    A. None   B. Complete   C. Short term

    D. Long term   E. Undetermined.

24. The function of antibodies in immunity is

    A. to neutralize toxins
    B. entirely bacteriostatic
    C. to produce more leukocytes
    D. to build up resistance against any infections
    E. A and D.

25. An antibody is chemically

    A. a protein   B. an amino acid   C. a polysaccharide

    D. any foreign substances in the body   E. none of the above.

26. Influenza vaccines seldom produces hypersensitivity because they are

    A. not prepared in eggs
    B. mixed with preservatives
    C. hypoallergenic extracts
    D. given in such low doses
    E. highly purified.

27. Passive immunity is the result of

    A. partial immunization
    B. recovery from a specific infection
    C. a lack of response to the antigen
    D. injection with the specific antigen
    E. injection with the specific antibody.

28. Bacterial antigens

    A. are vectors of disease
    B. are antibiotic substances
    C. never produce disease
    D. are used to produce active immunity
    E. may be demonstrated in the specific antibacterial serum.

29. A useful precaution when administering live virus vaccines is to have available

    A. whole blood   B. glucose solution   C. plasma expanders

    D. antiviral agents   E. epinephrine solution.

30. Smallpox vaccine

    A. is obtained from vaccinated horses
    B. is prepared by making a glycerol-water suspension of vesicles of vaccinia or cowpox.
    C. must be acid to bromocresol purple
    D. is injected intramuscularly
    E. is not stable when frozen.

31. Rabies vaccine

    A. provides permanent immunity
    B. must be tested for noninfectivity in rabbits

    C. is prepared from street virus

    D. is prepared from serum of infected rabbits

    F. may be stored at room temperature.

32. Rubella is another name for

    A. measles   B. meningitis   C. German measles

    D. mumps   E. scarlet fever.

33. The antitoxic effect of tetanus antitoxin lasts

    A. 4-6 hours   B. 24 hours   C. 10 days

    D. 2-3 years   E. indefinitely.

34. If symptoms of tetanus appear, the antitoxin should

    A. be given subcutaneously

    B. be given orally

    C. be given intramuscularly

    D. be given intravenously or intraspinally

    E. not be given.

35. Live rubella virus vaccines provide immunization for

    A. 1 year   B. 3 years   C. 6 years   D. 10 years   E. lifetime.

36. Antitoxins are usually associated with which of the following fractions of the blood?

    A. Euglobulin   B. Pseudo globulin   C. Albumin

    D. Fibrinogen   E. Leukocyte.

37. A common complaint after vaccination with live rubella virus vaccine is

    A. rash   B. sorethroat   C. headache

    D. polyneuritis   E. pain in the joints.

38. Poliomyelitis vaccine

    A. is made from type 1 and 2 strains only

    B. may be used if turbid

    C. should not be used if color changes

    D. should not be allowed to freeze and refreeze constantly

    E. contains polio virus killed with cresol.

39. Mumps in children usually involves

    A. salivary glands   B. sex glands   C. pancreas and liver

    D. CNS   E. tonsils and throat.

40. Toxoids are

    A. unofficial toxins

    B. non-antigenic toxins

    C. non-specific protein filtrates

    D. obtained from culture filtrates of viable organisms

    E. bacterial vaccines.

41. The proper interpretation of a positive reaction to a tuberculin test is that the person is

    A. suffering from active tuberculosis

    B. immune to invasion by the tubercle bacillus

    C. susceptible to invasion by the tubercle bacillus

    D. sensitive to tubercle-protein by virtue of previous or present infection

    E. none of the above.

42. Athlete's foot is caused by

    A. bacteria   B. viruses   C. rickettsia

    D. parasitic worms   E. fungi.

43. Antigen is :

    A. any foreign material introduced into the human body.

    B. only protein in nature.

    C. contained in serum injected in vaccination.

    D. any protein and few microbiological polysaccharides.

    E. all of the above.

44. An advantage of rabies immune globulin over antirabies serum is

    A. greater effectiveness

    B. lower incidence of adverse reactions

    C. greater immunity to all type of rabies

    D. faster action

    E. longer protection.

45. Reactions of antigens with antibodies are

    A. slow   B. rare   C. impossible

    D. controlled by temperature   D. highly specific.

46. Active immunization against diphtheria may be developed by injections with

    A. alum-precipitated culture

    B. antitoxin

    C. antidiphtheritic serum

    D. toxoid

    E. filtrates of *C. hoffmanni* and *C. xerosis* culture.

47. Interferon is

    A. an enzyme   B. a protein complex   C. an agglutinogen

    D. a precursor of amino acids E. none of the above.

48. Scabies is contagious skin disease caused by a

    A. mite   B. flea   C. fungus   D. tick   E. protozoa

49. Typhoid Vaccine IP is a sterile suspension or a freeze dried solid prepared from

    A. *Salmonella typhimurium*   B. *Salmonella paratyphi*   C. *Salmonella typhi*

    D. *Salmonella enteritidus*   E. all the above.

50. Which one of the following statements concerning Immune Serum Globulin is **true**?

    A. Immune Serum Globulin contains approximately 50% gamma globulin.

    B. Serum hepatitis is one of the most often reported adverse reactions.

    C. Skin tests should not be preformed before injecting any of the globulins.

    D. Virus infections attenuated by gamma globulin are non infectious.

    E. All of the above statements are true.

51. Special forms of gamma globulin such as tetanus or pertussis differ from immune gamma globulin in that they are
    A. obtained from humans hyperimmunized with either tetanus toxoid or pertussis vaccine
    B. effective after the onset of the disease symptoms
    C. administered by slow infusion
    D. prepared from foreign (animal) serum
    E. unsuitable for administration to children.

52. Which statement concerning mumps immune globulin is NOT true?
    A. Globulin is obtained from humans
    B. The i.m. route of administration is used
    C. Globulin provides passive immunity for the patient
    D. The globulin may also be used in larger doses to prevent complications of mumps such as orchitis (inflammation of a testis)
    E. The biological product is commercially available as immune serum globulin.

ANSWERS

1. C (Filtration and centrifugation will not be applicable; salting out and agglutination would damage it); 2. C (Others are to obtain immunity or to attenuate the severity of a disease); 3. C (Human immune serum is obtained from human blood and contains specific antibodies. Active immunity implies that the recipient of the biological will develop specific immunity due to an active response to the introduction of antigenic substances); 4. A [Here Diphtheria Toxin for Schick Test USP is injected intradermally (0.1 ml) into the forearm. The Schick test is based on the ability of circulating antitoxin to neutralise the diphtheria toxin given intradermally, and indicates immunity or susceptibility to the disease]; 5. E and F (Toxins are sometimes used as diagnostic aids for determining the state of immunity); 6. B; 7. A [Poliomyelitis is caused by poliovirus Type 1, 2 and 3. Some vaccines consist of only one type (monovalent) while others combine all three (trivalent). Sabin's vaccine is available in both forms. Salk's vaccine contains killed virus and is given by IM or SC injection. For this reason Sabin vaccine is superior to Salk vaccine]; 8. D [Another intra dermal test for detecting tuberculin sensitivity is the tuberculin tine test (multiple puncture method)]; 9. B [5 U/0.1 ml of purified protein derivative (PPD) i.e., specific bacterial protein antigen is used. The first strength (1U) generally used for individual suspected of being highly sensitive and the 250 U strength is exclusively for those who do not react to previous injections of either 1U or 5 units]; 10. E (Normal Human Serum Albumin USP is a protein in the plasma and used to control blood volume through its water-containing capacity in the treatment of shock or hemorrhage); 11. B; 12. C (To sustain immunity booster doses of the common toxoids are required. For example, a 0.5 ml dose of tetanus toxoid may be administered as a routine booster about every 10 years); 13. B (This is essential to produce high antibody titer. Recently developed colloidal dispersion of nanoparticles containing encapsulated toxoid is used for the same reason e.g., polymethyl methacrylate nanoparticles); 14.E (It is a bacterial infection); 15. C (It is a viral infection); 16. A (It is given as a single dose, being administered intradermally or placed on the skin followed by multiple skin puncturing. The other vaccines are administered SC or IM); 17. E

(For therapeutic effects, antitoxins are usually administered by the IM or IV routes. While the more slowly absorbed SC injection is generally preferred for prophylactic effects, the IM route is also used.); 18. B (Antitoxins are purified and concentrated antibody solutions derived from humans or animals that have been actively immunized against an antigen); 19. C; 20. A (Self generated vaccine); 21. B; 22. C; 23. C; 24. A; 25. A; 26. E; 27. E; 28. D; 29. E (This is essential as severe allergic reaction is not uncommon); 30. B (It contains living virus vaccinia) 31. B; 32. C; 33. C; 34. D; 35. C; 36. B; 37. E; 38. D; 39. A; 40. D (prepared from exotoxin); 41. D; 42. E (caused by Trichophyton group of fungi or *Epidermophyton floccosum*); 43. D; 44. B; 45. E (They are rapid, common and not temperature dependent); 46. D; 47. B (It is glycoprotein inhibits the replication of virus); 48. A; 49. C; 50. C (Intradermal skin tests with gamma globulin will cause a localized inflammation which may be incorrectly interpreted as a positive reaction. It is best to have epinephrine available to combat the occasional sensitivity reaction); 51. A; 52. E [Immune Serum Globulin (gamma globulin) is the general immune serum used to prevent or modify several disease, including measles, hepatitis A, poliomyelitis, and chickenpox. Mumps Immune Globulin (Human) is specific for the prevention or attenuation of mumps.]

Pharmaceutics II

CHAPTER 16

Prescriptions

- Prescriptions; Latin Terms Commonly Used
- Adoption of Metric System
- Calculations Involved in Dispensing.

The Prescription : A prescription is an order from a doctor, dentist or veterinary surgeon for the supply of a medicine, dressing or surgical appliance to a patient. It contains the following informations.

1. The patient's Name and Address.
2. A prefix (**superscription**) - This is the sign Rx. It is derived from 'R', an abbreviation for the latin word 'recipe', meaning "take thou", and possibly the letter 'j' - an invocation to Jove (Jupiter) the god of healing.
3. Inscription i.e., the body of the prescription containing the names and quantities of medicaments to be supplied.
4. Subscription i.e., the directions to the dispenser as well as the instructions for the patient through the dispenser.
5. The prescriber's signature and address.
6. The date on which the prescription was written.

Latin Terms Commonly Used

Abbreviation	English Translation	Abbreviation	English Translation
a.c.	Before meal	b.i.d = b.d.	Twice daily
a.m.	Before noon	c.	With
aa.	Of each	Calid	Warm

Abbreviation	English Translation	Abbreviation	English Translation
ad lib.	As much as desired	Caps.	Capsule
ad.	Upto, To	Cib.	Food
ag. aeratq	Carbonated water	Coch. parv.	Teaspoonful (5 ml)
agit	Shake	Coch.ampl.	One tablespoonful(15ml)
alt. hor	Alternate hour	Coch.mag.	A large spoonful
applic.	To be applied	Collun.	Nosewash
aq.	Water	Collyr.	Eye lotion
conc.	Concentrated	p.o.	Orally
collut (collutorium)	Mouthwash	p.r.n(pro re nata)	When required
consperg	Dust	Pig	Paint
d.t.d	Give of such dose	Pulv. (pulvis)	Powder
d.t.d. no. iv	Give four such doses	Pulv.consp	Dusting powder
dieb. alt	Every other day	q.d.=q.i.d.	Four times daily
dil.	Diluted	q.d.s	To be taken four times daily
duo	2	q.h.	Every hour
dup.	Double	q.q.h.	Every fourth hour
e.m.p.	As directed	q.s.	A sufficient quantity
ex.aq.	In water	Rx	You take or thou take
ft.	Let it be made	$\bar{s}$	Without
gtt.	Drop	s.o.s.	When need arises
h.s.	At bed time	sig.	Label
ht.	Draught	stat.	Immediately
liq.	Solution	sum.	To be taken
lot	Lotion	t.d.d.	Three times daily
m	Mix	t.i.d.	Three times a day
m.	In the morning	tuss. Urg.	When the cough troubles
m.d.	As directed	u.a.	As before
m.ft.m (mix, fiat, mist)	Mix and make mixture	ung (ungmentum)	Ointment
mist.	Mixture	unus	1
mitt.	Send	ut.dict.	As directed
n.	At night	utend	To be used
n.m.	Night and morning	vap.	Inhalation
narist	Nose drops	vitrell	Glass capsule (crushable)
neb.	Spray solution	1 minim =	0.062 ml
o.d.	Everyday	1fluid dram	= 4ml
o.d.	Right eye	s.a.	According to the art/ with pharmaceutical skill
o.u.	Both eyes		
o.m.	Every monrning		
o.n.	Every night		
o.s.	Left eye		
oculent	Eye ointment		
omn. hor	Every hour		
p.a.	To the affected part		
p.c.	After meals		
p.p.a	Bottle being first shaken		

Adoption of Metric System

(i) Units of mass (weights)   International Systems (SI)

1 gram (g)	=	1000 milligram (mg)
1 mg	=	1000 microgram (mcg, μg)
1 μg	=	1000 nanogram (ng) or millimicrogram (mμg)
1 ng	=	1000 picogram (pg)
1 pg	=	1000 femtogram (fg)
1 (fg)	=	1000 attogram (ag)

(ii) Units of Radiation

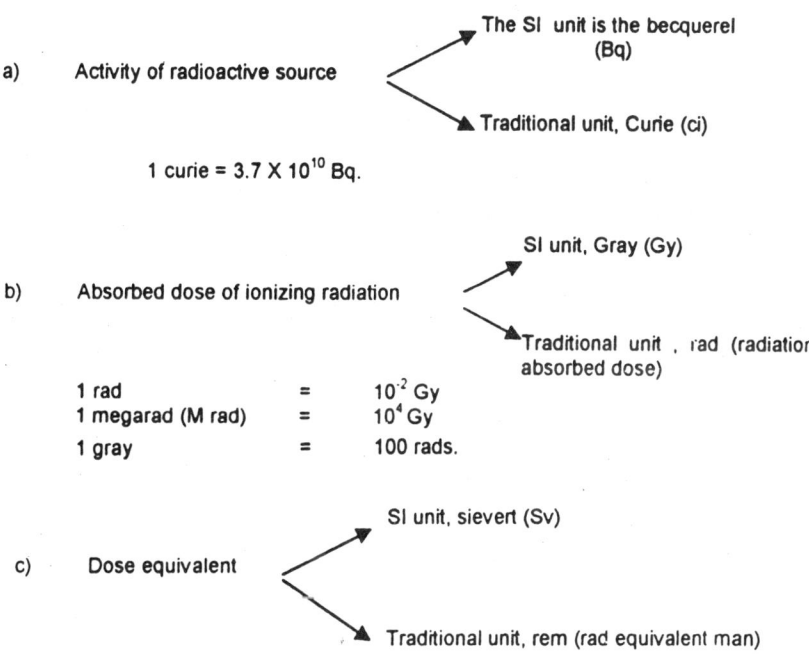

a)   Activity of radioactive source → The SI unit is the becquerel (Bq)

→ Traditional unit, Curie (ci)

1 curie = 3.7 X 10^{10} Bq.

b)   Absorbed dose of ionizing radiation → SI unit, Gray (Gy)

→ Traditional unit , rad (radiation absorbed dose)

1 rad	=	10^{-2} Gy
1 megarad (M rad)	=	10^{4} Gy
1 gray	=	100 rads.

c)   Dose equivalent → SI unit, sievert (Sv)

→ Traditional unit, rem (rad equivalent man)

Calculations involved in dispensing include multiplication, division, ratio, unitary methods, percentage, dilution etc. Some examples are already discussed in Chapter 3 (Metrology and Pharmaceutical Calculations chapter).

MODEL QUESTIONS

1. One picogram is equivalent to how many nanograms?

    A. 1×10^{-6} ng   B. 1×10^{-3} ng   C. 1×10^{-2} ng   D. 1×10^{3} ng   E. 1×10^{6} ng

2. The pharmacist uses both the apothecary and avoirdupois systems of weight measurement. Units that are quantitatively identical in both systems are the
   A. drachms
   B. grains
   C. ounces
   D. pounds
   E. grains and ounces.

3. One thousand nanograms equals one
   A. centigram
   B. gram
   C. kilogram
   D. microgram
   E. milligram.

4. The Angstrom equals
   A. 0.1 nanometer
   B. 1 nanometer
   C. 10 nanometers
   D. 100 nanometers
   E. 1000 nanometers.

5. Lugol's solution contains 5% of iodine. How much of Lugol's solution is administered to a patient thrice daily to provide 60 mg of iodine daily?
   A. 0.2 ml
   B. 0.3 ml
   C. 0.4 ml
   D. 0.5 ml
   E. 0.9 ml.

ANSWERS

1. B; 2. B (The apothecary system should be used for prescription compounding, while the avoirdupois system is employed for the purchase and selling of bulk chemicals); 3. D; 4. A; 5. C (60 mg of iodine daily through three doses. So, 1 dose contains 20 mg iodine. Strength of Lugol's solution is 5% i.e., 5000 ml iodine is present in 100 ml solution. So 20 mg iodine is present in 100 × 20/5000 ml solution = 0.4 ml).

CHAPTER 17

Incompatibilities in Prescriptions

• Study of Various Types of Incompatibilities -
Physical, Chemical & Therapeutic.

Incompatibility occurs when the components of a medicine interact in such a way that the properties of that medicine are adversely affected. Incompatibility may lead to changes in the physical, chemical and therapeutical qualities of the medicine. Such changes may affect the safety, efficacy and appearance of the medicine.

1. Physical incompatibility

Physical incompatibility is usually demonstrated in pharmaceutical formulations as immiscibility or insolubility, liquefaction etc. Such incompatibility can cause unsightly, non-uniform products from which it is difficult to remove the correct dose. Examples include :

(i) **Immiscibility :** Care is necessary when concentrated hydroalcoholic solutions of volatile oils, such as spirits and concentrated waters, are used as adjuncts (e.g., flavouring agents) in aqueous preparations. To prevent the oil separating in relatively large globules the hydroalcoholic solution should either be gradually diluted with the vehicle before admixture with the remaining ingredients or poured slowly in the vehicle with constant stirring. Addition of high concentrations of electrolytes to mixtures in which the vehicle is a saturated aqueous solution of a volatile oil causes the oil to separate.

(ii) **Insolubility :** Problems may be tackled by incorporation of a suitable wetting agent (HLB value 7-9) and suitable thickening agent.

Dispersions of hydrophilic colloids such as polysaccharide mucilages are precipitated by high concentrations of alcohol or salts but significant amounts are tolerated if well diluted and added in small amounts with vigorous stirring.

High concentrations of electrolytes cause cracking of soap emulsion by 'salting out' the emulgent.

(iii) **Liquefaction :** There are some compounds which are solid at room temperature and in most of the cases they can be powdered individually. But if two or more of such compounds are mixed together and triturated, the resulting m.p. of the mixture lowers down below the room temperature and as a result liquified to oily liquid and cannot be dispensed as powder dosage form. This phenomenon is known as **eutexia** and this mixture is known as **eutectic mixture**. Examples of such substances include, menthol, thymol, salol, camphor, naphthol, chloral hydrate etc.

(iv) **Precipitation**

(v) **Creaming and Cracking**

2. Therapeutic incompatibility

Therapeutic incompatibility arises when a medicine contains two or more antagonistic substances, the effects of which counteract or enhance each other, or when the action of one component in the body affects the action of another component. For example, a medicine containing an expectorant and a cough suppressant drug would be considered to be a therapeutic incompatibility.

3. Chemical incompatibility

(i) pH effects : If a solution of a salt of a weakly basic drug is made alkaline, the free base may be precipitated, while precipitation of free acid may occur if a solution of a weakly acidic drug is acidified.

(ii) pH and disperse systems : Emulsions made with soaps or emulgents, like self-emulsifying monostearin which contain soap, are incompatible with mineral acids which destroy the emulgent by precipitating the fatty acids. Below pH 3, alginic and strong acids precipitate carboxy methylcellulose from mucilages of the sodium derivative. The gelling property of bentonite is greatly reduced in acid media but improved by adding alkaline substances.

(iii) Soap emulsions and polyvalent cations : Emulsions prepared with alkali metal, ammonium and triethanol amine soaps are incompatible with salts producing polyvalent cations (Al^{+++}, Mg^{++}, Ca^{++}). Double decomposition yields a polyvalent soap, which inverts the emulsion.

(iv) Complexation of cationic and anionic compounds of high molecular weight.

(v) Reducing agents and oxidizing agents.

(vi) Alkaloidal salts (e.g., salts of strychnine, quinine, morphine, codeine, caffeine, cocaine etc.) with alkaline substances like spirit ammon aromate, ammonium bicarbonate, sodium or potassium bicarbonate, borax etc. There would be the precipitation of alkaloidal base.

(vii) Alkaloidal salts with salicylates.

(viii) Alkaloidal salts with tannins.

(ix) Soluble salicylates with alkali bicarbonates and ferric salts.

MODEL QUESTIONS

1. Foristal with paxum is incompatible. The type of incompatibility is
   A. physical   B. chemical   C. therapeutical
   D. no incompatibility.

2. Dispensing of carbonates and bicarbonates along with acid or acidic drug is an example of
   A. physical incompatibility
   B. chemical incompatibility
   C. therapeutical incompatibility
   D. eutexia
   E. synergism.

ANSWERS

1. C (Paxum contains diazepam which is hypnotic and foristal is antihistaminic, responsible for sedation. Alcohol, with antihistaminics are also incompatible - aggravate the sedation action); 2. **B.**

CHAPTER 18

Posology

- Dose and Dosage of Drugs
- Calculations of Doses on the **Basis** of Age, Sex and Surface Area
- Factors Influencing Dose and Effect of a Drug

'Posology' is a branch of science dealing with the dose of a drug The 'dose' of a drug is the quantity necessary to produce certain measurable biochemical or physiological changes in the body. It is expressed in terms of weight, volume, or unit.

ED_{50} or the median effective dose is the dose (mg/kg) that produces a desired response in 50% of the population. Similarly, **LD_{50}** or the median lethal dose is the dose (mg/kg) which is expected to kill 50% of a population of experimental animals of the same species and strain.

Therapeutic index is the ratio between LD_{50}/ED_{50}. Higher the index, greater is the margin of safety of the drug. This is an approximate estimation.

Uses of Drugs in Children—a guideline

For calculating dose of a drug, children may be considered into 3 or 4 groups such as :
(i) Neonate (first 30 days of life after birth)
(ii) Infant (upto 1 year of age)
(iii) 1 to 5 years age children, and
(iv) 6 to 12 years age children.

Before serving a prescription, the concerned pharmacist must be careful and confirmed about the age of the patient and dose should be adjusted accordingly in consultation with the concerned physician keeping in mind the following information.

Special care is always needed in case of neonates because they differ from adults in their response to drugs. The risk of toxicity is higher due to inefficient renal clearance, relative deficiencies of various enzymes, heightened sensitivity and inadequate detoxifying mechanism.

If possible, painful intramuscular injection should be avoided, particularly, in case of neonates. Even though liquid preparations are more easily accepted by children, may contain sucrose syrup as sweetening vehicle which can lead to dental decay. Therefore, after oral administration of such formulation, it is better to administer freshly boiled and cooled water in order a washing action to be effective.

Dose Calculation

The doses for children can be calculated from adult doses by using either age, or body weight or body surface area or by combination of these factors. Even though body surface area provides the most reliable method of determining doses, in practice it is exceedingly difficult.

Body weight can be easily used to calculate doses and are generally expressed in mg/Kg Because of their higher metabolic rate, children generally require higher dose per kilogram than adults. This method can pose problems while calculating dose for obese children since they are liable to be given higher than required dose. Under such circumstances, it is better to calculate dose based on ideal body weight of the child in that particular age.

Body Surface Area (BSA) is technically a better and more accurate method since many physical phenomena are more closely related to body surface area. The average body surface area of a 70 Kg Adult is about 1.7 - 1.8 sq. m. Thus, to calculate the dose for a child the following formula is used :

Approximate dose for child = Surface area of the child (m^2) × adult dose/1.8

The **percentage method** as given below can be conveniently used to calculate doses for children when there is wide margin between therapeutic and toxic dose.

Age	Ideal Body Weight (kg)	Height (cm)	Body Surface (m^2)	% of Adult Dose
Newborn	3.4	50	0.23	12.5
1 month	4.2	55	0.26	14.5
3 months	5.6	59	0.32	18.0
6 months	7.7	67	0.40	22.0
1 year	10.0	76	0.47	25.0
3 years	14.0	94	0.62	33.0
5 years	18.0	108	0.73	40.0
7 years	23.0	120	0.88	50.0
12 years	37.0	148	1.25	75.0

Besides these there are some formulae to calculate child dose. They are as follows :

1. Young's Formula $= \dfrac{\text{Age in years}}{\text{Age} + 12} \times$ adult dose

(Applicable for children under 12 years of age

2. Dilling's Formula $= \dfrac{\text{Age in years}}{20} \times$ adult dose

(Applicable for children between 4 to 20 years of age)

3. Cowling's Formula $= \dfrac{\text{Age in years} + 1}{24} \times$ adult dose

4. Clark's Formula $= \dfrac{\text{Wt. in pounds}}{150} \times$ adult dose

[Here the average weight of an adult is taken as 150 lb]

5. Fried's Formula $= \dfrac{\text{Age in months}}{150} \times$ adult dose

6. Bastado's Formula $= \dfrac{\text{Age in years} + 3}{30} \times$ adult dose

7. Gaubin's Formula : According to this formula the fraction of the adult dose for children of various ages and for the aged is as follows :

Under 1 year	1/12 of adult dose.
From 1-2 years	1/8 of adult dose.
From 2-3 years	1/6 of adult dose.
From 3-4 years	1/4 of adult dose.
From 4-7 years	1/3 of adult dose.
From 7-14 years	1/2 of adult dose.
From 14-20 years	2/3 of adult dose.
From 21-60 years	Full adult dose.
From 60-75 years	4/5 of adult dose.
From 70-80 years	3/4 of adult dose.
Over 90 years	1/2 of adult dose.

Factors Modifying the Dose and Effect of a Drug

In order to choose correct dose, the pharmacist must take into consideration of different factors that affect the action of a drug qualitatively or quantitatively. Such factors include :

1. Age : Children including the young infants are more sensitive to certain drugs because of the immaturity of the enzyme system which metabolizes and detoxicates drugs and incomplete development of the excretory system, blood-brain barrier and smaller tissue mass. However, doses of sera like anti-diphtheria, anti-tetanus and anti-gas gangrene do not depend on the age of the child but on the severity of the diseases and the amount of toxin that has to be neutralized.

2. Sex : Generally women require smaller doses than men because of smaller size and more fat, while prescribing for women one should take into consideration three conditions peculiar to them, namely, menstruation, pregnancy and lactation. Drugs like thalidomide if consumed as a hypnotic during the period of gestation may produce **phocomelia** (seal-like limbs) in the child born later. Thalidomide disasters is well known to everybody.

3. Body weight

4. Pathological condition
5. Time of administration
6. Channel of administration : Bismuth salts administered orally act as a sedative to the stom-ach, while used intramuscularly they are antisyphilitic. Magnesium sulphate given orally is a purgative, while given parenterally is a depressant of the CNS.
7. Rate of excretion and inactivation
8. Genetic factor
9. Cumulative effect
10. Frequency of administration

In drug combination the action of either drug is not altered, but the effectiveness may be enhanced or retarded :

(i) **Synergism :** The term literally means working in co-operation. If two or more drugs having similar actions when administered simultaneously, produce an effect not more than the sum of their individual actions, we can say the resultant action as synergism or summation, e.g., bromide and chloral hydrate; sulfamethoxazole and trimethoprim etc.

(ii) **Potentiation :** When the combined action of two or more drugs is more than the sum of their individual effects we call it potentiation.

(iii) **Antagonism :** This refers to the opposing or antagonising action of two or more drugs administered simultaneously; it means weakening or abolition of the action of one drug by others administered together. There may be chemical antagonism, physiological antagonism and biological antagonism.

MODEL QUESTIONS

1. Which of the following types of adverse drug reactions are not believed to be dose-related phenomena?
   A. Side effects and toxic reactions
   B. Toxic reactions and hypersensitivity
   C. Hypersensitivity and side effect
   D. Hypersensitivity and idiosyncracy
   E. Idiosyncracy and side effect.
2. The adult dose of a drug is 6 gr. What dose should be given to a 6 years old child according to Young's rule?
   A. 195 mg   B. 10 mg   C. 65 mg   D. 100 mg   E. 130 mg.
3. A prescription calls for 25 mM of potassium chloride. How many grams of KCl (MW 74.6) are needed?
   A. 7.46 g   B. 0.746 g   C. 8.86 g   D. 1.86 g   E. 0.186 g.

4. An IV order requires 5 million units of sodium penicillin G to be added to 1 litre of normal saline. How many mEq of sodium are available per litre of solution?

   A. 154   B. 1540   C. 8.4   D. 162   E. 1620

5. An order calls for 500 ml of solution of potassium sulfate to be made so that it contains 10 mEq of K^+. How many grams of potassium sulfate are required?

   A. 0.440   B. 4.44   C. 0.44   D. 0.870   E. 8.70.

6. How many millilitres of a 10% KCl (MW 74.6) solution contain 5.0 mEq of K^+?

   A. 2.10   B. 21.0   C. 3.73   D. 37.3   E. 0.373.

7. The dose of a drug is 0.5 mg per kilogram. What dose should be given a child of 6 who weighs 44 lb?

   A. 0.003 g   B. 0.033 g   C. 0.010 g   D. 0.100 g   E. 0.05 g.

8. The dose of a drug is 5 mg/kg of body weight, what dose should be given to a 110-lb women?

   A. 2 gr.   B. 4 gr.   C. 500 mg   D. 5 gr.   E. 0.5 gr.

9. A prescription calls for 500 mg of digoxin dissolved in enough solvent to make 3 fluid ounces. How much of their solution will contain approximately 1/30 gr. of digoxin?

   A. 5 minims   B. 4 minims   C. 8 minims   D. 10 minims   E. 6 minims.

10. How many millilitres of a 5% stock solution should be used to prepare 4 fluid ounces of a 1 : 200 solution?

    A. 1.2 ml   B. 4 ml   C. 10 ml   D. 12 ml   E. 48 ml.

11. How many cubic centimeters of 1 : 1000 epinephrine solution are necessary to make 30 c.c. of 1 : 5000?

    A. 6 c.c.   B. 8 c.c.   C. 10 c.c.   D. 15 c.c.   E. 60 c.c.

12. The USP contains a monograph for estimating body surface area for either children or adults. Which of the following measurements must be known in order to use this monograph?

    A. Age and height   B. Age and weight   C. Height only
    D. Height and weight   E. Weight only.

13. What would be the dose for a child weighing 40 lb if the adult dose is 50 mg? (Use Clark's rule)

    A. 15 mg   B. 20 mg   C. 25 mg   D. 30 mg   E. 35 mg.

14. The adult dose of a drug is 100 mg what is an approximate dose for a child whose body surface area is calculated to be 0.75 m^2?

    A. 25 mg   B. 40 mg   C. 50 mg   D. 75 mg   E. 80 mg.

15. One course of fluorouracil therapy is 6 mg/kg twice a day for 4 days. How many mg will be given daily to a 140 lbs patient?

    A. 48   B. 380   C. 760   D. 1480   E. 1975.

16. The loading dose of a drug is based upon the
    A. time taken for complete elimination
    B. percentage of drug excreted unchanged in urine
    C. percentage of drug bound to plasma protein
    D. apparent volume of distribution and the desired drug concentration in plasma
    E. all of the above.

17. Child doses of sera like antidiphtheria, antitetanus, etc., depend on
    A. the age of the child
    B. the severity of the diseases and the amount of the toxin that has to be neutralized
    C. the height of the child
    D. the excretory power of the child
    E. all of the above.

ANSWERS

1. D

2. E Young's Formula : Child dose $= \dfrac{\text{Age of child}}{\text{Age} + 12} \times$ Adult dose $= \dfrac{6}{6 + 12} \times 6$ gr

   $= 2$ gr. $= 2 \times 65$ mg $= 130$ mg (approx.)

3. D 1000 mM $= 74.6$ g $\therefore$ 25 mM $= 74.6 \times 25/1000$ g $= 1.865$ g

4. D 1 I.U. of sod. penicillin G $= 0.6$ μg

   $\therefore$ 5 million IU ,, ,, G $= 0.6 \times 5000000$ μg $= 3$ g

   Mol. wt. of sod. penicillin G $= 356.37$ g

   $\therefore$ 356.37 g ,, ,, ,, G $\equiv$ 1000 mEq of sod. penicillin G $\equiv$ 1000 mEq of sodium

   $\therefore$ 3 g ,, ,, ,, G $\equiv$ 1000 $\times$ 3/356.37 $\equiv$ 8.418 mEq of sodium

   1 litre normal saline solution contains 9 g of NaCl

   Now, 58.5 g of NaCl $\equiv$ 1000 mEq of NaCl $\equiv$ 1000 mEq of sodium

   $\therefore$ 9 g ,, ,, $\equiv$ 1000 $\times$ 9/58.5 $\equiv$ 153.846 mEq of sodium

   Therefore, total sod. present per litre of solution $= 8.418 + 153.846 = 162.26$ mEq.

5. D Mol wt of K_2SO_4 $= 174.2$ g

   $\therefore$ 2000 mEq of K^+ $\equiv$ 174.2 g

   $\therefore$ 10 mEq of K^+ $\equiv$ 174.2 $\times$ 10/2000 $= 0.871$ g.

6. C 1000 mEq of K^+ $= 1000$ mEq of KCl $= 74.6$ g

   $\therefore$ 5 mEq of K^+ $= 74.6 \times 5/1000 = 0.373$ g

   $\therefore$ 10% KCl solution, i.e., 10 g of KCl present in 100 ml

   $\therefore$ 0.373 ,, ,, ,, in 100 $\times$ 0.373/10 $= 3.73$ ml.

7. C For 1 kg i.e., 2.2 lb, the dose is 0.5 mg

   $\therefore$ for 1 lb, ,, ,, ,, 0.5/2.2 mg

   $\therefore$ for 44 lb ,, ,, ,, 0.5 $\times$ 44/2.2 $= 10$ mg $= 0.010$ g.

8. B For 2.2 lb (1 kg) body wt. the dose is 5 mg

   $\therefore$ 110 lb ,, ,, ,, is 5 $\times$ 110/2.2 mg $= 250$ mg

   Now, 65 mg $= 1$ gr.

   $\therefore$ 250 mg $= 1 \times 250/65$ gr. ≈ 4 gr.

9. E 500 mg digoxin is present in 3 fluid ounces $= 90$ ml.

1 gr. = 65 mg

1/30 gr. = 65 × 1/30 mg

Now, 500 mg digoxin is present in 90 ml. stock solution.

∴ 65/30 mg „ „ „ „ (90 × 65)/(30 × 500) ml.

1 ml = 15 minims

$$\therefore \frac{90 \times 65}{30 \times 500} \text{ ml} = \frac{15 \times 90 \times 65}{30 \times 500} \text{ minims} = 5.85 \text{ minims} \approx 6 \text{ minims}$$

10. D 200 ml contains 1 g material

  ∴ 4 fluid ounces i.e., 120 ml contains 1 × 120/200 g materials

Now, 5 g material is present in 100 ml

∴ 12/20 g material 100/5 × 12/20 = 12 ml.

11. A 5000 c.c. contains 1 unit

∴ 30 c.c. contains 1 × 30/5000 unit.

Now, 1 unit present in 1000 c.c.

∴ 30/5000 unit present in 1000 × 30/5000 = 6 c.c.

12. D The monograph in the USP consists of three parallel, vertical lines. The left line is calibrated with height measurements in both centimeters and inches, while the right line lists weights in kilograms and pounds. Using data based upon the patient's measurements, one draws a line between the two outside parallel lines. The intercept on the middle line, which is calibrated in square meters of body surface area, allows one to estimate the patient's body surface area.

13. A Child dose (according to Clarks rule) = [Child's wt (lb)/150] × Adult dose

$$= (40/150) \times 50 \text{ mg} = 13.3 \text{ mg} \approx 15 \text{ mg.}$$

14. B Child dose $= \dfrac{\text{Body surface area (child)}}{\text{Body surface area (adult)}} \times$ Adult dose

$$= \frac{0.75 \text{ m}^2}{1.8 \text{ m}^2} \times 100 \text{ mg} = 41.66 \approx 40 \text{ mg}$$

The average adult body surface in some literature is estimated to be 1.73 m^2.

15. C 2.2 lb = 1 kg

∴ 140 lb = 1 × 140/2.2 kg

For 1 kg, dose = 6 mg

∴ 140/2.2 kg, dose = 6 × 140/2.2 mg × 2 (twice daily) = 763 mg.

16. D

17. B

CHAPTER 19

Physico-Chemical Properties and Pharmaceutical Additives

Storage Conditions

I	Cold place	Above 0°C but within 8°C
II	Cool place	8-15°C (46° to 59°F)
III	Warm temperature	30-40°C
IV	Avoid excessive heating	Above 40°C
V	Protection from freezing	Protect from 0°C or less
VI	Room temperature	25°C

MODEL QUESTIONS

1. The USP specification of a "cool place" include the range
   A. –5° to + 5°C
   B. 0-10°C
   C. 0-20°C
   D. 8-15°C
   E. none of the above.

2. According to USP standards, a refrigerator may be used to store pharmaceuticals which specify storage in a
   A. cold place   B. cool place
   C. controlled room temperature
   D. dark place   E. both B and C.

3. The storage directions on a parenteral solution specify "Store in a cool place". This solution may be stored in
   A. an air-conditioned area at 68°F
   B. a refrigerator
   C. a cooler set at 59°F
   D. both A and C
   E. both B and C.

4. Storage conditions for Normal Human Serum Albumin USP are
   A. below 2°C   B. 2 to 4°C   C. 5 to 8°C
   D. 8 to 15°C   E. room temperature.

5. Storage conditions as per I.P. for different preparations are given. Match them with the correct temperature prescribed.
   (i)   Cold   A. Between 2°C to 8°C.
   (ii) Warm B. Below 2°C
                  C. Any temperature between 30° and 40°C
                  D. Above 40°C

ANSWERS

1. D; 2. A (A refrigerator is a cold place in which the temperature is maintained between 2° and 8°C. Controlled room temperature is 15 to 30°C); 3. E [It should be noted that articles specifying cool place storage may be stored in a refrigerator (cold place) unless otherwise specified in the individual monograph. But articles specifying cold place (2-8°C) storage must not be stored at 0°C or lesser temperature. This may damage the product]; 4. E (Normal human serum albumin is stable to heat and does not require special storage); 5. i - A, ii - C.

Solubility Profiles and Solubilization

In case of monophasic liquid dosage forms the solubility of the components should be considered primarily. To express about the solubility different descriptive terms are used as follows :

Descriptive terms	Parts of solvent for 1 part of solute
Very soluble	Less than 1
Freely soluble	From 1 to 10
Soluble	From 10 to 30

(Contd.)

Descriptive terms	Parts of solvent for 1 part of solute
Sparingly soluble	From 30 to 100
Slightly soluble	From 100 to 1000
Very slightly soluble	From 1000 to 10000
Practically insoluble or insoluble	More than 10000

The term HYDROTROPY is defined as the increase in aqueous solubility of a material by the inclusion of additives. Some examples are discussed below.

1. Inclusion of complexing agent like caffeine to form water soluble complex with drug

2. Inclusion of certain surface active agent which improves solubility by improving the wetability of the powdered drug [below the critical micelle concentration (CMC)] or by miceller solubilization technique (above CMC).

3. Co-solvency : Hydrophilic drugs are soluble in hydrophilic solvent whereas lipophilic drugs are soluble in lipophilic solvent. There are some molecules which has both hydrophilic as well as lipophilic moiety in the molecule (e.g., benzoic acid) and naturally is not freely soluble in any one solvent (either lipophilic or hydrophilic). But the solubility of such molecule will dramatically increases in a mixture of hydrophilic and lipophilic solvent (e.g., water + isopropyl alcohol). This phenomenon is known as co-solvency.

4. pH of the solution is also important. Therefore, pH solubility profiles of the drugs are to be kept in mind.

MODEL QUESTIONS

1. Solubility of a substance in a solvent may be expressed in several ways when a quantitative statement of solubility is given in the U.S.P., I.P., N.F, it is generally expressed as
   A. g of solute soluble in 1 ml of solvent
   B. g of solute soluble in 100 ml of solvent
   C. ml of solvent is required to dissolve 1g of solute
   D. ml of solvent is required to dissolve 100 g of solute
   E. ml of solvent is required to prepare 100 ml of saturated solution.

2. The solubility of a chemical in a given solvent is influenced by many factors. All of the following physicochemical constants may be useful in predicting the solubility of a chemical EXCEPT
   A. solubility parameters   B. pk$_a$ of the chemical   C. dielectric constants
   D. pH of solutions   E. valence of the chemical.

3. For many drugs in the U.S.P. - NF and I.P., exact solubility limits are not listed. Instead descriptive terminology is employed. MATCH the lettered solubility limits with the correct numbered solubility expression.

	Parts of solvent required for 1 part of solute
(i) Freely soluble	A. Less than 1
(ii) Slightly soluble	B. 1 to 10
(iii) Soluble	C. 10 to 30
(iv) Sparingly soluble	D. 30 to 100
(v) Very soluble	E. 100 to 1000

ANSWERS

1. C; 2. E (Dielectric constants and solubility parameters of solutes and solvents reflect relative polarities. The closer the solute and solvent values, the greater the potential solubility). 3. i - B; ii - E; iii - C; iv - D; v - A.

Surface Active Agents

Molecules and ions that are adsorbed at surface and interfaces and reduce the surface tension of the solvent or reduce the interfacial tension between two immiscible phase are termed surface active agents, or surfactants. Because of their affinity for both polar and non-polar solvents they are also known as amphiphile. These amphiphile are utilized in a wide variety of fields as (i) emulgents, (ii) detergents, (iii) solubilizing agents, (iv) wetting agents, (v) foaming agents, (vi) anti foaming agents, (vii) flocculants and (viii) deflocculants etc.

It is the amphiphilic nature of surface-active agents that causes them to be adsorbed at the interfaces.

Synthetic surface-active agents may be classified as following on the basis of the nature of the polar group.

(i) Anionic	Sodium or potassium stearate, sodium lauryl sulphate, sodium cetyl sulphonate etc.
(ii) Cationic	Cetyl trimethyl ammonium bromide (cetrimide), dodecyl pyridinium chloride etc.
(iii) Ampholytic	N-dodecyl alanine etc.
(iv) Non-ionic	Spans (i.e., span 80, span 40, span 20) (Sorbitan mono oleate/laurate etc.); Tweens (Polyoxyethylene sorbitan mono oleate/laurate etc.)—Tween 80, Tween 40, Tween 20. They are also known as polysorbates.

Surfactant molecules above a certain concentration which is also known as critical micelle concentration (CMC), form small aggregates/micelles **as an alternative means of protecting the hydrophobic part of the molecule from aqueous environment**. Within the inner environment of the micelles a considerable amount of oil or oil soluble drug may be incorporated to get a homogeneous transparent aqueous solution. This technique is known as miceller solubilization. The diameter of the micelles are less than the wave length of white light and naturally the solution becomes transparent or translucent.

HLB values of some amphiphilic agents are given below.

	HLB values
Oleic acid	1
Glyceryl monostearate	3.8
Sorbitan mono oleate (span 80)	4.3
Sorbitan mono laurate (span 20)	8.6
Triethanol amine oleate	12.0
Polyoxyethylene sorbitan monooleate (Tween 80 or Polysorbate 80)	15.0
Polyoxyethylene sorbitan monolaurate (Tween 20 or Polysorbate 20)	16.7
Sodium oleate	18.0
Sod. lauryl sulphate	40.0

MODEL QUESTIONS

1. HLB is
   A. hydrophobic lyophilic balance
   B. hydrophilic lipophilic balance
   C. hydrophilicity and lipophilicity of bases
   D. none of the above.
2. HLB of sodium lauryl sulphate is
   A. 4.3   B. 11.1   C. 20.5   D. 40.0
3. Surface-active agents tend to enhance absorption due to
   A. effects on biological membrane
   B. effects on dissolution rate of drugs.
   C. reduction of interfacial tension.
   D. B and C.
   E. A, B and C.
4. Tween 20 is a
   A. deflocculant   B. lipophilic surfactant   C. preservative
   D. hydrophilic surfactant   E. none of the above.
5. Brij is a trade name for a
   A. suspending agent   B. surfactant   C. deflocculant
   D. propellant   E. flavour.
6. Benzalkonium chloride solution is partially inactivated by
   A. soap   B. warming the solution   C. methyl cellulose
   D. acetone   E. none of the above.
7. The HLB system is used to classify

   A. flavors   B. colours   C. surfactants

   D. organic ring structures   E. perfumes.

8. Which of the following should be classified as deflocculating agent?

   A. Tween 20   B. Tween 80   C. Marasperse

   D. Sodium lauryl sulfate   E. Carbowax.

9. When nonpolar substances are dissolved in a polar solvent using surfactants, the process is called

   A. gelation   B. emulsification   C. solubilization

   D. HLB   E. none of the above.

10. Polysorbate is the synonym for

   A. brij   B. tween   C. span

   D. sodium lauryl sulfate   E. polyvinyl pyrrolidone.

11. Which of the following is not a category of surfactant?

   A. Cationic   B. Amphoteric   C. Non-ionic   D. Anionic   E. Lympholytic.

12. Surfactants are characterized by the presence of

   A. water solubilizing groups

   B. negative charges

   C. positive charges

   D. fat-solubilizing groups

   E. water-solubilizing and fat-solubilizing group in the same molecule.

13. The HLB system is most applicable for the classification of which surfactants?

   A. Anionic   B. Ampholytic   C. Cationic

   D. Non-ionic   E. Either cationic or anionic.

14. An example of nonionic surfactant would be

   A. ammonium laurate

   B. cetyl pyridinium chloride

   C. sorbitan monopalmitate

   D. dioctyl sodium sulfosuccinate

   E. triethanolamine stearate.

15. Given below (A-F) are the HLB range of surfactants. Match them with their appropriate categories (i-vi).

   (i)   Solubilizing agents   A. 1-3

   (ii)   Detergents   B. 7-9

   (iii)   O/W emulgents   C. 16-19

   (iv)   Wetting and spreading agents   D. 13-16

   (v)   W/O emulsifying agents   E. 8-16

   (vi)   Antifoaming agents   F. 3-8

ANSWERS

1. B; 2. D (It is an anionic surfactant, having the HLB value 40 and used as foaming and wetting agent); 3. E (All three mechanisms listed here contributes significantly in the absorption process); 4. D (HLB value = 16.7); 5. B (It is product of Atlas company);

6. A [Benzalkonium chloride is a germicidal surfactant and is positively charged whereas soap (anionic surfactant) is negatively charged. So there would be precipitation due to reaction between (+)vely charged and (-)vely charged molecules. Soaps are sodium or potassium salts of higher fatty acids. Examples include, sodium/potassium stearate (or palmitate, oleate etc.)];

7. C; 8. C; 9. C (It is more specifically known as miceller solubilization); 10. B; 11. E; 12. E;

13. D (Although some anionic and cationic emulsifiers have been assigned HLB values, the system's prime use is to classify the thousands of nonionics that are commercially available. Anionic and cationic surfactants are predominantly hydrophilic but non-ionic surfactants may be hydrophilic as well as lipophilic. Subsequently HLB values are assigned to the ionic surfactants to express their degree of hydrophilicity.); 14. C (It is also known as span 40);

15. i - C; ii - D; iii - E; iv - B; v - F; vi - A.

Commonly Used Vehicles, Bases and Diluents Used as Additives in Different Dosage Forms

These additives are included in the dosage forms either to dissolve a drug or to give it a bulk or alternately to act as a vehicle for the proper use and effectiveness of the formulation. These may be liquids, semisolids or solids.

A. Liquids

(i) Aqueous : Different waters official in I.P. and other pharmacopoeias (discussed in chapter 10 of pharmaceutics-I); various aromatic waters like cinnamon water, peppermint water, camphor water, rose water. Like other solvents, water is also not an universal solvent, there is the possibility of hydrolysis and microbial growth.

(ii) Non-aqueous : Oils and oily materials, e.g.,
   a. Vegetable oils, viz., castor oil, peanut oil, cotton seed oil, corn oil etc. Vegetable oils have a possibility of rancidity.
   b. Mineral oil - liquid paraffin;
   c. Synthetic esters - ethyl oleate, iso-propyl myristate etc.

(iii) Alcohol : It is also a good solvent for a number of drugs and also has anti microbial action.

(iv) Propylene glycol : It must not be contaminated with ethylene glycol which is very toxic and can be responsible for death of the patient.

(v) Glycerol

(vi) Syrups like Simple Syrup I.P.

B. Semisolid bases

These are used in the preparation of ointments, suppositories, pessaries etc., for example, yellow and white soft paraffin (also known as petroleum jelly or vaseline) discussed in Chapter 23.

C. Solids

The solid materials which are included in formulation of tablets, capsules, powders, granules etc. in appreciable quantities are called diluents. The most common diluent used for internal preparation is lactose. Other examples include—sucrose, mannitol (it is a desirable additive for chewable tablets), starches (also used as binder and disintegrants) and celluloses, dibasic calcium phosphate, calcium sulphate, sodium chloride, talc as diluent.

MODEL QUESTIONS

1. The usual purpose of chilling medication prior to administration is to increase
   - A. absorption
   - B. palatability
   - C. stability
   - D. ionization
   - E. gastric motility.
2. The nonaqueous vehicle used in injections is
   - A. alcohol
   - B. glycerol
   - C. alcoholic sodium stearate
   - D. vegetable oils
   - E. wax or liquid petrolatum.
3. Preserved water is made by adding which of the following to purified water?
   - A. Phenol
   - B. Benzoic acid
   - C. Zephiran
   - D. Parabens
   - E. None of the above.

ANSWERS

1. B (Chilled solution do not interact with the taste bud quickly); 2. D; 3. D.

Stabilizers

When a dosage form is said to be stable it should be stable in its physical form, chemical composition and also stable against microbial spoilage. The materials that ensure stability of chemical composition or which help to prevent microbial growth are called stabilizers.

I. Destabilization due to hydrolysis

Aspirin (Acetyl salicylic acid) with water to form salicylic acid and acetic acid.

Precautions :

(i) To use non-aqueous vehicle in case of liquid preparation.

(ii) To apply a waterproof protecting coating over tablets.

(iii) To use tightly closed container.

(iv) To supply as dry powder which has to be reconstituted before use.

(v) To formulate the product, if possible, at a pH of maximum stability (Because pH has great influence on the hydrolytic decomposition of drug).

(vi) To store the product at low temperature

(vii) To use suitable desiccant along with solid dosage form in the sealed container.

II. Destabilization due to oxidation

Precautions :

(i) To use suitable antioxidants as follows.

    a. Chelating agents (to form chelate with traces amount of Cu, Mn, Fe etc. which are responsible for catalytic oxidative degradation) - EDTA (ethylene diamine tetra acetic acid), citric acid, tartaric acid, phenyl alanine, phosphoric acid, tryptophane etc.

    b. Preferentially oxidized compounds : Ascorbic acid, sodium bi-sulfite, sodium sulfite etc.

    c. Chain terminators

        Water soluble : Thiols (cysteine hydrochloride, thioglycerol, thioglycolic acid, thiosorbitol).

        Lipid soluble : Alkyl gallates (octyl, propyl, dodecyl), ascorbyl palmitate, t-butyl hydroquinone (TBHQ), butylated hydroxy anisole (BHA), butylated hydroxy toluene (BHT), nordihydro guaiaretic acid (NDGH) (α-tocopherol).

(ii) To use certain gas such as N_2 in the container of liquid preparation to replace headspace air.

(iii) To seal the drug powder under vacuum.

(iv) To remove the dissolve oxygen from the manufacturing vat of the liquid preparation by N_2 sparging or by using freshly, boiled and cooled water or by the application of vacuum during ultrasonic agitation.

(v) To use opaque or light resistant containers in case of light catalyzed oxidation.

(vi) To use U.V. light absorbing compounds (e.g., benzophenones) to prepare container.

(vii) To formulate the product at a pH of maximum stability, if possible (like hydrolysis, pH can also influence oxidative degradation).

(viii) To store the product at low temperature.

MODEL QUESTIONS

1. Which vitamin is used occasionally as an antioxidant?

    A. Vitamin D   B. Vitamin K   C. Vitamin B_1 D. Vitamin E   E. Vitamin B_3.

2. The presence of sodium bi-sulfite in a drug solution implies that the drug

    A. is heat labile

    B. is susceptible to oxidation

    C. has poor water solubility

    D. requires an alkaline media

E. will sustain growth of microorganisms.

3. In salicylate mixture sodium metabisulphite is used as

A. preservative   B. antioxidant   C. therapeutic agent

D. viscosity builder   E. emulsifier.

ANSWERS

1. D (Like ascorbic acid, vitamin E is also preferentially oxidizable compound); 2. B (Sodium bisulfite is a very good antioxidant. It is preferentially oxidised. But unfortunately it may be responsible to cause asthma like reaction in a certain number of patient); 3. B.

Preservatives

A preservative is, in the common pharmaceutical sense, a substance that prevents or inhibits microbial growth and may be added to pharmaceutical preparations for this purpose to avoid consequent spoilage of the preparations by microorganisms.

An ideal preservative should have wide spectrum of activity (i.e., effective against all types of microorganisms) be non-toxic and compatible to other formulation ingredients including containers and closures, be equally soluble in aqueous and oily media and be organoleptically acceptable.

No single antimicrobial compound possesses all the above properties and hence combination of two or more preservatives is used in practice.

Example of some preservatives : Chlorocresol, benzoic acid and sodium benzoate, propyl parahydroxy benzoate (propyl paraben), phenyl mercuric nitrate/acetate, methyl parahydroxy benzoate (methyl paraben), benzalkonium chloride (also used as cationic surfactant), thiomersal, chlorhexidine acetate, chlorobutanol, monothioglycerol, potassium sorbate etc.

If any ingredient of the formulation has similar antimicrobial effect at least equal to that of preservative, then extra preservative addition may not be essential. e.g., 10% (v/v) or more alcohol containing preparations, some radiopharmaceutical preparations etc.

In case of single dose injectable containers no preservative is recommended but in case of multi-dose injectables, preservative addition is mandatory unless it is not prescribed by the individual monograph.

In case of injectables intended for intraatrium, intracisternal, intracardiac, intraocular, intrathecal or any other route of injection giving access to the cerebrospinal fluid, no preservative in any case is recommended and naturally they are packed in single dose container.

Organoleptic Additives

The additives used to improve the colour, flavour and taste of the preparations intended for oral administration are known as organoleptic additive. Among them are colouring, flavouring and sweetening agents.

Coloring Agents or Colorants

The certified colors are classified into three groups as follows (1) F, D and C dyes which may legally be used in foods, drugs and cosmetics (2) D and C dyes which may legally be used in drugs and cosmetics and (3) External D and C dyes which may legally be used only in externally applied drugs and cosmetics.

Pharmaceutical preparations are coloured for the following reasons :

(i) To mask an unpleasant appearance.

(ii) To increase their acceptability to patients.

(iii) To prepare products of a consistent colour.

(iv) To aid identification.

(v) To give warning.

Selection of the appropriate coloring agent is based on the principle that a color should appropriate to the flavour of the medicine and vice versa.

A list of the colors recommended for incorporation to medicines and cosmetics is given ir Forensic Pharmacy (Chapter 30).

Flavoring Agents

One of the aims of formulation is to produce a palatable and hopefully pleasant-tasting medicine. The flavoring agents should matched with the four primary tastes—sweet, bitter, sour and saline.

People are more sensitive to odor than to taste. There are about 10,000 to 30,000 identifiable scents, of which the average person can identify about 4000. Women are more sensitive to odors than men.

Some examples of flavouring agents are given below : Aromatic oils, Pineapple, Cardamom, Ginger, Cinnamom, Peppermint, Rose, Jasmine, Lavender, Orange, Cherry, Tolu balsam, Vanilla, Spearmint, Raspberry, Methyl salicylate (oil of wintergreen), Fennel oil, Ethyl acetate, Coriander oil, Clove oil, Caraway oil, Anethole, Anise oil.

Sweetening Agents

(i) Sugars : Sucrose, lactose, mannitol (about 72% as sweet as sucrose) etc.

(ii) Sorbitol

(iii) Glycerol

(iv) Saccharin (artificial 300 to 500 times sweeter than sucrose) - it has bitter after taste.

(v) Cyclamates.

(vi) Licorice liquid extract (*Glycyrrhiza glabra*). The root of *G. glabra* contains 5 to 7% of the sweet principle glycyrrhizin, or glycyrrhizinic acid which is 50 times as sweet as cane sugar.

(vii) Liquid glucose.

(viii) Honey.

(ix) Aspartame : It is approximately 200 times sweeter than sucrose. It is a synthetic sweetener, that is, a dipeptide of L-aspartic acid and L-phenylalanine. If heated aspartame breaks down into its respective amino acids, with a corresponding decrease in sweetness.

Hydrocolloids Used as Additive (Suspending Agents, Emulsifying Agents etc.)

These are high molecular weight materials of colloidal dimensions which in water produce highly viscous solutions, suspensions or gels. Examples :

(i) Natural hydrocolloids :

    a. Plant source : Polysaccharides such as, agar, acacia, tragacanth, alginates, psyllium, seedhusk.

    b. Animal source : gelatin - Pharmagel A and B (these are protein in nature).

    c. Mineral source : Attapulgite - veegum (aluminium magnesium silicate), bentonite, collidal alumina, colloidal silica.

(ii) Semisynthetic : Methyl cellulose, hydroxy methyl cellulose, carboxy methyl cellulose (CMC) and its sodium salt, hydroxy propyl methyl cellulose (HPMC), etc.

(iii) Synthetic : Carbopol, poloxamer, carbomer (carboxy vinyl polymer), colloidal silicon dioxide.

Dry hydrocolloids like acacia powder etc. are known as **xerogel**.

Bentonite, a complex silicate, obtained from mineral source is a very good suspending agent. Suspensions or sol of bentonite magma during undisturbed storage converted to gel (having higher viscosity) which on stirring or agitation again converted to sol (having lower viscosity). This sol to gel or gel to sol conversion properties are known as **Thixotrophy**. This character is due to the "**house of cards**" formation by the bentonite particles which in hydrated condition are flat flake like structure, the flat surface of which is negatively charged whereas the sharp edges are positively charged. Naturally in suspension they orient themselves due to the attractive forces between these two different charges to form the house of cards.

Bentonite, veegum, graphite, $Mg(OH)_2$ etc. are wetted by both oil and water and naturally these finely divided solids are adsorbed at the interfaces and act as emulsifying agents.

Hectorite is used industrially in suspensions for external use. It absorbs more water than bentonite and a 1% or 2% dispersion is a clear highly thixotropic gel.

Acacia gum is obtained from some species of Acacia. Since it is a natural product, it may be contaminated with microorganisms and may need to be sterilized before use. It also contains PEROXIDASE enzymes which may affect susceptible products but which are destroyed by heating to 100°C.

Tragacanth is a dried extract from some species of Astragalus Compound **Tragacanth Powder** BP 1980 consists of acacia (20%), tragacanth (15%), starch (20%) and sucrose (45%) and is used in quantities of 2 g per 100 ml of product.

Sodium alginate is the sodium salt of alginic acid and is derived from seaweed. Heating above 70°C cause depolymerization with consequent loss of viscosity. At pH 3 the alginic acid precipitated and is incompatible with heavy metals, calcium salts and phenyl mercuric salts.

Methyl cellulose : These are methyl ethers resulting from the methylation of cellulose. The varying degrees of methylation and chain length produce various characteristics and the name is usually followed by a number that gives an indication of the viscosity of a 2% aqueous solution at 20°C. The high viscosity grades (2500 and 4500) are used as thickening and dispersing agents.

MODEL QUESTIONS

1. A synthetic sweetening agent which is approximately 200 times sweeter than sucrose and has no after taste is
 A. saccharin B. aspartame C. cyclamate D. sorbitol E. glycerol.

2. Ostwald pipettes are used to measure
 A. specific gravity   B. samples for assay   C. density
 D. osmotic pressure   E. viscosity.

3. Veegum is a (an)
 A. polyol   B. organic gum   C. synthetic gum
 D. clay   E. nonionic surfactant.

4. Polyvinyl alcohol is commonly employed in pharmaceutical systems as a
 A. preservative   B. buffer   C. viscosity builder
 D. lubricant   E. solvent.

5. The Munsell system is associated with
 A. flavor   B. odour   C. chemical classification
 D. colour   E. incompatibilities.

6. Povan could be classified as a
 A. deflocculant B. lubricant   C. cyanine dye D. disintegrator E. surfactant.

7. The Crocker-Henderson system is used to classify
 A. flavours   B. dyes   C. odours   D. surfactants E. deflocculants.

8. A disadvantage of sodium saccharin as sweetening agent is
 A. its bitter after taste
 B. its solubility in water
 C. its poor strength compared to glucose
 D. its poor strength compared to dulcin
 E. its toxicity.

ANSWERS

1. B; 2. E (Ostwald pipettes are used to measure the relative viscosity compared to water); 3. D (It is aluminium - magnesium silicate); 4. C; 5. D (Munsell system is a classification system of color); 6. C (It is a red dye and stains the stool brownish red); 7. C; 8. A.

Powders

Undivided (bulk) oral powders usually contain non-potent medicaments such as antacids (light magnesium carbonate, heavy magnesium carbonate and magnesium trisilicate) where the accuracy with which the patient measure the dose is not critical.

Note : Light magnesium carbonate and heavy magnesium carbonate is chemically same. The difference is in their particle size and bulk density. The light variety is separated from the heavy by way of **elutriation**.

Divided oral powders are packaged individually (minimum quantity 20 mg, with or without diluent) each dose is separately wrapped in paper or sealed (in case of air sensitive and hygroscopic material) in a sachet.

Dusting powders for external use are free-flowing very fine powders for application to the body surfaces but not to open wounds unless sterilized. This may be non-medicated and used as cosmetics or medicated where active medicament(s) are mixed up with pre-sterilized inert diluent like talc (also known as French chalk, soap stone, steatite).

Granules for oral administration are small irregular particles (0.5-2 mm in diameter) often supplied in single dose sachets.

Geometric dilution : In case of dilution the potent drugs (having small volume) with suitable inert diluent like lactose (having bulk or high volume), the entire drug if mixed in one step with the entire amount of diluent all at a time, there is a high chance of non-homogeneity in the preparation. Therefore, the potent drug is to be mixed up in the first step with an equal volume of diluent to make the volume nearly double which is again mixed up with the double i.e., equal volume of diluent. This gradual dilution is known as geometric dilution process.

Advantages of Powders

1. Adsorption is faster than from corresponding tablets or capsules. In case of tablets or capsules, after disintegration the material never attain that state of subdivision as achieved from powder dosage form.
2. Dry powders are more stable than liquid preparation.

Disadvantages of Powders

1. Difficult to mask unpleasant tastes and odor, if any.
2. Inconvenient to carry.
3. In case of bulk powder the measurement of dose may be inaccurate.
4. As surface area is increased so chances of oxidative degradation is high.

Containers : Wide mouth glass container with close-fitting closures may be used for undivided (bulk) powder. In case of divided powder moisture proof sachets may be used which may be packed in wide mouth screw-capped plastic jar or paper board boxes.

Special Labels and Advice for Patients

1. In case of bulk powder : Patients should be advised that the powders should be dissolved or dispensed as appropriate in a little water before taking.
2. In case of divided powder : Patients should be instructed that individual powders should be dispersed in a little water or placed on the back of the tongue before swallowing.

Powders for mixtures

There are powders mixed in the proportion of standard, suspension type mixtures, e.g., Magnesium Trisilicate Mixture B.P. The mixed powders may be conveniently stored in the dry form and the mixture prepared by the pharmacist when required for dispensing, by suspension of the powders in the appropriate vehicle with addition of any liquid ingredients.

Cachets

The shells of cachets are moulded from rice paper and are used to enclose quantities of medium-density dry powder upto 2 g in weight, cachets are now rarely dispensed but in the past were used to administer unpleasantly tasting powder drugs in a tasteless form. Because of the large size, cachets should be immersed in water for a few seconds before swallowing with a draught of water.

Tablet Triturates or Moulded Tablets

These are powders moulded to form a tablet. They may be swallowed whole or crushed to powder or placed under the toungue.

Powders for Injection

These are sterile, solid substances (including freeze-dried materials) which are distributed in their final containers and which, when shaken with the prescribed volumes of the appropriate sterile liquid, rapidly form clear and practically particle-free solutions or uniform suspensions.

Insufflations

Insufflations are very fine (60 μ or less) impalpable (not perceivable by touch) powdered medicament intended to be administered with the help of an insufflator to the areas to which the powder could not be applied directly, e.g., pulmonary tree.

Powder Containing Eutectic Mixture (Liquefiable Substances)

Some substances like menthol, thymol, camphor, phenol, salol etc which are solid at room temperature, but when any two or more of these are mixed together and powdered, becomes liquefied to oily liquid. This is due to the lowering of the m.p. of the resulting mixture below the room temperature. This phenomenon is known as 'eutexia' and this mixture is known as 'eutectic mixture'.

For dispensing of the eutectic mixture the individual components are pulverized separately and mixed up thoroughly with suitable inert diluent like talc, dry starch etc. and finally all are mixed together very loosely and supplied.

Camphor may be better pulverized by first addition of small amount of alcohol and immediately grinding before the evaporation of the alcohol.

Effervescent Mixture/Powder/Citro-Tartarate of Soda/Granule/Tablet

Along with the active constituents the effervescent preparations must contain a carbon dioxide source like sodium bicarbonate ($NaHCO_3$), which reacts with an equivalent amount of tartaric acid or citric acid or a mixture of both in presence of water to produce water and carbon di-oxide along with corresponding sodium salts. This liberated CO_2 is actually responsible for effervescent action and helps in administration of unpalatable drugs by preventing direct contact with the taste buds

$$
\begin{array}{l}
\text{H} \\
| \\
\text{HO - C - COOH} \\
| \\
\text{HO - C - COOH} \\
| \\
\text{H} \\
\text{Sod. bi-carbonate}
\end{array}
\; + 2NaHCO_3 \longrightarrow
\begin{array}{l}
\text{H} \\
| \\
\text{HO - C - COONa} \\
| \\
\text{HO - C - COONa} \\
| \\
\text{H}
\end{array}
\; + 2H_2O + 2CO_2 \uparrow
$$

Tartaric acid   Sod. tartrate   Carbon dioxide

$$
\begin{array}{l}
\text{H} \\
| \\
\text{H - C - COOH} \\
| \\
\text{HO - C - COOH} \\
| \\
\text{H - C - COOH} \\
| \\
\text{H}
\end{array}
\; .H_2O + 3NaHCO_3 \longrightarrow
\begin{array}{l}
\text{H} \\
| \\
\text{H - C - COONa} \\
| \\
\text{HO - C - COONa} \\
| \\
\text{H - C - COONa} \\
| \\
\text{H}
\end{array}
\; +4H_2O + 3CO_2 \uparrow
$$

Citric acid   Sod. citrate   Carbon dioxide and also helps in solubilization or dispersion of certain drugs formulated as effervescent tablet. The evolved gas also responsible for carminative action.

In practice, for the preparation of effervescent granule a mixture of both tartaric and citric acid is used. If only tartaric acid is used, then the powder mass will not be converted to granule via soft coherent dummy mass. The citric acid containing one molecule of water of crystallization which liberates at the high working temperature to make the powdered mass to soft dummy mass which is immediately passed through suitable sieve to make moist granules, which is then dried at about 60°C.

If only citric acid is used the liberated water would be too high to complete the reaction.

MODEL QUESTIONS

1. Dental powder is an example of
   A. effervescent powder   B. bulk powder   C. simple powder
   D. divided powder   E. none of the above.
2. Which of the following operation is not applicable to powders?
   A. Levigation   B. Trituration   C. Spatulation
   D. Resolution   E. Pulverization.
3. Common equipment used for powder mixing is
   A. sigma blender   B. triple roller   C. hammer mill
   D. colloid mill   E. fluid energy mill.
4. Effervescent granules usually contain following acid as one component.
   A. Tartaric or citric acid B. Sulphuric acid   C. Benzoic acid
   D. Barbituric acid   E. Lactic acid
5. Atropine sulphate 15 mg in lactose is an example of
   A. potent powder   B. simple powder   C. compound powder
   D. effervescent powder   E. bulk powder.
6. Fill in the blanks
   (i) A gas is produced from effervescent preparations during administration due to the reaction between ...... (1) ...... and ...... (2) ...... or ...... (3) ....
   (ii) In fusion method for preparation of effervescent granules water of crystallisation present in citric acid acts as ....

ANSWERS

1. B; 2. D; 3. A; 4. A; 5. A; 6. (i) 1. sodium bicarbonate, 2. citric acid, 3. tartaric acid (ii) binding agent.

CHAPTER 21

Monophasic Liquid Dosage Forms

- Solutions for Oral Administration
- Solutions Instilled into Body Cavities
- Solutions for External Use
- Syrups.

Solutions as Oral Dosage Forms

Elixirs : Elixirs are solutions for oral administration. The vehicle usually contains syrup, ethanol or other co-solvents to give a clear solution and a pleasant taste.

Linctuses : These are formulated with syrup as the vehicle and are designed to soothe sore mucous membranes in the treatment of cough.

Special information in label : Should be sipped and swallowed slowly without the addition of water.

Mixtures : These are liquid preparations for oral administration and contain medicaments dissolved and/or suspended in water.

Advantages of Solutions as an Oral Dosage Form

(i) Absorption of the medicine from the g.i. tract is rapid

(ii) Easy to swallow

(iii) Uniform distribution of medicament.

Disadvantages

(i) Medicaments are less stable in solution than in a dry dosage form.

(ii) Unpleasant flavours may be difficult to mask.

(iii) Bulky.

(iv) Container is breakable.

(v) Dose measurement is required.

Mouthwashes are used to clean and refresh the buccal cavity. They contain antiseptics or astringents in a pleasantly flavoured vehicle.

Gargles are used to relieve soreness in mild throat infections and contain antiseptic, analgesic and weak astringents.

Gargles and mouthwashes are usually diluted by the patient with warm water before use and most are not intended to be swallowed in significant amounts. They should be dispensed in amber fluted bottles.

Special information in the label : Not to be swallowed in large amount.

Solution Instilled into Body Cavities

Nasal drops and sprays : Solutions of medicaments designed to be applied to the nasal mucosa in a small volume are usually formulated to be iso-osmotic with nasal secretions and if necessary buffered slightly to the acid side of neutral (pH 6.5) in order to minimize damage to the nasal cilia. Nasal solutions are used commonly to relieve nasal irritation and congestion, although antimicrobial substances may also be included. The nasal route can be used to introduce drugs required to produce a systemic effect, e.g., the peptide hormones of the posterior lobe of the pituitary gland and their synthetic analogues.

Containers for nasal and ear drops : Nasal drops are supplied in hexagonal amber fluted glass bottles with a rubber teat and dropper closure. Some commercially produced nasal drops are also supplied in glass dropper bottles which may or may not be fluted.

Special information in the label :

(i) Avoid excessive use.

(ii) Avoid use in very young babies unless under medical advice.

Ear drops : These are usually simple solutions of medicaments designed to exert a local effect in the ear, to soften wax, to treat local inflammation and infection, or to relieve pain. The vehicle may be water although glycerol and propylene glycol may also be used.

Enemas : Enemas are aqueous or oily solutions or suspensions that are introduced into the rectum for cleansing, therapeutic or diagnostic purpose. Enemas prior to administration should be warm up to 37°C.

Container : Amber fluted glass bottles.

Special information in the label : For rectal use only.

Douches : A douche is a medicated solution for rinsing a body cavity. This includes all irrigation solutions, enemas etc.

Solutions for External Use

Liniments are solutions formulated with an alcoholic or an oily vehicle and are intended for rubbing into unbroken skin.

Lotions are also intended to be applied to unbroken skin but without friction. For lotions intended to evaporate quickly on the skin surface the vehicle is usually alcoholic and acetone may also be included.

Paints are usually applied to the skin with a brush. The solvent may be water or an organic solvent where rapid evaporation is required. Throat paints are applied in the inner mucosa of the throat during infection.

Containers : Fluted amber

Special information in the label : Liniments and lotions should not be applied to broken skin. Flammable products must carry a warning to avoid naked flames.

Antiseptic (used in living tissue site) and **disinfectant** (used in case of inanimates) solutions : These contain antimicrobial substances and may be used to reduce the numbers of microorganisms on the skin surface (antiseptic) or on inanimate objects (disinfectant) such as equipment or work surfaces. Examples include benzalkonium chloride solution, cetrimide solution, potassium permanganate solution and proflavine solution.

Special information in the label :

(i) Dilution direction.

(ii) Patient should be warned to discard the stock solutions after 7 days and to discard any diluted solution immediately after use.

Rideal-Walker Coefficient (R.W.C) value is used to express the germicidal power of disinfectants. Higher the R.W.C. value higher is the germicidal action.

Syrups

Syrups are viscous oral liquids that may contain one or more active ingredients in solution. The vehicle usually contains large amounts of sucrose or other sugars to which certain polyhydric alcohols (e.g., glycerol, sorbitol etc.) may be added to inhibit crystallization or to modify solubilisation, taste and other vehicle properties. **Sugarless syrups** may contain sweetening agents and thickening agents. Syrups may contain ethanol (95%) as a preservative or as a solvent to incorporate flavoring agents. Antimicrobial agents may also be added to syrups.

The solubility of sucrose in water is 66.9% (w/w). The Simple Syrup I.P. '85 contains 66.7% (w/w) sucrose and prepared by hot process. This syrup is concentrated enough to act as self preservative due to osmotic effect. In the closed container the superficial layer of the syrup may be diluted by condensed water. Due to this surface dilution the surface layer becomes susceptible to microbial growth. The presence of ethanol may prevent this growth due to its preferential accumulation at the superficial layer, alcohol being the more volatile component evaporated at a faster rate and condensed back to the superficial layer. Simple Syrup B.P. is also produced by hot process and contains 66.7% (w/w) sucrose, but Simple Syrup USP is prepared by cold process (percolation) and contains 85% (w/v) sucrose. Syrups prepared by cold process is colorless whereas syrups prepared by hot process is slightly yellowish brown colour due to **caramelization** of sucrose during heating.

Simple syrup is actually the concentrated solution of sucrose and used as pharmaceutical aid (sweetening agent), on the other hand medicated syrup contains pharmacologically active ingredients dissolved in simple syrup.

MODEL QUESTIONS

1. Elixirs are
   A. sweetened hydroalcoholic solutions

    B. plain hydroalcoholic solutions

    C. sweetened aqueous solutions

    D. none the above.

2. Aromatic elixirs contain

    A. aromatic flavouring agent

    B. orange spirit

    C. hydroalcoholic soluble aromatic compounds

    D. none of the above.

3. Gargle prior to use to be

    A. undiluted

    B. diluted

    C. diluted with equal volume of water only

    D. boiled

    E. refrigerated.

4. Potassium bromide mixture is an example of

    A. simple mixture

    B. diffusible mixture

    C. indiffusible mixture

    D. emulsion

    E. none of the above.

5. Mist Alba (Alba mixture) is an example of

    A. simple mixture

    B. diffusible mixture

    C. indiffusible mixture

    D. mixture containing precipitate forming liquids

    E. none of the above.

6. Bismuth compound mixture is an example of

    A. simple mixture

    B. diffusible mixture

    C. indiffusible mixture

    D. effervescent mixture

    E. none of the above.

7. Syrups cannot be sterilized by autoclaving because

    A. they decompose by heat

    B. they contain flavoring agents

    C. they are filled in glass bottles

    D. they are used by common people.

8. The purpose of parabens in syrup is as

    A. stabilizers   B. preservatives   C. buffers

    D. tonicity adjusters   E. thickeners.

9. Syrup USP contains 85% w/v sucrose and has a specific gravity of 1.313. Express the concentration of sucrose in terms of % w/w.

    A. 55%   B. 65%   C. 75%

  D. 85%   E. Impossible to calculate with the given data.

10. Which of the following is NOT suitable as sweetening agent for inclusion in an elixir or syrup formula?

  A. Glycerin   B. Aspartame   C. Lactose   D. Sorbitol   E. Saccharin.

11. The concentration of sucrose in Simple Syrup B.P. is

  A. 40.74% w/w   B. 60.70% w/w   C. 66.70% w/w

  D. 70.50% w/w   E. 85% w/v.

12. Invertion of sucrose in syrup due to heat is known as

  A. isomerization   B. epimerization   C. tautomerization

  D. caramelization   E. ionization.

13. A vehicle for nasal medication should possess all of the following properties except

  A. an acid pH   B. high buffer capacity   C. isotonicity

  D. ability to resist growth of microorganisms

  E. all of the above are important properties no exceptions.

14. An antimicrobial preservative commonly used for nasal solution is

  A. benzalkonium chloride   B. sorbic acid   C. thiomersal

  D. phenylmercuric acetate   E. benzyl alcohol.

15. Phenol glycerin ear drop to be diluted as directed by the physician by using
  A. freshly boiled and cooled water
  B. alcohol
  C. glycerin
  D. phenol
  E. all of the above.

16. Iodine is soluble in water in the presence of

  A. sodium citrate   B. sodium sulfate   C. lactose

  D. PVP   E. PEG.

17. Which of the following statements concerning wild cherry syrup is not true?
  A. Contains both glycerin and sucrose
  B. Tannins are present in the final preparation
  C. Has some expectorant activity
  D. Has a pleasant cherry flavor
  E. Manufacturing procedure includes percolation.

18. Match the lettered ingredients with the numbered official product of which they are constituents

  (i)   Cherry Syrup NF 14   A. benzoic acid and cinnamic acid
  (ii) İpecac Syrup USP 19   B. emetic and cephaeline
  (iii) Tolu Balsam Syrup NF 14   C. emodin and aloe emodin
  (iv) Wild Cherry Syrup USP 18   D. malic and citric acid
                                    E. prunase and emulsion

ANSWERS

1. A; 2. B; 3. B; 4. A; 5. B; 6. C; 7. A; 8.B [Methyl paraben (methyl parahydroxy benzoate) and propyl paraben (propyl parahydroxy benzoate) both are used as preservative]; 9. B [85% w/v means 100 ml (i.e., 100 × 1.313 = 131.3 g syrup contains 85 g sucrose. ∴ 100 g syrup containing (85 × 100)/131.3 = 64.7% (w/w)]; 10. C [Lactose (milk sugar has only a slight degree of sweetness)]; 11. C; 12. D; 13. B (Both opthalmic and nasal preparations should have only mild buffer capacity so that the organ's natural buffer system can overcome any pH differences. Otherwise irritation might result. pH range is usually 5.5 to 7.5); 14. A; 15.C (The strength of phenol is reduced as desired by diluting with glycerol); 16 D [Polyvinyl pyrrolidone (PVP) or povidone form a soluble complex with iodine. Iodine is incorporated within the big spiral structure of povidone]; 17. D (Wild cherry syrup has a somewhat bitter taste mainly because of the tannins present, and as a result it shows incompatibility with most of the prescription ingredients, forms insoluble salt with alkaloids, discoloration will occur in presence of iron salt. Cherry syrup is often a better choice as a vehicle of cough syrup. Cherry syrup is manufactured by percolation of the bark of a tree that is a member of the plum family. Sucrose is added to the syrup as a sweetener. Glycerin is included to prevent precipitation of the tannins); 18. (i) - D; (ii) - B; (iii) - A; (iv) - E.

CHAPTER 22

Biphasic Liquid Dosage Forms

• Suspensions and Emulsions

SUSPENSION

A pharmaceutical suspension is a type of disperse system in which one (or more) substance (the dispersed phase) is distributed in particulate form throughout another (the continuous phase).

Formulation additives

The additives of a suspension formulation such as vehicles, thickeners, buffers, stabilizers, preservatives, colours and flavors are already discussed in Chapter 4.

In case of suspension formulation of hydrophobic drugs, it is very difficult to disperse the drug particle in aqueous media. The surface of such drug particles is better wetted by the incorporation of a suitable **wetting agent** having the HLB value 7 to 9. This wetting agent by reducing the "contact angle" between the spreading liquid and the solid surface of the drug particles help in wetting the particle with the vehicle. The contact angle between a liquid and a solid may be 0°, signifying complete wetting, or it may approach to 180°, at which wetting is insignificant.

Dispersing Agents

These agents help in causing the dispersion of the solid particles to be evenly distributed in the suspension. Especially in deflocculated suspensions, the individual particles should remain dispersed. In some materials where the quantum of surface charge is not sufficient, the particles tend to come together. To overcome this tendency some materials which carry good charge and can get easily adsorbed into the dispersed phase particle can be added. These are the dispersing agents, e.g., Darvans, Daxods, etc. They increase the *"Zeta* potential" considerably, thus, discouraging the particles in the suspension to come together.

The surface of the dispersed drug particles may be charged due to preferential adsorption of a particular ion (cation or anion) or due to ionization of a particular ionizable group attached to the solid surface of the drug particles. Naturally a potential known as *"Nernst* potential" or electrothermodynamic potential is developed at the surface of the solid, which will attract oppositely charged counterion or **gegenion** in the tightly bound solvent layer around the surface of the solid. Now depending upon the number of ions adsorbed at the surface of the solid and the counterion in the tightly bound solvent layer, the surface of the tightly bound layer may be charged. The *zeta* potential is defined as the difference in potential between the surface of the tightly bound layer and the electroneutral region of the solution. This may be positive, zero or negative. **Good dispersing agents increase the magnitude of zeta potential** and thereby help the individually dispersed solid particles to retain their individuality due to the repulsive force experienced between two approaching particles.

A good pharmaceutical suspension should possess the following characters :

(i) After shaking, the medicament stays in suspension long enough for a dose to be accurately measured.

(ii) It is easily pourable.

(iii) The sediment formed on standing is bulky, easily redispersed and do not form cake.

(iv) The particles in suspension are small and relatively uniform in size so that the product is free from a gritty texture.

Difference Between Flocculated and De-Flocculated Suspensions

Non/De-flocculated	Flocculated
a. Dispersed particles exist in suspension as separate entities.	a. Particles form loose aggregate.
b. Rate of sedimentation is slow, since each particle settles separately and particle size is minimal.	b. Rate of sedimentation is high, since particles settle as a floc which is a collection of particles.
c. Sediment is formed slowly.	c. Sediment is formed rapidly.
d. Repulsive forces between particles are overcome and a hard cake is formed which is difficult to redisperse.	d. Loosely packed sediment is easy to redisperse.
e. Suspension has a pleasing appearance since the suspended material remains suspended for a relatively long time. The supernatant also remains cloudy even when settling is apparent.	e. Rapid sedimentation and supernatant is relatively clear.

There are several methods of preparing flocculated suspensions. For instance, in the preparation of the oral suspension of a drug, clays such as diluted bentonite magma are commonly employed as the flocculating agent. Electrolytes can also act as flocculating agents, apparently by reducing the electrical barrier between the particles of the suspensoid and forming a bridge so as to link them together.

Levigation (wet grinding) process is followed in small scale manufacturing of suspension whereas in industry the mixture is passed through **colloid mill** to break the clumps and to produce a homogeneous suspension.

Suspensions Containing Diffusible Solids

Some insoluble powders are light and easily wettable; hence, they readily mix with water and, on shaking, diffuse evenly through the liquid for long enough to ensure even distribution in each dose. Such substances are known as diffusible or dispersable solids. e.g., Calcium carbonate, light kaolin, light magnesium carbonate, magnesium trisilicate, rhubarb powder etc.

Suspensions Containing Indiffusible Solids

Indiffusible solids will not remain evenly distributed in a vehicle long enough to ensure uniformity of dose. The simplest way of correcting the problem is to increase the viscosity of the vehicle by adding a thickening agent. Some examples of indiffusible solids are aspirin, chalk, phenobarbitone, succinyl sulphathiazole, sulphadimidine, calamine, hydrocortisone, sulphur, zinc oxide etc.

In case of suspensions containing poorly wettable solids such as sulphur, hydrocortisone etc., incorporation of a suitable wetting agent is a must in order to prepare an elegant suspension.

Suspensions of Precipitate-Forming Liquids

Some liquid preparations contain resinous matter that is precipitated on addition to water. The following are examples : Compound Benzoin Tincture, Benzoin Tincture, Lobelia Ethereal Tincture, Myrrh Tincture, Tolu Tincture, etc.

Suspensions Produced by Chemical Reaction

Very occasionally the insoluble active constituent of a lotion etc. is formed by a chemical reaction. A finer precipitate is obtained if dilute solutions of the reactants are mixed; hence, the reacting substances should be dissolved separately in approximately half volumes of the vehicle and the two parts mixed. Prepared in the manner the precipitate is diffusible and no suspending agent is necessary. An official example of this kind of preparation is Zinc Sulphide Lotion B.P.C. which is used to treat acne and scabies.

Formula :

Sulphurated potash

Zinc sulphate

Concentrated camphor water

Water q.s.

To produce diffusible precipitate of zinc sulphide, the solution of sulphurated potash is added to the zinc sulphate solution with stirring and not vice versa.

Physical Stability of Suspension

In most cases suspension formulations are not physically stable due to the sedimentation of the dispersed particles. Hydrocolloids used as suspending agents are very susceptable to microbial growth resulting in gas and odour formation, discoloration and loss of viscosity along with others. Therefore, suitable preservative(s) should be incorporated along with other necessary stabilizers.

The factors influencing the rate of sedimentation is expressed by Stoke's law as follows :

$$V = \frac{d^2(\rho_1 - \rho_2)g}{18\eta} = \frac{2r^2(\rho_1 - \rho_2)g}{9\eta}$$

where,

v = velocity of the settling particles

g = acceleration due to gravity

d = average diameter of the particle

r = average radius of the particle

ρ_1 = density of the particle

ρ_2 = density of the liquid/dispersed medium

η = the viscosity of the dispersion medium.

As 'ρ_1' and 'ρ_2' are the inherent properties of the material concerned and 'g' is also constant at a particular place, therefore, the rate of sedimentation may be minimized only by decreasing the particle size and increasing the viscosity of the media.

The special information mentioned in the label is 'SHAKE WELL BEFORE USE'

MODEL QUESTIONS

1. Suspensions and emulsions are coarse dispersions when particle size is usually
   A. 1-100 micron (μ)   B. 50-100 micron (μ)   C. 0.05-10 micron (μ)
   D. 100-500 micron (μ)
2. An ideal suspension should contain
   A. particles of identical size with no agglomeration
   B. a distribution of particles from fine to coarse
   C. particles with 10% fines
   D. particles with 30% fines.
3. Stoke's formula for sedimentation velocity 'v' is given by
   A. $\dfrac{d^2(\rho_1 - \rho_2)g}{18\eta}$ B. $\dfrac{d^2(\rho_1 + \rho_2)g}{18\eta}$ C. $\dfrac{d^2(\rho_1 - \rho_2)g}{9\eta}$
   D. $\dfrac{d^2(\rho_1 + \rho_2)g}{9\eta}$ E. $\dfrac{r^2(\rho_1 - \rho_2)g}{18\eta}$
4. The principal limiting factor in the rate of absorption from suspensions is
   A. dissolution rate   B. viscosity   C. the suspending agent
   D. chemical stability   E. physical stability.
5. In the suspensions, for stability considerations
   A. agglomeration are preferred   B. flocs are preferred
   C. particles that do not floc are preferred   D. none of the above.

6. Commonly used flocculating agent is
   A. soaps
   B. sodium benzoate
   C. tween 80
   D. bentonite magma.

7. The study of flow characteristics of fluids is termed
   A. surface science.
   B. oncology
   C. rheology
   D. micromeritics.

8. Packing and storage of suspensions preferred in containers with adequate airspace above.
   A. to keep sufficient nitrogen to enhance stability
   B. to facilitate shaking before use
   C. to allow for expansion due to heat
   D. to allow sufficient breathing space.

9. Caking at the bottom of suspension indicates
   A. suspension is good
   B. suspension has failed
   C. suspension shelf life is very good
   D. none of the above.

10. A suspension is not a suitable dosage for what type of injection?
    A. Intra-articular (within joint)
    B. Intramuscular
    C. Intravenous
    D. Subcutaneous
    E. Intradermal.

11. Which of the following properties is desirable in a pharmaceutical suspension?
    I. Caking; II. Pseudoplastic flow; III. Thixotropy
    A. I only
    B. III only
    C. I and II only
    D. II and III only
    E. I, II and III

12. Compound powder of tragacanth is used in
    A. simple mixture
    B. diffusible mixture
    C. indiffusible mixture
    D. none of the above
    E. all of the above.

13. Fill in the Blanks

    A suspension is said to be colloidal when its particles fall between ...... I ...... and about ...... II ...... millimicrons.

ANSWERS

1. A; 2. A; 3. A; 4. A; 5. B; 6. D; 7. C; 8. B; 9. B; 10. C (There is a chance of blockage of a blood vessel by suspended particles); 11. D [If the flow rate of any formulation increase due to agitation then this type of flow is known as pseudoplastic flow (the reverse is known as dilatant flow). Thixotropy is characterized by a gel that forms a flowable sol when shaken and upon undisturbed standing the reformation of the gel will slow sedimentation of the dispersed particles. Both these properties are desirable in pharmaceutical suspension. In case of caking, it is very difficult to break this cake by shaking and to reconstitute the original suspension]; 12.C (Acacia is also used to prepare mixture containing indiffusible solids); 13. I -1; II - 500

EMULSION

1. An emulsion is
   A. a thermodynamically unstable dispersed system
   B. consisting of at least two immiscible liquid phases
   C. stabilized by the presence of emulgent(s)
   D. all of the above
   E. none of the above.
2. Ordinary emulsions are white/off-white in colour. This is due to
   A. the particle diameter of the dispersed phase generally extends from about 0.1 to 10 μm
   B. the components used to make emulsion are white in colour
   C. the dispersed globule diameter is higher than the wave length of light
   D. all of the above
   E. A and C.
3. Among the following which is/are the example of an oil-in-water (o/w) type emulsion?
   A. Milk   B. Vanishing creams   C. Cold creams
   D. A and B   E. Butter.
4. Following is/are the example of water-in-oil (w/o) type emulsion.
   A. Butter   B. Cold creams   C. Salad creams
   D. All of the above   E. None of the above.
5. Multiple emulsions are
   A. three phase emulsions
   B. emulsions with in emulsion
   C. always microemulsion
   D. A and B
   E. A, B and C.
6. Multiple emulsions may be used
   A. for prolongation of drug action
   B. localization of drug in the body
   C. in the overdose treatment of certain drugs
   D. A, B and C
   E. A and B
   F. B and C.
7. The surfactant and co-surfactant content of microemulsions are
   A. much higher than that of macroemulsions
   B. equal with macroemulsions
   C. less than that of macroemulsions
   D. none of the above
   E. all of the above.
8. Which of the following is not a method of determining the type of an emulsion?
   A. Dye-solubility test
   B. Viscosity measurement test
   C. U.V. fluorescence test

  D. Dilution test

  E. Electrical conductivity test.

9. Total Parenteral Nutrition (TPN), a product recently available in the market to maintain debilitated patients belongs to the class of

   A. solution   B. suspension   C. emulsion

   D. none of the above.

10. Following are the example of finely divided solid particle used as emulgents, except

   A. bentonite   B. veegum   C. polysorbates

   D. graphite   E. magnesium hydroxide.

11. Which of the following is not a method of cracking or splitting or breaking of an emulsion?

   A. Centrifuging   B. Filtering   C. Addition of electrolytes

   D. Heat   E. Addition of a liquid in which both phases are soluble

   F. Addition of a chemical that is incompatible with the emulsifying agent like calcium and magnesium salts to emulsion stabilized with anionic surfactants

   G. Bacterial growth   H. Freezing

   I. Addition of higher percentage of alcohol to an emulsion stabilized with hydrocolloids.

12. Total Parenteral Nutrition (TPN) includes amino acids, carbohydrates, fats, electrolytes, minerals and

   A. animal protein   B. vitamins   C. dehydrocholic acid ·

   D. cholinesterase   E. none of the above.

   Phase inversion means changing the type of an emulsion from w/o to o/w and vice-versa. Any change (external or internal) which is responsible for changing the H.L.B value of the emulgent may be responsible for phase inversion if phase volume ratio permits e.g., (i) the addition of an electrolyte to anionic and cationic surfactants may suppress their ionization due to common ion effect and thus a w/o emulsion may result even though normally an o/w emulsion would be produced, (ii) an o/w emulsion having sodium stearate as the emulsifier can be inverted by the addition of calcium chloride, because the calcium stearate formed is a lipophilic emulsifier and favours the formation of a w/o product.

13. Which one is not related with the physical instability of an emulsion?

   A. Phase inversion

   B. Creaming or sedimentation

   C. Ostwald ripening

   D. Oxidation of the components

   E. Cracking of the emulsion.

   Emulsion preservation : A blend preservative [(e.g., mixture of methyl paraben (hydrophilic) and propyl paraben (lipophilic)] should be used to preserve the both oil and water phase of an emulsion system.

14. Emulsion can also be

   A. transparent   B. solid   C. gaseous   D. none of the above.

15. Surfactant type emulsifiers act by reducing

   A. globular size   B. surface tension   C. interfacial tension

   D. sedimentation.
16. Emulsions are always
    A. highly viscous preparation
    B. medium viscous preparation
    C. non-viscous preparation
    D. none of the above.
17. Emulsions may not be used as
    A. oral preparation
    B. parenteral preparation
    C. topical preparation
    D. none of the above.
18. Creaming may occur
    A: upward   B. downward   C. both ways   D. none of the above.
19. Emulsion made with tweens are usually
    A. unstable   B. w/o   C. o/w   D. clear   E. reversible.
20. According to Stoke's law, the creaming of emulsions is indirectly proportional to
    A. density of the dispersed phase
    B. gravity
    C. radius of dispersed phase
    D. viscosity of the medium
    E. none of the above.
21. Agglomeration of particles in emulsion is, often called
    A. grouping   B. coalescence   C. dimerization
    D. polymerization   E. dichromalism.
22. In Stoke's law
    A. rate of settling is directly proportional to particle diameter
    B. viscosity is directly proportional to particle diameter
    C. temperature is important
    D. concentration of suspended phase is unimportant
    E. none of the above.
23. Which one of the following ions will always present an incompatibility problem when added
    to TPN formulations?
    A. Bicarbonate   B. Calcium   C. Magnesium   D. Sulfate   E. Phosphate.
24. The maximum amount of dispersed liquid of uniform sized globules occupying a given space
    irrespective of the size of the globules is
    A. 55%   B. 66%   C. 74%   D. 82%   E. 90%
25. Addition of sodium chloride to sodium oleate emulsion will
    A. stabilize emulsion
    B. destabilize emulsion
    C. decrease the globule size of the emulsion
    D. none of the above.
26. Which one of the following is a synthetic emulsifying agent?

A. Gelatin   B. Bentonite   C. Cetrimide

D. Acacia   E. Methyl cellulose

27. Emulsion formulations are intended for
    A. oral administration
    B. parenteral administration
    C. topical administration
    D. administration into the mucous membrane
    E. all of the above.

28. Following is an example of inorganic emulsifying agent.

    A. Pectin   B. Gelatin   C. Bentonite   D. Acacia   E. CMC.

29. Given below (A to D) are the principle mechanism of action of the following categories of emulsifying agents. Match them correctly.

    (i)   Surface-active agents   A. Form a multimolecular, strong, rigid film around the dispersed droplets.

    (ii) Hydrophilic colloids   B. Adsorbed at oil/water interfaces to form monomolecular films and reduce interfacial tension.

    (iii) Finely divided solids   C. Adsorbed at the interphase and form film of particles around the dispersed globules.

                                     D. Increase mutual solubility of oil and water.

30. Given below (A to E) are the ratio of oil : water : gum for preparing primary emulsion of different oils (i-iv). Match them correctly.

    (i)   Fixed oil   A. 1 : 2 : 1
    (ii) Mineral oil   B. 2 : 2 : 1
    (iii) Volatile oil   C. 3 : 2 : 1
    (iv) Oleo-resin   D. 4 : 2 : 1
                           E. 2 : 1 : 2

31. Fill in the blanks :
    (i)   Chemically veegum is "..........".
    (ii) ".........." is an ideal example of naturally occouring emulsion.
    (iii) The full form of TPN is ....
    (iv) Creaming (upward movement) and sedimentation (downward movement) of droplet or particle is governed by "..........".

32. True or False?
    (i)   The bioavailability of an oily drug would be higher when administered as an oil-in-water emulsion than when administered as an oily solution.
    (ii) Microemulsions are either o/w type or w/o type
    (iii) The dispersed globule diameters in case of microemulsions, may range from 10 to 200 nm i.e., less than the wave length of light
    (iv) Micro-emulsions are transparent or translucent
    (v)   Some oil-soluble compounds such as some of the vitamins are absorbed more completely when emulsified than when administered orally as oily solution.

ANSWERS

1. D; 2. E; 3. D; 4. D; 5. D; 6. D; 7. A; 8. B; 9. C; 10. C; 11. B; 12. B; 13. D; 14. A; 15. C; 16. D; 17. D; 18. C; 19. C (Because of high HLB of tweens; tween 20-16.7, tween 80-15.0); 20. D; 21. B; 22. A; 23. A [The addition of alkaline sodium bicarbonate to TPN (having pH 5 to 6) will cause a loss of bicarbonate through the formation of carbon dioxide]; 24. C [An assembly of close-packed monodisperse (all particles have the same size) spherical droplets as the internal phase can occupy no more than approximately 74% of the total volume of an emulsion. It is evident, however, that the internal phase can exceed 74% if the spherical particles are not monodisperse]; 25. B; 26. C (Cetrimide i.e., cetyl trimethyl ammonium bromide is a cationic surfactant. Most of the surfactants are synthetic in nature. Methyl cellulose is a semisynthetic emulsifying agent and viscosity builder); 27. E; 28. C (Bentonite, veegum, magnesium hydroxide etc. are inorganic emulsifiers); 29. i - B, ii - A, iii - C; 30. i - D, ii - C, iii - B, iv - A. 31. (i) magnesium-aluminium silicate (ii) milk (iii) total parenteral nutrition. (iv) Stoke's law. 32 (i) - true, (ii) - true, (iii) - true, (iv) - true, (v) - true.

CHAPTER 23

Semi-Solid Dosage Forms

- Ointments
- Pastes
- Gels
- Poultice
- Suppositories and Pessaries.

OINTMENTS, PASTES and GELS are semi-solid preparations for application to the skin. Ointments are greasy preparations, the base is usually anhydrous and immiscible with skin secretions. Gels are transparent or translucent, non-greasy, aqueous preparation. Pastes contain a higher proportion of finely powdered medicament than ointments or gels but have similar bases.

Bases for Ointments and Ointment Type Pastes

These may be classified into four main groups as follows :

1. Hydrocarbon bases

These being immiscible with water, inhibit water loss from the skin by forming a waterproof film and by improving hydration, may encourage absorption of the medicaments through the skin.

The constituents of hydrocarbon bases include :

a. Soft paraffin [yellow and white (bleached)] also known as yellow/white petrolatum or petroleum jelly. There is no chemical difference between yellow and white variety. Yellow variety is bleached to form white variety, which may contain residual amount of bleaching agent.

b. Hard paraffin

c. Liquid paraffin

All paraffins are hydrocarbon having different melting point due to different molecular weights. Paraffin Ointment B.P. is an official hydrocarbon ointment base.

2. Absorption bases

a. Non-emulsified - These bases absorb water and aqueous solution to produce water-in-oil (w/o) emulsions.

The constituents include :

(i) Wool fat (anhydrous lanolin) : It is a semisolid, fat like substance obtained from the wool of sheep (*Ovis aries*). It can absorb about 50% of its weight of water and is used in ointments in which the proportion of aqueous fluid is too large for incorporation into a hydrocarbone base.

(ii) Wool alcohols.

(iii) Bees wax and cholesterol - Bees wax is obtained from the honey coomb of *Apis melifera*.

(iv) Lanolin (hydrous wool fat) - It is a water-in-oil emulsion that contains between 25 and 30% water.

Absorption bases are less occlusive than the hydrocarbon bases and are easier to spread. They are good emollients.

3. Water-miscible bases

Ointments made from these bases are easily removed after use. The three emusifying ointments from water-miscible bases, i.e.,

- Emulsifying Ointment B.P.(anionic),
- Cetrimide Emulsifying Ointment B.P. (cationic), and
- Cetomacrogol Emulsifying Ointment B.P. (non-ionic).

These contain paraffin and an o/w emulgent and have the general formula :

Anionic, cationic or non-ionic emulsifying wax	30%
White soft paraffin	50%
Liquid paraffin	20%

Other advantages of this type of base include miscibility with exudates, good contact with skin, high cosmetic acceptability and easy removal from the hair.

4. Water-soluble bases

Example, macrogols [polyethylene glycols (PEG)] - Products with ointment like consistency can be obtained by mixing low molecular weight liquid PEG with high molecular weight waxy solid PEG The water soluble bases have the advantages of being non-occlusive miscible with exudates, non-staining and easily removed by washing

Other Ingredients of Ointment Bases

(i) Vegetable oils - arachis, castor, coconut, olive oil, etc.

(ii) Synthetic esters of fatty acids - isopropyl myristate etc.

(iii) Higher fatty alcohols - cetyl, stearyl and cetostearyl alcohols etc.

(iv) Silicones

(v) Propylene glycols.

Other additives include Antioxidants and preservatives etc.

Ointments may be prepared by (i) trituration, (ii) fusion, (iii) chemical reaction and (iv) emul-sification.

After manufacturing, ointments at room temperature may contain some agglomeration. This may be due to earlier congealing of high melting fraction of the base. Therefore, prepared ointment before filling in container is passed through **tripple roller mill** for better homogenization.

The consistency of the prepared ointment should not change from batch to batch. The consistency i.e., the 'yield value' of the viscoelastic materials like ointments, pastes, gels, etc. is measured with the help of a **'penetrometer'**

Non-staining Iodine Ointment

Iodine is a good antiseptic, but free iodine is irritating to the skin, produces burning sensation and stains clothing. It is also degraded in presence of light and lost due to its volatility by way of sublimation. These problems are solved by making iodine 'non-staining'. Iodine is first solubilized in lowest possible volume of chloroform, which is then added to the required amount of arachis oil or other vegetable oils, which are chemically triglycerides i.e., ester of glycerol with fatty acids. These fatty acids contain double bonds i.e., point of unsaturation. On heating in a closed iodine bottle, iodine will enter into these unsaturated points by addition reaction and would be bounded. This iodinated oil is then mixed up with suitable base and sometimes with other components to give non-staining iodine ointment. As iodine is now in bound form the above mentioned problems are no longer there but on application to the skin by rubbing the iodine would be slowly liberated to exert antiseptic action.

Another non-staining iodine preparation is povidone iodine. Povidone [polyvinyl pyrrolidone, PVP)] having an average molecular weight of 40,000 is heated with elemental iodine in the presence of a lit'le water whereby a small amount of the iodine enters into loose organic union with the polymer to form a compound which contains approximately 10% of available iodine.

Bases of pastes, their preparation and preservation are similar to those of ointments.

MODEL QUESTIONS

1. Determination of iodine value depends upon
   A. substitution with iodine for the hydrogen in the fatty acids
   B. addition of iodine at the double bond of fatty acids
   C. oxidation of the fatty acids by iodine
   D. analysis of the iodine content of a fatty acid
   E. none of the above.
2. Which form of sulfur should a pharmacist use when extemporaneously preparing an ointment?

   A. Cake of sulfur   B. Flowers of sulfur   C. Precipitated sulfur
   D. Sublimed sulfur   E. Washed sulfur.
3. The most hygroscopic of the following liquids is
   A. acetone   B. alcohol   C. glycerin   D. PGE 400   E. mineral oil.

4. Plastibase is a common ointment vehicle. It is a/an
   A. oil in water emulsion base
   B. polyethylene glycol type base
   C. polyethylene gelled mineral oil
   D. mixture of mineral oil and hydrocarbon waxes
   E. undisclosed patented formula.

5. Which one of the following procedures would not improve the absorption of a drug into the skin?
   A. Application of the ointment and covering the area with an occlusive bandage or saran wrap.
   B. Incorporating an oil-soluble drug in polyethylene glycol ointment rather than white ointment.
   C. Applying the medicated ointment on the back of the hand rather than on the palms.
   D. Increasing the concentration of the active drug in the ointment base.
   E. Using an ointment base in which the active drug has excellent solubility.

6. All of the following substances have been shown to increase the permeability of the skin EXCEPT
   A. sodium lauryl sulfate   B. propylene glycol   C. benzene
   D. dimethyl sulfoxide   E. chloroform.

7. Aqueous solutions may be incorporated into all of the following ointment bases except
   A. lanolin   B. aquaphor   C. unibase
   D. polysorb   E. white ointment.

8. Silicones are useful in ointment formulas since they are good
   A. surfactants   B. non-polar solvents   C. humectants
   D. preservatives   E. water repellents.

9. Lassar's paste is
   A. zinc oxide ointment
   B. zinc oxide paste
   C. zinc oxide paste with salicylic acid
   D. benzoic acid and salicylic acid ointment
   E. none of these.

10. Hydrophilic petrolatum contains what as an emulsifier?
   A. Span 80   B. Tween 80   C. Glyceryl monostearate, self emulsifying
   D. Cholesterol   E. Sodium lauryl sulfate.

11. A synonym for cold cream USP is
   A. Galen's cerate
   B. rose water ointment
   C. petrolatum rose water ointment
   D. vanishing cream
   E. wool fat emulsion.

12. A physician requests a 0.1% strength of a steroidal cream that is commercially available as

a 0.25% strength in a "vanishing cream" base. Which one of the following ointment bases is the best choice as a diluent for this order?

A. Lanolin   B. PEG ointment   C. Vaseline
D. Hydrophilic ointment   E. Cold cream.

13. Iodine value may be defined as
   A. the weight of iodine absorbed by 100 parts by weight of the sample of fat or oil
   B. the number of milligrams of KOH required to neutralize the fatty acids resulting from complete hydrolysis of 1 g of the sample of fat or oil
   C. the number of milligrams of KOH required to neutralise the acetic acid capable of combining by acetylation with 1 g of the sample of fat or oil
   D. the number of milligrams of KOH required to neutralise the free acids present in 1 g of the sample of fat or oil
   E. the number of milligrams of KOH required to combine with fatty acids which are present in glyceride form in 1 g sample of oil or fat.

14. Given below are the types of ointment bases. Match them with the correct ointments in A to E

   (i)   Absorption base   A. Emulsifying ointment
   (ii) Oleogenous base   B. Hydrophilic ointment
   (iii) Emulsion base   C. Oily cream
   (iv) Water soluble base   D. Kaolin poultice
                                E. Simple ointment

ANSWERS

1. B (Iodine value is the number of grams of iodine required to saturate 100 grams of fat or oil. Iodine is absorbed in direct proportion to the degree of unsaturation); 2. C; 3. C [Because of very high hygroscopicity (ability of a substance to attract and retain moisture) glycerin is used as a humectant to keep creams or other semi-solid formulations from drying out. A humectant is an ingredient that will either absorb water from the air or retain water in a formula]; 4. D (This jelly like base maintains a good consistency over a wide temperature range. It appears to be compatible with many active ingredients); 5. E [Drugs that are very soluble in a vehicle (i.e., partition coefficient in favour of vehicle is high) will tend to remain in the vehicle and will show slower rates of penetration than less soluble drugs. Covering the area is responsible for sweat accumulation at the skin-vehicle interface induces hydration of the skin, a condition which facilitates penetration of drug. Poorer solubility of the drug in PEG ointment than in white ointment may lead to faster diffusion. The thicker epidermis of the palms will result in slower drug penetration than that which will occur on the back of the hands. Higher drug concentrations will increase the rate of diffusion and penetration]; 6. B [This is used as solvent and/or a humectant. Many non-polar solvents such as benzene and chloroform increase the skin permeability by removal of lipids from the stratum corneum (i.e., the outer most layer of the skin). Dimethyl sulfoxide (DMSO) has been used as a penetration enhancer. It may solvate the stratum corneum and also causes swelling of the cells, thereby opening channels for drug penetration. Certain surfactants such as sodium lauryl sulfate,

appear to cause a reversible denaturation of skin protein, thereby interrupting the barrier nature of the stratum corneum]; 7. E [White ointment (composed of white wax and white petrolatum) being hydrocarbon in nature is hydrophobic and having very low "water number" (i.e., the largest amount of water that 100 g of ointment base will hold at 20°C)]; 8. E (They will form a thin occlusive film on the skin, producing an emollient effect because water loss by evaporation from the skin surface is reduced. The film also can protect the skin from irritants); 9. C (It is used as astringent and protective); 10. D (It is a steroidal alcohol which is available from several sources, including wool fat. Usually w/o emulsions are formed when cholesterol is the emulsifier); 11. C; 12. D (Both vanishing cream and hydrophilic ointment are o/w type emulsion); 13. A ['B', 'C', 'D' and 'E' are respectively known as saponification value, hydroxyl value, acid value and ester value]; 14. i) - A; ii) - E; iii) - C; iv) - B (Emulsion base usually consider as superior base).

GELS

Gels may be defined as semisolids, being either suspensions of small inorganic particles or large organic molecules interpenetrated with liquid.

Uses of Gels in Pharmaceutical and Cosmetic Fields

(i) As gels proper, or as capsule shells made from gelatin.
(ii) As topical preparation intended to be applied to the skin, mucous membranes, or eye.
(iii) As long-acting forms of drugs injected intramuscularly.
(iv) As binders in tablet granulations, protective colloids in suspensions, thickeners in oral liquids, and as suppository bases.
(v) Cosmetically, in shampoos, fragrance products, dentifrices, and skin-and-hair care preparations.

Classification

(i) On the basis of the nature of the colloidal phase :
  a. Inorganic gels, e.g., bentonite magma.
  b. Organic gels like natural gums (acacia, carrageenan, xanthan gum, anionic polysaccharides etc.), polyethylenes and metallic stearates, polypeptides (gelatin) and synthetic block copolymers (poloxamers).
(ii) On the basis of nature of solvents :
  a. Hydrogel (i.e., water bases) e.g., bentonite magma and gelatin.
  b. Organogels (with nonaqueous solvent) e.g., low molecular weight polyethylene dissolved in mineral oil and shock cooled metallic stearates in oils.

Solid gels with very low solvent concentration are known as **xerogel**, e.g., dry gelatin, tragacanth ribbons and acacia tears etc.

Characteristics of gels

The inclusion of gelling agent in a formulation should provide a reasonable solid like nature during storage that can be broken easily when subjected to shear forces generate in shaking a bottle, squeezing a tube, or during topical application.

(i) Swelling : Gels can swell, absorbing liquid with an increase in volume. Swelling can be looked on as the initial phase of dissolution. Solvent penetrates the gel matrix, gel-gel interactions are replaced by gel-solvent interactions.

(ii) Syneresis : Many gel systems undergo a contraction upon standing. The interstitial liquid is expressed, collecting at the surface of the gel. This phenomenon is referred to as "syneresis". The mechanism of contraction has been related to the relaxation of elastic stresses developed during the setting of the gel. As these stresses are relieved, the interstitial space available for solvent is reduced, forcing the expression of fluid.

(iii) Structure : Inorganic particles are capable of gelling a vehicle due to the formation of a **"house of cards"** structure. Clays such as bentonite or kaolin possess a lamellar structure that can be extensively hydrated. The flat surfaces of bentonite particles are negatively charged, while the edges are positively charged. The attraction of face to edge of these colloidal lamellae creates a three-dimensional network of particles throughout the liquid, immobilizing the solvent. The interactions between the particles are fairly weak, being broken by stirring or shaking, i.e., the gel structure would converted to sol structure which again during undisturbed storage converted to gel structure due to above mechanism. The phenomenon is also known as **Thixotropy**.

Salts may attract part of the water of hydration of the polymer, allowing the formation of more intermolecular secondary bonds, leading to gelation and precipitation. This is known as "salting out". Multivalent cations have a strong effect on the solutions of anionic polymers. Bridging of the polymers by di- or trivalent cations, as in the addition of copper to solutions of sodium carboxymethyl cellulose or calcium to sodium alginate, leads to gel formation.

Alcohols have a similar effect. In addition, alcohols alter the solvent's characteristics, changing the solubility parameter. The addition of alcohol often brings about coacervation rather than gelation. **Coacervation** is the production of a viscous, solvated, polymer-rich phase leaving behind a phase that is mostly solvent and therefore, polymer poor.

Molecular weight is an important consideration in gel formation. Very long polymers can entangle to a greater extent, leading to higher viscosity at a given concentration. Thus, lower concentration of a high molecular weight polymer may be required to gel the solvent.

(iv) Rheology : Solutions of gelling agents and dispersions of flocculated solids are, typically, pseudoplastic, exhibiting a non-Newtonian flow behavior characterized by a decreasing viscosity with increasing shear rate.

(v) Stability testing : The stability of visco elastic material can be measured by measuring the yield value with the help of a **penetrometer**. The depth of penetration resulting from the contact of the cone of penetrometer with the product under conditions of known force is measured.

POULTICES (CATAPLASMS)

Poultices are pastes like preparations used externally to reduce pain and inflammation because they retain heat well. After heating, the preparations is spread thickly on a dressing and applied as hot as the patient can bear, to the affected area. Poultices represent one of the most ancient classes of pharmaceutical preparations:

SUPPOSITORIES AND PESSARIES

"Suppositories" are solid medicated preparations designed for insertion into the rectum where they melt, dissolve or disperse and exert a local or systemic effect.

"Pessaries" are similar solid medicated preparation designed for insertion into the vagina, usually to exert a local effect.

"**Bougies**" are urethral suppositories.

Suppository bases : There are two main classes of suppository base

I. Fatty bases designed to melt at body temperature. These include, Theobroma oil (cocoa butter), synthetic hard fat etc.

II. Water-soluble or water-miscible bases designed to dissolve or disperse within the body. These include, Glycero-gelatin, Macrogols [Polyethylene glycols (PEG)] like Macrogol 400, 1000, 1540, 4000, 6000.

An ideal suppository base should melt at body temperature or dissolves in body fluids, non-toxic, non-irritant, compatible with medicament, releases any medicament rapidly, easily moulded and removed from the mould, stable to heating above the m.p. resistant to handling and stable on storage.

Other additives : Antioxidants, preservatives, emulsifiers, hardening agents, viscosity modifiers etc.

Displacement Values

The volume of suppositories from a particular mould will be constant but the weight will vary because the densities of the medicaments usually differ from the density of the base with which the mould calibrated.

The density of the medicament affects the amount of base required for each suppository. One part by weight of a medicament with density equal to the base will 'displace' an equal volume of the base. A medicament with twice the density of the base will 'displace' half the volume, while medicament with five times the density of the base will 'displace' only one-fifth of the volume of base. It is necessary therefore to make an allowance for each medicament in terms of the particular base, this allowance is the "displacement value".

The displacement value may be defined as "the number of parts by weight of medicaments that displaces one part by weight of the base."

Stages Involved in the Preparation of Suppositories

(i) Calculate the quantities required.

(ii) Prepare the mould.

(iii) Prepare the base.

(iv) Prepare the medicament.

(v) Melt the base and heat treatment of the base, if required.

(vi) Incorporate the medicament.

(vii) Fill the mould.

(viii) Remove the excess.

(ix) Open the mould.

Medicaments are prescribed in the form of suppositories mainly for three reasons :

(i) To exert a local effect on the rectal mucosa.

(ii) To promote evacuation of the bowel.

(iii) To provide a systemic effect.

Medicaments like anti-infectives, anti-inflammations, anti- prurities, hormones and spermicides are prescribed in the form of pessaries.

Special information in the labels

(i) Store in a cool place

(ii) For rectal use only or for vaginal use only.

Disadvantages of Glycerogelatin Base

(i) A physiological effect - Glycerol suppositories have laxative action.

(ii) Unpredictable solution time.

(iii) Hygroscopic.

(iv) Microbial contamination likely.

(v) Long preparation time.

Advantages of Macrogol Bases

(i) No laxative effect.

(ii) Microbial contamination less likely.

(iii) Preparation is convenient.

(iv) Melting point generally above the body temperature.

(v) Produce high-viscosity solutions.

(vi) Good solvent properties.

(vii) Give products with clean smooth appearance.

Disadvantages of Macrogol Bases

(i) Hygroscopic.

(ii) Poor bioavailability of medicaments.

(iii) Incompatibilities with some medicaments.

(iv) Brittleness.

(v) Crystal growth of certain medicaments in the base.

MODEL QUESTIONS

1. Glycerin suppositories contain 92% glycerin and are solidified by the use of

   A. white wax   B. stearic acid   C. sodium stearate

   D. PEG 4000   E. glyceryl triacetate.

2. A group of substances used as suppository bases that dissolve rather than melt are

   A. esters   B. saturated acids   C. carbowaxes

   D. unsaturated fatty acids   E. none of the above.

3. Rectal suppsitories are suitable for the treatment of many diseases or symptoms. For which one of the following is a commercial suppository dosage form not available?

   A. Epilepsy   B. Fever   C. Asthma   D. Migraine   E. Insomnia.

4. Characteristics of rectal drug administration include all of the following EXCEPT

   A. drugs may avoid first-pass hepatic inactivation

   B. neutral pH of colon fluids lessens possible drug inactivation by stomach acidity

   C. irritating drugs have less effect on the rectum than on the stomach

   D. the release and absorption of drug is predictable

   E. drugs intended for systemic activity can be administered.

5. Most commercial vaginal suppositories use a base of

   A. bees wax   B. glycerin   C. cocoa butter

   D. glycerinated gelatin   E. polyethylene glycols.

6. Norforms suppositories may be used as a/an

   A. antitrichomonal agent   B. tampon   C. mild laxative

   D. deodorant   E. contraceptive.

7. The rectal route of administration may be preferred over the oral route of some drugs because

   A. the dissolution process is avoided

   B. inert binders, diluents and excipients can not interfere with absorption

   C. the drug does not have to be absorbed

   D. a portion of the absorbed drug does not pass through the liver before entering the systemic circulation

   E. absoption is predictable and complete.

8. A pharmacist should suggest to the patient that suppositories made with what substance as the base, be moistened with water before insertion?

   A. Hydrogenated vegetable oils

   B. Theobroma oil

   C. Carbowax

   D. Glycerinated gelation

   E. Both C and D.

9. Which of the following suppository bases melt rather than dissolve when inserted into the rectum?

   I. Cocoa butter; II. Witepsols; III. PEGs

   A. I only   B. III only   C. I and II only

   D. II and III only   E. I, II and III only.

10. The term "displacement value" is related with the preparation of

   A. tablet   B. capsule   C. ointment   D. suppository   E. injectable.

11. Shrinkage of gels by extrusion of liquid is called

   A. syneresis   B. coacervation   C. ebullition   D. dilatancy   E. plasticity.

ANSWERS

1. C; 2. C (Others melt at body temperature); 3. A (Asthma may be treated with aminophylline suppositories. For fever, migraine and insomnia suppositories of aspirin, ergotamine tartrate and chloral hydrate are available respectively); 4. D [The extent of drug release and absorption will vary depending upon the properties of the drug, the suppository base, and the condition of the colon. Drugs absorbed from the buccal cavity and lower part of the rectum directly enter into the general circulation by 'by-passing' the liver. Whereas, the drugs absorbed from the region starting from the oesophagus to the upper part of the rectum pass directly through the portal vein into the liver first (where metabolism to inactive products can occur) and then to the general circulation]; 5. E (This permits easy insertion without prior refrigeration); 6. D (This vaginal suppositories contain quaternary ammonium germicide, methyl benzethonium chloride, which will have the tendency to decrease odor-producing microbes); 7. D; 8. E (Because of their hygroscopic nature, these may cause a stinging sensation when first inserted. This can be avoided by dipping the suppository into water just prior to insertion); 9. C [Different molecular weight polyethylene glycols (PEGs) can be blended and formed into suppositories by fusion using molds which do not melt in the body; instead, they slowly dissolve in the limited amount of water in the colon]; 10.D; 11. A.

CHAPTER 24

Dental and Cosmetic Preparations

• Dentifrices	• Antiperspirants and Deodorants
• Fluoride and Dental Health	• Hair Care Preparations.
• Facial Cosmetics	

Dentifrices are agents used for cleansing the teeth. Although they exert effect only for a short period, their use is nevertheless helpful in keeping the teeth clean, if used after every meal. However, they should be used in the morning and evening and also after each principal meal. Dentifrice may be in the form of powder or paste and applied preferably by means of a suitable brush.

An ideal dentifrice should have the following properties :

(i) It should not contain substances harmful to the teeth, mucous membrane of the mouth or if swallowed, to the stomach, e.g., gritty substances, caustic substances, strong antiseptics, fermentable substances, strong acids or alkali etc.

(ii) It should not inactivate the enzymes of the saliva or gastric juice, or inhibit their secretion.

(iii) It should not stain the teeth, rather should make them sparkling white.

(iv) It should have pleasant odour and taste.

(v) It should not be too acidic or too alkaline.

Usually dentifrices contain the following ingredients :

(i) Detergents e.g., hard-soap, synthetic detergents.

(ii) An antiseptic, e.g., phenol, menthol, thymol, benzoic acid, boric acid, etc.

(iii) An abrasive agent which cleans the teeth mechanically, e.g., calcium carbonate, calcium phosphate, magnesium oxide, chalk, kaolin, calcium sulfate, sodium metaphosphate, hydrated aluminium oxide, magnesium carbonate and phosphate etc.

(iv) A sweetening (usually noncarbohydrate) agent like saccharin sodium and a flavouring agent with or without any colouring matter.

(v) Preservatives.

(vi) Occasionally therapeutic agents.

Fluorides and dental health

Fluorides are protoplasmic poisons and tissues are destroyed by it. But for our dental health it is required. Fluoride ion enters the surface layers of the enamel and becomes parts of the enamel structure. Excess fluoride can reduce serum calcium ion levels due to formation of calcium fluoride and finally the bone becomes brittle.

The average value of optimum level of fluoride in drinking water is 1.0 ppm. If this value exceeds 1.5 ppm then it causes fluorosis. It is of two types : (i) Skeletal fluorosis, and (ii) Dental fluorosis. In case of skeletal fluorosis the excess fluride replace phosphate ion form the ca-combination of the bones and the bones become brittle and dental caries occur.

In fluoride deficiency, sodium fluoride tablet is available. One such tablet in 1 litre water gives 1 ppm. Tin fluoride treatment is more effective than sodium fluoride treatment. By this technique, the cleaned dry teeth are kept moist for four minutes with freshly prepared 8% solution of tin (II) fluoride. The mouth must not be rinsed and no food or drink taken for 30 minutes after this application. A single application is required every 6 to 12 months. Tin (II) fluoride in a stabilized form is available in fluoridated toothpastes also.

Facial Cosmetics

(i) **Face powder :** A face powder is a cosmetic preparation, which is applied to the face by means of a powder puff. It is generally applied at the end of the make up process, as a finishing touch.

(ii) **Compact powder :** A compact powder is simply a face powder, which is pressed in the form of a cake and is applied on the face with powder puff.

(iii) **Rouges :** A rouge is a preparation which is applied to the cheeks for enhancing the face beauty and to impart and stimulate the rosy freshness of the young and healthy skin. Various types of rouges such as liquid, cream and solid rouges are available in numerous shades. Solid rouges are stable and easy to apply. Dry compact rough is applied by means of a puff.

(iv) **Cold creams :** Cold creams are the cosmetic preparations, which are applied on the face. The name cold cream is given because of cooling effect of such products on the skin. It is a w/o type emulsion.

(v) **Vanishing creams :** Vanishing creams are oil-in-water (o/w) type emulsions which are prepared by emulsification of stearic acid and water by means of alkalies such as sodium hydroxide, potassium hydroxide, triethanolamine, etc. Glycerin is also added

(vi) **Preparations for eye make-up :**
a. *Eye shadow :* Eye shadow is used to give a background of colour to the eyes and is applied to the eyelids.
b. *Eyebrow pencils*
c. *Mascara :* Mascara is a pigmented preparation used on the eyelashes and eyebrows to darken and thicken their appearance. It is applied with a brush.

(vii) **Lipsticks :** Lipstick is the most widely used item of cosmetics by the women to brighten the colour of the lips.

(viii) **Shaving media** including brushless shaving creams, lather shaving creams and shaving soaps. After-shave products include lotions and gels used to refresh the skin after shave.

Antiperspirants and Deodorants are cosmetic products which are used to reduce underarm and body odour. Antiperspirants inhibit the flow of perspiration and deodorants inhibit the formation of mal odour in perspiration by suppressing bacterial growth or cover the mal odour with a more pleasing one (masking effect). Many products have both antiperspirant and deodorant action.

The astringent action is accompanied by contraction and wrinkling of the tissue and by blanching. The cement substances of the capillary endothelium is hardened, so that pathological transcapillary movement of plasma protein is inhibited and local edema, inflammation and exudation are hereby reduced. Mucus or other secretions may also be reduced, so that the affected area becomes drier.

Astringents are used therapeutically to arrest hemorrhage by coagulating the blood and to check diarrhoea, reduce inflammation of mucous membranes, promote healing, toughen the skin, or decrease sweating. The antiperspirant effect is the result both of the closure of the sweat ducts by protein precipitation to form a plug and peritubular irritation that promotes an increase in inward pressure on the tubule. Astringents also possess some deodorant properties by virtue of interaction with odorous fatty acids liberated or produced by action of bacteria on lipids in sweat, and by an action suppressing bacterial growth, partly because of a decrease in pH.

The principal astringents are (1) the salts of aluminium, zinc, manganese, iron, and bismuth, (2) certain other salts that contain these metals (such as permanganates) and, (3) tannins or related polyphenolic compounds. Acids, alcohol, phenols and other substances that precipitate proteins may be astringent in the appropriate amount or concentration; however, such substances generally are not employed for their astringent effects, because they readily penetrate cells and promote tissue damage. Strongly hypertonic solutions dry the affected tissues and are thus often but wrongly called astringents, unless protein precipitation also occurs.

Examples : Alum - Ammonium Alum [$AlNH_4(SO_4)_2 . 12H_2O$] or Potassium Alum [$AlK(SO_4)_2 . 12H_2O$], Aluminium Acetate Topical Solution, Aluminium chloride, Aluminium chlorohydrates, Aluminium subacetate Topical Solution, Aluminium sulphate, Calamine, Zinc chloride, Zinc oxide etc.

The liquid antiperspirants consist of an aqueous or hydroalcoholic solution of an astringent salt to which a small amount of humectant, a perfume, a dispersing agent for the perfume and a deodorant is added.

Shampoos

Shampoo may be defined as preparation containing surface active agents which when used will remove grease, dirt and debris from the hair and scalp without seriously affecting the hair, scalp and other parts of the body. Apart from cleansing action it must leave the hair fragrant, lustrous, soft and manageable. Though the shampoos act as detergents like that of detergent cakes but along with these properties they behave as cosmetics. Among the formulation ingredients there are opacifier, solubilizing agent, thickening agent, conditioning agent, preservatives, flavouring and colouring agents etc.

Hair Dressing

Healthy hair not only acts as a protective covering for the head but is also an attractive feature of men and women. Hair dressing was used by men and women to impart good appearance to the hair. The preparation used for the hair include :

(i) Brilliantines : Used to impart lustre to the hair and also for keeping the hair in place.

(ii) Hair conditioners : Used to make the hair manageable glossy and of soft texture.

(iii) Hair tonics : Used for curing baldness, relieving oily or dry skin and to prevent or cure dandruff.

(iv) Hair waving and hair-straightening preparations

(v) Hair dyes

(vi) Depilatories (Hair removers) : Depilatory products are used to soften unsightly human hair so that it can be easily removed by wiping or rinsing a short time after application. When the hair are removed by chemical methods it is known as **depilation** and when the relatively intact unwanted hair are removed by plucking, electrolysis and x-ray etc. it is known as **epilation**. The chemicals most commonly used for preparation of depilatories include metallic sulphides or barium, calcium and strontium. Other chemicals like tin salts, calcium thioglycerol and calcium thioglycollate are also used. Out of all these chemicals barium sulphide is the most popular depilating agent because it has excellent depilating properties without serious effects.

(vii) Antidandruff preparations : They contain selenium disulphide, Betanaphthol etc.

MODEL QUESTIONS

1. Disclosing solutions are used to
   A. stain plaque   B. act as abrasives
   C. dissolve food particles   D. wash away food dabris
   E. sterilize the oral cavity.

2. Selsun blue is used mainly as a/an
   A. ointment   B. aerosol   C. skin lotion
   D. shampoo   E. bath additive.

ANSWERS

1. A (This makes plaque on teeth more visible); 2. D (It is selenium sulfide).

CHAPTER 25

Sterile Dosage Forms

- Parenteral Dosage Forms, Their Standards
- Sterility Testing
- Pyrogen Testing
- Faulty Seal Packaging
- Routes of Administration of Parenteral Products
- Irrigation and Dialysis Solutions
- Ophthalmic Products.

Note : The following discussion do not necessarily apply to Blood Products or Immunological Products because of their special nature and licensing requirements.

Injectable Preparations are sterile products intended for administration by injection, infusion or implantation into the body. There are five main types of Injectable Preparations namely Injections, Powders for Injection, Intravenous Infusion, Concentrated Solutions for Injection and Implants.

Injectable Preparations should be prepared by methods designed to ensure their sterility and to avoid the introduction of foreign contaminants, the presence of pyrogens or of bacterial endotoxins and the growth of microorganisms.

Injectable Preparations, which are solutions or suspensions, require vehicles in which the medicaments are incorporated. The most commonly used vehicle is Water for Injection. Any other suitable vehicles may be used provided they are safe in the volume of injections administered and also do not interfere with the therapeutic efficacy of the preparation or with its response to the prescribed tests and assays of the pharmacopoeia. It may be necessary to include auxiliary substances to increase the stability or usefulness of the preparation, unless otherwise specified in the individual monograph. No coloring agent may be added solely for the purpose of coloring the finished preparation.

Aqueous Injectable Preparations for administration by the subcutaneous, intradermal, intramusculer, or in the case of large volumes intravenous route, should if possible be made isotonic with blood by the addition of sodium chloride or other suitable substances. Buffering agents should not be used in preparations intended for intraocular or intracardiac injection, or in products that may gain access to the cerebrospinal fluid.

Injectable Preparations that are packaged in **multiple dose** containers, regardless of the method of sterilization employed may contain suitable antimicrobial preservatives in appropriate concentration, unless otherwise directed in the individual monograph, or unless the active ingredients themselves are bacteriostatic. Preservatives **should not be added** when the volume to be injected as a single dose exceeds 15 ml, unless otherwise justified, or when the preparation is intended for administration by the intraocular, intracardiac or intracisternal routes (or other routes giving access to the cerebrospinal fluid).

Where the active ingredients are susceptible to oxidative degradation a suitable antioxidant may be added and/or the air in the container may be evacuated or displaced by oxygen-free nitrogen or other suitable inert gas.

Injectable Preparations must be sterile and the methods of sterilization are already discussed under Pharmaceutics I.

Containers

Containers for injectable preparations are made as far as possible from materials that (1) are sufficiently transparent to permit visual inspection of the contents, except for implants; (2) do not adversely affect the quality of the preparation under the ordinary conditions of handling, shipment, storage, sale and use; (3) do not permit diffusion into or across the walls of the container or yield foreign substances into the preparations. Injectable Preparations may be supplied in glass ampoules, vials or bottles or in other containers such as plastic bottles or bags etc.

The multiple dose containers may be used for intramascular, subcutaneous or intracutaneous administration, but no multiple dose container may contain a total volume of injection sufficient to permit the withdrawal of more than **ten doses**, unless otherwise stated in the individual monograph. The period of time between the withdrawal of the first and final dose should not be unduly prolonged.

Closures

Vials or bottles are fitted with suitable closures which ensure a good seal, prevent the access of microorganisms and other contaminants and usually permit the withdrawal of a part of the whole of the contents of the container without removal of the closure. The plastic or rubber materials of which the closure is composed must be compatible with the preparation and be sufficiently firm and elastic to allow the passage of a needle with minimal shedding of particles and to ensure that the puncture is resealed when the needle is withdrawn.

Before use, closures should be washed with a suitable detergent and rinsed with and boiled in several changes of Purified Water. Closures made from rubber and synthetic materials are liable to absorb the ingredients of the injectable preparation with which they are used, e.g., the preservative or any other added substances. When an antimicrobial preservative is used, the closure, when necessary, should be placed in a solution of that preservative in Purified Water containing **at least twice the concentration** to be used in the preparation; the quantity of solution used should be sufficient to cover the closure and should be at least 2 ml for each 8 of the material. The vessel should then be closed and heated at an appropriate combination of time and temperature. After heating, the closures should be kept in the sealed container until required for use. Closures intended for containers of oily preparations should be made of oil resistant materials.

Inspection : All injectable preparations should be physically inspect and that every container the contents of which show evidence of contamination with visible foreign material be rejected. The unlabelled containers are held by the neck against strongly illuminated screen of which **white surface is used for dark colour particles and black surface for the detection of light coloured particles.**

Injections

Injections are sterile solutions, emulsions or suspension should comply with the following prescribed standards :

I. Particulate Matter

Injections that are solutions, when examined under suitable conditions of visibility, are clear and practically free from particles that can be observed on visual inspection by the unaided eye. **Injections that are supplied in containers with a nominal content of 100 ml or more comply with the limit test for particulate matter.** The limits **do not apply** to multiple dose injections, to single dose small volume parenterals and to injectable solutions constituted from sterile solids. All the manipulative procedures should be carried out in a laminar air- flow cabinet or hood (of the horizontal type), equipped with HEPA (high efficiency particulate air) filters and preferably located in a separate room which is supplied with filtered, air-conditioned air and maintained under positive pressure with respect to the surrounding area.

The preparation meets the requirements of the test if it contains particles within the maximum limits shown below.

Particle size in μm (equal to or larger than)	Maximum number of particles per ml
10	50
25	5
50	Nil

II. Uniformity of Content

Unless otherwise stated in the individual monograph, suspensions for injection that are presented in single dose containers and that contain less than 10 mg or less than 10% of active ingredient comply with the following test. For suspensions for injection containing more than one active ingredient carry out the test for each active ingredient that corresponds to the above conditions. The content of the active ingredients should be within prescribed limits. The test for uniformity of content is not applicable to suspensions for injection containing multivitamins and trace elements.

III. Extractable Volume

The average content of 5 containers is not less than the nominal volume and not more than 115% of the nominal volume, where the nominal volume does not exceed 5 ml and the average content of 3 containers is not less than the nominal volume and not more than 110% of the nominal volume where the nominal volume is greater than 5 ml.

IV. Tests for Sterility

The tests for sterility are intended for detecting the presence of viable forms of bacteria, fungi and yeasts in or on pharmacopoeial preparations. The tests are based upon the principle that if bacteria or fungi are placed in a medium which provides nutritive material and water, and kept at favourable temperature, the organisms will grow and their presence can be indicated by a turbidity in the originally clear medium.

The sample under test is collected randomized. Moreover, if contamination is not uniform throughout the batch, random sampling cannot detect contamination with certainty. Compliance with the tests for sterility alone cannot therefore constitute absolute assurance of freedom from microbial contamination. Greater assurance of sterility must come from reliable manufacturing procedure and here is the importance of following good manufacturing practices (G.M.P.). It is only by following these practices a manufacturer would be able to build up the quality of a product during its manufacture.

Culture Media :

a. For aerobic and anaerobic bacteria
  (i) Fluid thioglycollate medium - For use in testing of clear fluid products.
  (ii) Alternative thioglycollate medium - For use with turbid and viscid products and for devices having tubes with small lumina.
b. For fungi and aerobic bacteria
  (i) Soyabean-casein digest medium.
      The media used should comply with the following tests carried out before or in parallel with the test on the preparation being examined.
      (i) Sterility
      (ii) Growth - promotion test
      (iii) Tests for bacteriostasis and fungistasis.

Test Procedure : The tests can be carried out using method A, Membrane Filtration or Method B, Direct Inoculation, Method A is to be prefered where the substance being examined is (a) an oil, (b) an ointment that can be put into solution, (c) a non- bacteriostatic solid not readily soluble in the culture medium and (d) a soluble powder or a liquid that possesses inherent bacteriostatic and fungistatic properties. For liquid products where the volume in a container is 100 ml or more; Only method A should be employed.

Precautions During the Tests : The tests for sterility should be carried out under conditions designed to avoid accidental contamination of the product during the test using, for example, a laminar sterile air flow cabinet. The precautions taken to avoid contamination must be such that they do not affect any microorganisms that should be revealed in the test. Laminar sterile airflow cabinet is fitted with High Efficiency Particulate Air (HEPA) filter which arrest all suspended microorganisms in air adhere to dust particles.

Observation and Interpretation of Results : After inoculation of the product under test asceptically into sterile culture media (direct inoculation method) or the membrane filter into the sterile culture media (filtration method), the inoculated plates are incubated separately for specified periods at 30° to 35°C (for bacterial growth) and 20° to 25°C (for fungal growth).

At intervals during the incubation period, and at its conclusion, examine the media for macroscopic evidence of microbial growth. If no evidence of growth is found, the preparation being examined passes the tests for sterility. If evidence of microbial growth is found, observe the container showing this and, unless it is demonstrated by any other means that their presence is due to causes unrelated to the preparation being examined and hence that the tests for sterility are invalid and may therefore be recommended, perform a retest using the same number of samples, volumes to be tested and the media as in the original test. If no evidence of microbial growth is then found, the preparation being examined passes the tests for sterility. If evidence of microbial growth is found, isolated and identify the organisms. If they are not readily distinguishable from those growing in the containers reserved in the first test, the preparation being examined fails the tests for sterility. If they are readily distinguishable from those growing in the containers reserved in the first test, perform a second retest using twice the number of samples. If no evidence of microbial growth is found in the second retest, the preparation being examined passes the tests for sterility. If evidence of growth of any microorganisms is found in the second retest the preparation being examined fails the tests for sterility. **Injections comply with the tests for sterility.**

V. Pyrogens

Unless otherwise stated in the individual monograph when the volume to be injected in a single dose is **10 ml or more**, Injections comply with the test for pyrogens, unless the test for bacterial endotoxins is prescribed.

Test for pyrogens involves measurement of the rise in body temperature of **rabbits** following the i.v. injection in the **marginal vein of the ear** of a sterile solution (preheated to 38.5°C) of the substance being examined. It is designed for products that can be tolerated by the test rabbit in a dose not exceeding 10 ml per kg (limit 0.5-10.0 ml) injected intravenously within a period of not more than 10 minutes.

All the glassware, solvent etc. used to carryout the experiment must be apyrogenic. Animals are housed according to the prescribed condition and the fluctuation of body weight and temperature are recorded as prescribed. Test is carried out using healthy, adult rabbits of either sex, preferebly of the same variety, weighing not less than 1.5 kg

Before the main test a "Preliminary Test (**Sham Test**)" is performed by injecting pyrogen free saline solution **to acclimatized the animal with the testing**. Any animal showing a temperature variation of 0.6°C or more must not be used in the main test. The **rectal** temperature is recorded as prescribed with the help of a thermometer or suitable electrical devices like thermocouple.

The "Main Test" is performed using three rabbits, which are acclimatized through Sham Test. If the sum of the responses of the group of three rabbits does not exceed 1.4°C and if the response of any individual rabbit is less than 0.6°C, the preparation being examined passes the test. If the response of any rabbit is 0.6°C or more, or if the sum of the responses of the three rabbits exceeds 1.4°C, continue the test using five other rabbits. If not more than three of the eight rabbits show individual responses of 0.6°C or more, and if the sum of responses of the group of eight rabbits does not exceed 3.7°C, the preparation being examined passes the test.

At present an *in vitro* test for pyrogen is developed which is known as **LAL-Test** (Limulus Amoebocyte Lysate Test) and much more sensitive than rabbit test. This lysate is used in BACTERIAL ENDOTOXINS TEST as prescribed by the Indian Pharmacopoeia.

The bacterial endotoxins test (BET) measure the concentration of bacterial endotoxins that may be present in or on the sample of the article to which the test is applied using a lysate derived from the hemolymph cells or amoebocytes from the horse shoe crab, *Limulus polyphemus*. The Indian also yields amoebocyte lysate having similar activity. The addition of a solution containing endo-toxin to a solution of the lysate produces turbidity, precipitation or gelation of the mixture. The rate of reaction depends on the concentration of endotoxin, the pH and the temperature.

VI. Leaker Test (For Faulty Seal Packaging)

All the ampoules, which have been sealed by fusion, must be subjected to leaker test to check that there should not be any passage for leaking of the contents from the containers. This test is performed by dipping the ampoules in a deeply colored dye solution for which 1% solution of methylene blue is used. The whole process is carried out in a vacuum chamber under negative pressure. When the vacuum is released the coloured solution will enter the ampoules with defective sealing. After careful washing of ampoules from outside, the dye can be seen in the leaker ampoules.

This test is **not performed** on vials and bottles because of flexibility of rubber, moreover the dye will badly stain the rubber stoppers.

Routes of Administration of Parenteral Products

Parenteral preparations must be introduced through the same route for which they are intended, for example, if an oily suspension meant for i.m. injection is introduced by i.v. injection may prove fatal. Similarly potent drugs meant for administration through intramuscular injection may lead to even death if given by intravenous injection.

(i) *Intracutaneous or intradermal injections :* These injections are given in between dermis and epidermis. This route is mainly used for testing the sensitivity of the injectables and for diagnostic purposes.

(ii) *Subcutaneous or hypodermic injections :* These injections are given in the subcutaneous tissue under the skin of the upper arm. The volume of the injectables is within 1ml usually.

(iii) *Intramuscular injections :* These injections are usually given in three muscles viz *deltoid* (arm), *glutious maximus* (buttocks) and *vastus lateralis* (thigh). The volume of injectables should be within 4 ml. For i.m. injection the drug may be dissolved or suspended in an aqueous or oily vehicle but the drugs dissolved in aqueous vehicles are absorbed faster than the drugs in oily solutions or suspensions in oily vehicle.

(iv) *Intravenous injections/drip/infusion :* Drip means the slow, drop-by-drop infusion of a liquid. The infusion is the slow therapeutic introduction of fluid other than blood into a vein. Large volumes of solutions ranging from 1ml. to 500 ml or even more can be injected but volumes of more than 15 ml should be isotonic with blood. Oily injections and suspensions cannot be injected by this route.

(v) *Intraarterial injections :* These injections are given to a particular artery carrying blood to a peripheral tissue. This route is employed to localize a toxic drug to a desired particular tissue (e.g., cancer chemotherapy) or for radio imaging of a particular organ (radiotracer technique).

Besides these there are some less commonly used routes such as :

(vi) *Intracardiac injections :* Directly into the heart muscles or ventricle and are used in emergency only.

(vii) *Intrathecal injections :* They are given into the subarachnoid space surrounding the spinal cord. This route is used for giving spinal anaesthesia.

(viii) *Intracisternal injections :* Given in between the first and second cervical vertebrae. This route is principally used to withdraw cerebrospinal fluid for diagnostic purposes.

(ix) *Peridural injections :* These injections are given between the duramaters and the inner aspects of the vertebra.

(x) *Intraarticular injections :* Given into the liquid that lubricates the joints.

(xi) *Intracerebral injections.*

(xii) *Intrasynovial injections :* Given into a joint fluid area

(xiii) *Intraocular.*

Essential Qualities of a Parenteral Product

(i) It should be free from living microorganisms and microbial products.

(ii) It should be free from pyrogen.

(iii) It should be free from foreign particles such as dust, fibres, etc.

(iv) It should be free from chemical contaminants.

(v) It should be isotonic with body fluids.

(vi) It should have matching specific gravity with respect to some body fluids.

(vii) Multidose injections must contain preservative(s).

(viii) Container/closure must not affect the product.

Vehicles for Injectables

The commonly used vehicle is water for injection. When water free from dissolved gases (CO_2, O_2) is required, it should be freshly boiled, cooled and stored in a well closed container to avoid reabsorption of oxygen and carbon di oxide.

Oily vehicles or non-aqueous vehicles include fixed oils from vegetable origin (cotton seed oil, pea nut oil, olive oil, sesame oil, corn oil etc.), propylene glycol, polyethylene glycol (PEG), glycerol, isopropyl myristate, dimethylacetamide etc.

Added substances : These substances are added to increase the stability or quality of the product and may include solubilising agents, antibacterial agents, antifungal agents, antioxidants, chelating agents, buffers, isotonicity factors, hydrolysis inhibitors, wetting, suspending and anti-foaming agents, etc.

Common examples of large volume parenterals which are generally used include :

(i) Dextrose injection : 2.5, 5, 10, 20% or other concentrations of dextrose and used as fluid and nutrient replenisher.

(ii) Dextrose and sodium chloride injection : 2.5 to 25% dextrose and 0.11 to 0.9% sodium chloride. This solution is used as fluid, nutrient and electrolyte replenisher.

(iii) Fructose injection : It contains 10% fructose and is used as fluid replenisher and nutrient.

(iv) Fructose and sodium chloride injection : It contains 10% fructose and 0.9% sodium chloride. This solution is used as fluid, nutrient and electrolyte replenisher.

  (v) Mannitol injection : It contains 5, 10, 15, 20 and 25% mannitol and is used as diagnostic aid in renal function determinations and diuretic.

 (vi) Mannitol and sodium chloride injection : It contains 5,10 and 15% mannitol and 0.45% sodium chloride and is used as diuretic.

(vii) Ringer's injection : It contains 0.86% sodium chloride, 0.03% potassium chloride and 0.033% calcium chloride. This solution is used as fluid and electrolyte replenisher.

(viii) Lactated Ringer's injection : It contains 2.7 mEq calcium, 4 mEq potassium, 130 mEq sodium and 2.45 gm lactate per litre. This solution is used as systemic alkalizer, fluid and electrolyte replenisher.

 (ix) Sodium chloride injection : It is also known as **normal saline** and contains 0.9% sodium chloride. This solution is used as fluid and electrolyte replenisher and isotonic vehicle.

Incorporation of drugs like antibiotics, vitamins etc. into packed infusion bottles by injecting the drug through the rubber closure is unscientific and even dangerous in many cases. Because that may lead to bacterial growth as no infusion contains a preservative rather sugars present in infusions provide good medium for bacterial growth. On the other hand it may be responsible for drug-drug, drug excipient, excipient -excipient interactions leading to certain visible changes such as haziness, precipitation, crystallization, discolouration, etc., or may affect the efficacy or potency of the therapeutic agent, which is not desirable.

Hypotonic solution is more harmful than hypertonic solution because in hypotonic media the blood cells swell rapidly and bursts (hemolysis) but in hypertonic solution the blood cells shrink and these cells attain normal size after isotonicity is reached.

Total Parenteral Nutrition (TPN) or Parenteral Hyper Alimentation : In order to maintain debilitated patients who are running with negative nitrogen balance, a total parenteral nutrition in the form of large volume emulsion type i.v. infusion is already available in the market. This solution contains high concentrations of dextrose, proteins, lipids/fats, vitamins and minerals/electrolytes and are administered slowly through a large vein and near to the heart for rapid dilution of the concentrated hyper alimentation fluid so as to minimize the risk of tissue or cellular damage due to hyper tonicity of the solution.

Irrigation and Dialysis Solutions

Irrigation and dialysis solutions are quite similar to parenteral solutions as they are subjected to some standards. The difference is in their use. These solutions are not injected into the vein but are used outside of the circulatory system. Since these types of solutions are generally used in large volumes so they are packed in large volume plastic containers.

Irrigation solutions are used for bathing or washing the wounds, surgical incisions or body tissues. A large number of officials and patent irrigation solutions are available in the market. Some of them include Ringer's Irrigation USP, Sodium Chloride Irrigation USP, and Sterile Water for Irrigation USP.

Dialysis solutions : Dialysis may be defined as the process by which the substances are separated from one another due to their difference in diffusibility through membranes. The solutions used in dialysis are known as dialysis solutions. In cases of poisoning or kidney failure or in cases where kidney transplantation is to be done, dialysis is an emergency life-saving procedure.

In the case of renal failure, the removal of waste products and the maintenance of electrolyte balance are done either by haemodialysis or intraperitoneal dialysis.

Haemodialysis is used to remove toxins from the blood. In this method blood from a convenient artery is shunted through a polyethylene catheter through an artificial dialyzing membrane bathed in dialyzing fluid. The dialyzing membrane is permeable to urea, electrolytes and dextrose but not to plasma proteins and lipids. Substances such as urea, which are in excess in the blood, pass out in the fluid. After the dialysis the blood is freed from air bubbles and clots and is returned back to the body circulation through a suitable vein. The fluids used in the artificial kidney are called haemodialysis solutions.

Ophthalmic Products

Drugs are administered to the eye for local effects such as myosis, mydriasis and anesthesia. Steroids and anti-infective drugs are also frequently used in the eye. Unlike skin preparation, the ophthalmic preparation must be free from grittiness, should be nonirritant and must be sterile because cornea has no barrier to microorganism due to very low blood flow. Ideally eye drops, eye lotions should be isotonic with lachrymal secretion. Similarly the pH of eye preparation should ideally be equal with the lachrymal pH. But from the stability or solubility viewpoint if it is essential to deviate from this pH, then it should not be strongly buffered to minimize irritation.

Although the eye is not a route for systemic drug administration, systemic absorption can occur probably from the entry of the drug into the lachrymal duct, which drains lachrymal fluid into the nasal cavity and ultimately into the G.I. tract.

Drugs may be applied to the eye in the form of sterile aqueous solutions, suspensions, ointments or inserts intended to reside in the conjunctival cul-de-sac. Solutions used during surgery should not contain any preservatives and supplied in single-use containers and solution remaining at the end of the operation must be discarded.

Usually all eye preparation must not be used after one month of first opening the seal (whatever may be the expiratory date). As aqueous solutions are much susceptible to microbial growth, the eye drops must be used within two weeks after first opening of the container. In the hospital ward or out-patient departments, eye drops should not be used after one week after first opening of the container and in the operation theatre a new unopened container should be used for each patient.

The volume of the instilled solution is important because a major fraction of liquid are lost by drainage and not only this but also it causes irritation and higher lachrymal secretion. Under normal conditions the human eye can hold about 10 µl of fluid. The normal dropper used in commercial ophthalmic preparation delivers approximately 50 to 75 µl. The use of smaller drops (5 to 10 µl) of somewhat higher concentration would reduce costs, increases efficacy and might reduce the side effect.

Sometimes patients are directed to instill more than one drops of an ophthalmic preparation at a time. Also in other cases more than one preparation are administered at the same time. But because of limited accommodation capacity of the eye, the above fact should be taken into consideration and if possible, a comparative concentrated combined formulation should be prepared. **The viscosity-increasing agent in an ophthalmic solution will increase ocular drug bioavailability by prolonging the contact time of drug with eye tissues.**

Usually suspension type eye preparations give higher as well as a prolonged effect because particles present in a dose of suspension are retained within the cul-de-sac of the eye.

The major advantage in case of the ointment is increased contact time and sustained effect, but the major disadvantage is the mixing problem between ointment vehicle and the tears that may limit the penetration rate. The drug levels persisted for far longer than observed after instillation of suspension or a solution of the drug But the onset of action is delayed in case of ophthalmic ointment.

Ocusert is a membrane-controlled system that is placed in the conjunctival cul-de-sac to release the drug continuously at an essentially uniform and predetermined rate for 1 week. Clinical studies suggest that the once weekly placement of the ocusert - pilocarpine system produces hypotensive effects in glaucomatous patients comparable to those achieved by the use of 1 to 4 percent pilocarpine eye drops, four times daily.

Contact Lens Solutions

Contact lenses are generally made from hard hydrophobic plastic known as polymethyl methacrylate but nowadays some softer hydrophobic lenses are also used.

The wearers of hard contact lenses generally use two types of solutions.

(i) One before inserting the lenses into the eyes which is known as wetting solution the formulation of which includes a wetting agent, buffering agent, a thickening agent, a substance for adjusting the osmotic pressure, a preservative and a vehicle which is generally a purified water.

(ii) The other one used for overnight cleaning, soaking and storage which is known as storage solution and usually contains a non-ionic surfactant and a blend of preservatives along with other excipients.

MODEL QUESTIONS

1. Sterility tests for molds and yeasts should be conducted with
   A. thioglycollate medium   B. agar plates   C. honey media
   D. glucose broth   E. none of these above.
2. Solutions that contain bacteriostatic agents
   A. cannot be tested for sterility
   B. must be cultured on agar plates for sterility tests
   C. must be diluted beyond the bacteriostatic level for sterility tests
   D. do not require a sterility test
   E. none of the above.
3. The sterility test for liquids involves
   A. colorimetric assay
   B. rabbit test

   C. injection into guinea pigs
   D. culturing in fluid thioglycollate medium
   E. none of the above.
4. The minimal effective flow rate of air in laminar flow hoods should be not less than how many cubic feet per minute?
   A. 10   B. 50   C. 100   D. 500   E. 1000.
5. The Chick-Martin test is used to test the efficiency of
   A. coumarins   B. heparin   C. antibiotics
   D. blood clotting   E. analgesics.
6. Sterility test for the materials meant for surgical suture requires incubation for
   A. 7 days   B. 14 days   C. 21 days   D. 28 days   E. 3 months.
7. Name equipment that can give limited asceptic area.
8. Unless otherwise stated in the individual monograph the antimicrobial preservative is used in
   A. single dose container
   B. multi-dose container
   C. large volume parenterals (LVP)
   D. intracardiac preparation
   E. all of the above.
9. Anticoagulant acid citrate dextrose injection is required to be pyrogen-free. Pyrogens are
   A. organic catalysts formed in living cells
   B. antigens contained in bacteria
   C. nonspecific globulins
   D. products which stimulate hematopoietic organs
   E. products causing febrile reaction upon injection.
10. The limulus test is rapid *in vitro* method for
   A. determining the pH of blood
   B. checking the tonicity of i.v. solutions
   C. determining the sterility of i.v. solutions
   D. pyrogen testing in parenteral solutions
   E. testing for specific antibodies.
11. Insulin preparations are usually administered by
   A. intradermal injection   B. intravenous injection   C. subcutaneous injection
   D. intramuscular injection   E. intrathecal injection.
12. Which one of the following needles is most suited for the administration of insulin solutions?
   A. 16 G 5/8″   B. 21 G 1/2″   C. 21 G 5/8″   D. 25 G 5/8″   E. 25 G 1″
13. "Winged" needles are most closely associated with which type of injections?
   A. Intradermal   B. Intramuscular   C. Intrathecal
   D. Intravenous   E. Subcutaneous
14. Hypodermic needle sizes are expressed by gauge numbers. The gauge number refers to
   A. the bevel size

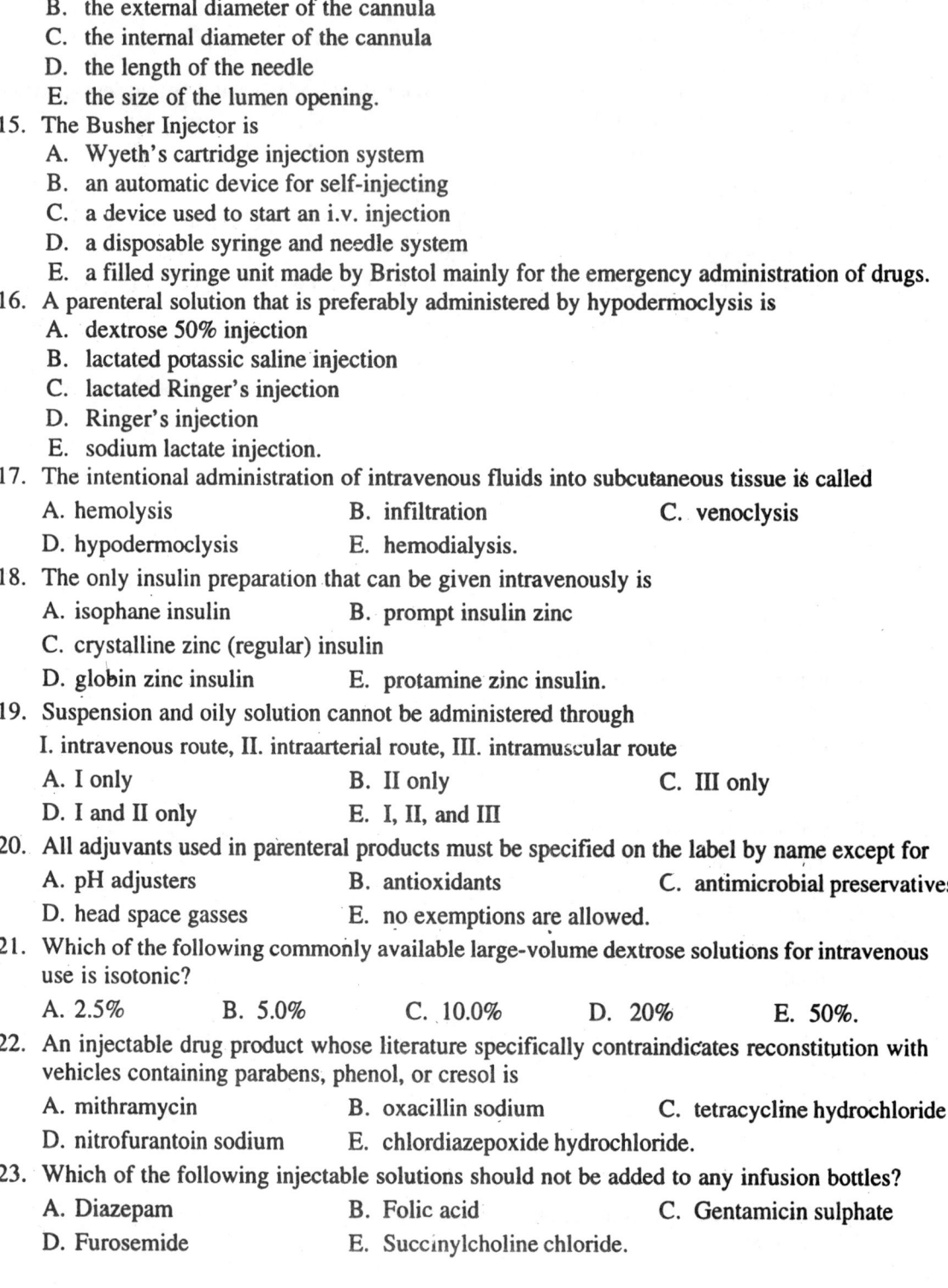

B. the external diameter of the cannula
C. the internal diameter of the cannula
D. the length of the needle
E. the size of the lumen opening.

15. The Busher Injector is
   A. Wyeth's cartridge injection system
   B. an automatic device for self-injecting
   C. a device used to start an i.v. injection
   D. a disposable syringe and needle system
   E. a filled syringe unit made by Bristol mainly for the emergency administration of drugs.

16. A parenteral solution that is preferably administered by hypodermoclysis is
   A. dextrose 50% injection
   B. lactated potassic saline injection
   C. lactated Ringer's injection
   D. Ringer's injection
   E. sodium lactate injection.

17. The intentional administration of intravenous fluids into subcutaneous tissue is called
   A. hemolysis   B. infiltration   C. venoclysis
   D. hypodermoclysis   E. hemodialysis.

18. The only insulin preparation that can be given intravenously is
   A. isophane insulin   B. prompt insulin zinc
   C. crystalline zinc (regular) insulin
   D. globin zinc insulin   E. protamine zinc insulin.

19. Suspension and oily solution cannot be administered through
   I. intravenous route, II. intraarterial route, III. intramuscular route
   A. I only   B. II only   C. III only
   D. I and II only   E. I, II, and III

20. All adjuvants used in parenteral products must be specified on the label by name except for
   A. pH adjusters   B. antioxidants   C. antimicrobial preservatives
   D. head space gasses E. no exemptions are allowed.

21. Which of the following commonly available large-volume dextrose solutions for intravenous use is isotonic?
   A. 2.5%   B. 5.0%   C. 10.0%   D. 20%   E. 50%.

22. An injectable drug product whose literature specifically contraindicates reconstitution with vehicles containing parabens, phenol, or cresol is
   A. mithramycin   B. oxacillin sodium   C. tetracycline hydrochloride
   D. nitrofurantoin sodium E. chlordiazepoxide hydrochloride.

23. Which of the following injectable solutions should not be added to any infusion bottles?
   A. Diazepam   B. Folic acid   C. Gentamicin sulphate
   D. Furosemide   E. Succinylcholine chloride.

24. Product literature often suggests that sterile water for injection be used as the reconstituting solvent for injectable antibiotic powders. However, sodium chloride injection (normal saline) is frequently used. Normal saline would not be used to reconstitute

A. ampicillin sodium   B. erythromycin lactobionate   C. penicillin G potassium

D. methicillin sodium   E. polymyxin B sulfate.

25. Of the following vehicles, which is the most appropriate for an IV admixture of ampicillin (500 mg per 50 ml)?

A. Dextrose 5% injection.

B. Dextrose 5% and sodium chloride 0.9% injection

C. Dextrose 2.5% and sodium chloride 0.9% injection

D. Sodium chloride 0.9% injection

E. All of the above.

26. The quantities of all ingredients present in parenteral solutions must be specified on the label EXCEPT for I. chelating agents; II. antimicrobial preservatives; III. pH adjustors; IV. isotonicity adjustors

A. I only   B. II only   C. III only

D. IV only   E. III and IV only.

27. Which one of the following statements concerning Sodium Chloride Irrigation USP is NOT true? The solution

A. may contain an antimicrobial preservative

B. is intended for either topical or rectal administration

C. is sterile

D. contains the same concentration of sodium chloride as present in Sodium Chloride Injection USP

E. may be packaged in bottles as large as three litres.

28. The bevel length of a hypodermic needle may vary from very short to long (regular). A short bevel is preferred for injections by which route of administration?

A. Intradermal   B. Subcutaneous   C. Intramuscular

D. Intravenous   E. Intrathecal.

29. The manufacturing formula of Ascorbic Acid Injection USP may include

A. hydrochloric acid   B. acetic acid   C. propylene glycol

D. tetracycline hydrochloride   E. sodium hydroxide.

30. The usual expiration dating that should be placed on a parenteral admixture prepared in a hospital pharmacy is

A. 1 hour   B. 24 hours   C. 48 hours   D. 72 hours   E. 1 week.

31. Plastic parenteral bottles and bags differ from glass units in that the plastic units have I. an air tube in the unit; II. a vacuum; III. two entry ports.

A. I only   B. III only   C. I and II only

D. II and III only   E. I, II and III.

32. Commonly used bulking agent in parenteral formulation is

A. mannitol   B. cellulose   C. starch

D. lecithin   E. all of the above.

33. Ascorbic acid is sometimes added in parenteral preparations mainly as
    A. vitamin   B. antioxidant   C. antimicrobial preservative
    D. tonicity adjustor   E. all of the above.

34. Which one of the following is used as sustained release ophthalmic preparation?
    A. Implants   B. Ophthalmic suspension   C. Niosomes
    D. Ocusert system   E. Iontophoretic system.

35. For opthalmic use, boric acid solution should be
    A. diluted with an equal volume of isotonic distilled water
    B. undiluted
    C. diluted with an equal volume of saline solution
    D. diluted with an equal volume of sterile distilled water
    E. diluted with an equal volume of sterile isotonic saline solution.

36. The advantage(s) associated with ophthalmic ocusert system is/are
    A. improved patient compliance
    B. improved overnight therapy
    C. reduced side effects
    D. non-fluctuation of the drug level during therapy
    E. all of the above.

37. The incorporation of methyl cellulose or similar agent in an ophthalmic solution is due to
    A. increase the viscosity of the preparation
    B. increase ocular drug bioavailability by prolonging the contact time of drug with eye tissues
    C. stabilize the ophthalmic solution
    D. improve the pourability of the solution
    E. all of the above.

38. On the basis of duration and intensity of action the eye preparations of a particular drug may be arranged as
    A. ocusert > suspension > saturated solution > ointment
    B. ocusert > ointment > suspension > saturated solution
    C. saturated solution > suspension > ointment > ocusert
    D. suspension > ocusert > ointment > saturated solution.

39. Glycerin is used in the eye primarily
    A. to constrict the pupil   B. to dilate the pupil   C. to clear the corneal haze
    D. as a contact lens solution   E. to prevent itching.

40. Which of the following solutions should be sterile when dispensed?
    A. Tincture   B. Ophthalmic solutions   C. Spirit
    D. Syrups   E. None of the above.

41. Storage of soaking solutions for hard contact lenses should be
    A. heated prior to use   B. acidified with weak acids   C. replaced weekly
    D. replaced daily   E. none of the above.

42. Liquifilm is a vehicle used in preparing
    A. topical gels
    B. ophthalmic solutions
    C. topical aerosols
    D. otic solutions
    E. none of the above.

43. The most popular commercial combination of preservatives that appears to be effective for ophthalmic use is
    A. phenylmercuric nitrate and phenylethyl alcohol
    B. benzalkonium chloride and EDTA
    C. benzalkonium chloride and chlorobutanol
    D. methyl and propyl paraben
    E. chlorobutanol and EDTA.

44. All of the following viscosity builders have been used in ophthalmic solutions EXCEPT
    A. veegum   B. methylcellulose   C. polyethylene glycols (PEG)
    D. polyvinyl pyrrolidone (PVP)   E. polyvinyl alcohol.

45. The function of papain in soft contact lens product is to
    A. remove grease
    B. keep the lens soft
    C. disinfect
    D. remove proteinaceous residues
    E. prevent dehydration of the lens.

46. Which of the following would be most irritating to the eye?
    A. Purified water
    B. 0.7% sodium chloride solution
    C. 0.9% sodium chloride solution
    D. 1.2% sodium chloride solution
    E. Both B and D.

47. A microorganism that is particularly dangerous to the eye is
    A. *Streptococcus thermophilus*
    B. *Escharichia coli*
    C. *Aspergillus niger*
    D. *Pseudomonas aeruginosa*
    E. *Bacillus subtilis*

48. Which one of the following is used as preservative in ophthalmic preparations?
    A. Benzalkonium chloride   B. Phenol   C. Benzoic acid
    D. Chlorocresol   E. All of the above.

49. Which one is important for ophthalmic preparation?
    A. sterility   B. isotonicity   C. viscosity
    D. pH   E. all of the above.

ANSWERS

1. C; 2. C (A false negative result is common if tested without dilution); 3. D; 4. C; 5. C [Reidal Walker Coefficient (R.W.C.) value is estimated to determine the efficacy of disinfectants (to kill the microorganisms in case of inanimates). Chick-Martin test actually a modification of this which is performed in presence of organic matter. Because in actual practice disinfectants have to work in presence of organic matter. This C.M. test is also done to test the efficiency of antibiotics]; 6. A; 7. [A cubiclized table fitted with laminar air flow system (through High Efficiency Particulate Air (HEPA) filter]; 8. B; 9. E; 10. D; 11. C [This route is convenient and safe for self administration of the drug]; 12. D [Insulin solutions have low viscosities and only small volumes are injected. Therefore small-bore needles (25 G or 26 G) may be used short (1/2″ to 5/8″) needles are adequate for usual subcutaneous route of insulin administration]; 13. D; 14. B (The larger the gauge number the smaller the diameter of the needle); 15. B; 16. B (This is preferred to avoid potassium overdose); 17. D (Hypodermoclysis is used on rare occasions in infants or obese patients in whom veins are inaccessible. Venoclysis refers to the administration of solutions by rapid i.v. injection or infusion); 18. C (used when rapid onset and brief duration of action are desired as in the treatment of diabetic ketoacidosis. It is often used in conjuction with subcutaneously administered longer acting insulin preparations); 19. D; 20. D (In case of oxygen sensitive material, the head space gasses containing oxygen should also be removed and replaced by suitable inert gas); 21. B; 22. D (Nitrofurantoin is precipitated by certain commonly used preservatives. Suitable vehicles include sterile water for injection and 5% dextrose injection); 23. A (Because of precipitation even when added to normal saline or 5% dextrose solution); 24. B (A precipitate develops in solutions made with normal saline and or other containing inorganic salts); 25. D (Ampicillin is more stable in sodium chloride solution than dextrose solution); 26. E [The amount of acid (HCl) or base (NaOH) used to adjust the pH may vary from batch to batch. Therefore, the label can not specify an exact quantity. Name of the isotonicity adjuster and their purpose are mentioned but not their quantity]; 27. A (It is intended for unit dose administration, and unused portions must be discarded); 28. D (A short bevel needle reduces the possibility of perforating the back wall of the vein, very short bevel is preferred for intradermal injection); 29. E (Solution of ascorbic acid would be too acidic for injection purposes. Therefore, an alkali such as NaOH, NaHCO$_3$, or Na$_2$CO$_3$ is used to adjust the pH to between 5.5 and 7); 30. B (An expiration date of 24 hours is considered to be safest unless the solution is known to be less stable chemically. Refrigeration helps to retard microbial growth); 31. B (Advantages of the plastic units in comparison to glass units, include their lighter weight and resistance to breakage as compared to glass and their ability to collapse as solution flows out, thus, precluding the need for a method to add air as the solution exits. Glass bottles require either an air tube or air filter); 32. A; 33. B; 34. D; 35. D; 36. E; 37. B; 38. B; 39. C; 40. B; 41. D; 42. B (Liquifilm is a name used for an ophthalmic vehicle containing polyvinyl alcohol. The polyvinyl alcohol increases the viscosity of the ophthalmic solutions, there by prolonging the contact with the corneal surface); 43. B; 44. A [Veegum is not an organic gum but is an inorganic clay (magnesium-aluminium silicate) though hydrated by water but is insoluble]; 45. D (Papain is proteolytic enzyme); 46. A (0.5 to 2.0% solution can be put into either normal or inflamed eyes without causing pain or detectable tissue change. Purified water will sting because it has such a low tonicity); 47. D; 48. A (It is germicidal cationic surface active agent, usual concentration used is 0.013%); 49. A.

CHAPTER 26

Miscellaneous Questions

• Miscellaneous Questions

1. Barrier creams are quite useful in preventing
   A. drug allergies
   B. poison sumac
   C. food allergies
   D. psoriasis
   E. dry skin.
2. Which of the following is contained in a number of sun screening lotion?
   A. Benzocaine
   B. PABA
   C. Zinc oxide
   D. Benzoic acid
   E. Salicylic acid.
3. The ideal antiseptic concentration of ethyl alcohol is
   A. 100%   B. 95%   C. 75%   D. 70%   E. 50%
4. Which of the following is the most effective sunscreen?
   A. Baby oil
   B. PABA
   C. Titanium dioxide
   D. Methyl salicylate
   E. Methoxysoralen.
5. What imparts the pink color to calamine?
   A. Zinc oxide
   B. FDC red no. 3
   C. Ferric oxide
   D. Titanium dioxide
   E. Carmine.
6. Another name for polyethylene glycol polymers is
   A. sodium alginate
   B. silica gel
   C. carbowax
   D. Friar paste
   E. none of the above.
7. PEG 4000 monostearate is NOT miscible with
   A. water
   B. alcohol
   C. ether
   D. benzene
   E. isopropyl alcohol.

8. An ophthalmic preparation should have which of the following pHs to conform to that of lacrimal fluid?

  A. 6.2 - 6.8   B. 7.2 - 8.0   C. 8.4 - 9.0
  D. 9.2 - 10.0   E. None of these.

9. Which of the following is a stabilizer in magnesia magma?

  A. Benzoic acid   B. Citric acid   C. Oxalic acid
  D. Lactic acid   E. Mandelic acid.

10. The active ingredient in Desenex solution is

  A. salicylic acid   B. glyceryl triacetate C. basic fushsin
  D. undecylenic acid   E. none of the above.

11. Betadine contains

  A. benzocaine   B. gentian violet   C. betamethionine
  D. surfacaine   E. povidone-iodine complex.

12. Sorbitol is useful mainly as a (an)

  A. solubilizer   B. surfactant   C. emulsifier
  D. counter-irritant   E. humectant.

13. If a bottle of tablets has an expiration date of "June 1999" the pharmacist may
  A. continue to dispense the product if he has already opened the container
  B. dispense the tablets only until June 1, 1999
  C. dispense the tablets through June 15, 1999
  D. dispense the tablets through June 30, 1999
  E. dispense the tablets if he informes the patients to discard unused tablets in six months (December 1, 1999).

14. The expiration date on a pharmaceutical container states "Expires June 1999". This statement means that by July 1, 1999, the product will have lost

  A. 5% of its activity   B. 10% of its activity   C. 20% of its activity
  D. 50% of its activity
  E. suffieient activity to be outside USP or NF or other official monograph requirements as the case may be.

15. The USP and NF specifies that almost all measurements and tests that are temperature dependent must be conducted at

  A. 15.6°C   B. 20°C   C. 25°C   D. 60°F   E. 98.6°F

16. The monograph for Strong Ammonia Solution NF contains a note pertaining to
  A. the method of manufacturing
  B. the incompatibility of ammonia
  C. proper dilutions for use
  D. its reaction with strong acids
  E. the manner of handling and opening of bottles

17. Ringer's solution is an aqueous solution containing
  A. sodium, potassium, and magnesium cations
  B. dextrose and sodium chloride

    C. fructose and sodium chloride

    D. dextrose and sodium bicarbonate

    E. sodium, potassium and calcium chloride

18. Fleet's Enema differs from Fleet's Pediatric Enema in that

    A. Fleet's Enema contains magnesium sulfate while the Pediatric form does not.

    B. Fleet's Pediatric Enema contains magnesium sulfate while Fleet's Enema does not

    C. a bottle of Fleet's Enema contains twice as much enema as a bottle of the pediatric form

    D. Fleet's Enema is twice as concentrated as the pediatric form

    E. none of the above statements are true.

19. Rectal clinical thermometers differ from oral thermometers in

    A. stem shape   B. stem length   C. bulb shape

    D. distance between graduation marks on the stem   E. standards for accuracy.

20. A basal thermometer is

    A. used to estimate time of ovulation

    B. a rectal thermometer.

    C. graduated only in celsius degrees

    D. used vaginally

    E. used to determine basal metabolic rate.

21. What length crutch would usually be correct for a person who is 5' 11" tall?

    A. 42 inches   B. 48 inches   C. 54 inches   D. 58 inches   E. 71 inches

22. The product inserts for many drug products contain cautionary statements. Which one of the following sequences lists the three types of cautions in the order of least serious to most serious?

    A. Contraindication, warning, precaution

    B. Precaution, warning, contraindication

    C. Contraindication, precaution, warning

    D. Warning, precaution, contraindication

    E. Warning, contraindication, precaution

23. A unit dose package always contains

    A. one discrete pharmaceutical dosage form (i.e., one tablet, one capsule, one ampoule, etc.)

    B. a single dose of a drug intended to be administered by hospitalized patient

    C. the exact amount of drug ordered by physician in a dosage form ready for administration

    D. solid dosage forms only

    E. the exact amount of drug that is to be administered to a patient during one complete nursing shift.

24. The best emergency advice that a pharmacist could give an individual who has just suffered a minor burn is to

    A. immerse the burn area in cold water

    B. immerse the burn area in warm water followed by cold water

    C. contact a physician immediately

    D. apply butter to the burn

    E. apply vaseline to the burn.

25. Stomatitis refers to an inflammation of the
    A. tongue   B. oral mucosa   C. stomach wall
    D. eyelid   E. nasal passages.

26. Parenteral administration of one litre of 5% dextrose in water provides the patient with approximately how many calories?
    A. 100 to 125   B. 170 to 200   C. 400 to 450   D. 800 to 850   E. 1000

27. The level of potassium chloride usually included in each hyperalimentation solution bottle is
    A. 2 mEq/L   B. 5 mEq/L   C. 10 mEq/L   D. 40 mEq/L   E. 80 mEq/L

28. Which of the following is considered effective in the treatment of accidental drug poisoning?
    I. Activated charcoal; II. Ipecac syrup; III. "Universal antidote"
    A. I only   B. III only   C. I and II only
    D. II and III only   E. I, II and III

29. Basal thermometers and rectal thermometers are similar in that both
    I. have the same degree of accuracy; II. can be used to determine ovulation; III. can be used orally.
    A. I only   B. III only   C. I and II only
    D. I and III only   E. I, II and III

30. Prior to administration enema should be kept at
    A. refrigerator   B. room temperature   C. body temperature
    D. boiling water   E. cool temperature.

31. Match the following
    (i)   Long-release tablet   A. Medihaler
    (ii)   Sublingual tablet   B. Glosset
    (iii) Aerosol device   C. Abboject
    (iv) Color-flecked tablet   D. Gradumet
    (v)   Disposable syringe   E. Medilet

32. Match each substances with its pharmaceutical use
    (i)   Freon   A. Flavouring agent
    (ii)   Sodium metabisulfite   B. Antioxidant
    (iii)   Ethyl acetate   C. Aerosol propellant
    (iv)   Alcohol USP   D. Diluent
    (v)   Lactose   E. Solvent
    (vi)   Theobroma oil   F. Lubricant
    (vii) Magnesium stearate   G. Suppository base
    (viii) Potassium metaphosphate   H. Buffering agent.

33. Match each active ingredient with the appropriate product containing this ingredient
    (i)   Sodium metabisulfite   A. Collodion
    (ii)   Cholesterol   B. Rubbing alcohol

    (iii) Methyl isobutyl ketone   C. Ascorbic acid injection

    (iv) Cellulose acetate phthalate   D. Hydrophilic petrolatum

    (v) Pyroxylin   E. Enteric-coated tablets.

34. Match the following

(i)	Aerosol propellant	A. Ainsworth
(ii)	Gum	B. Du Bose
(iii)	Cyanine dye	C. Strong-Cobb
(iv)	Carbohydrate mixture	D. Stormer
(v)	Viscometer	E. Povan
(vi)	Balance	F. Acacia
(vii)	Colorimeter	G. Emetrol
(viii)	Tablet hardness tester	H. Patterson-kelly
(ix)	Blender	I. Freon II
(x)	Mill	J. Fitz

35. Match the following

(i)	Continental method	A. Rheology
(ii)	Granulation	B. Buffers
(iii)	Freezing-point depression method	C. Tableting
(iv)	Vanslyke equation	D. Isotonic solutions
(v)	Newtonian	E. Emulsions.

36. Match the lettered term concerning hypodermic needles with the associated numbered description.

(i)	Extension of needle that fits onto the syringe	A. Bevel
(ii)	Portion of needle that is ground for sharpness	B. Cannula
(iii)	Shaft portion of the needle	C. Hub
(iv)	The needle hole	D. Heel of bevel
		E. Lumen.

37. Match the lettered pH value that is nearest to the pH usually found in the numbered body areas. Answers may be used once, more than one, or not at all.

(i)	Blood	A. 4.0 - 4.5
(ii)	Eye	B. 5.5
(iii)	Skin	C. 6.4
(iv)	Vagina	D. 7.0
		E. 7.4

38. Choose the instrument or apparatus, listed from A to E to study the following

(i)	Rheology of semisolids	A. Andreasen pipette
(ii)	Hardness of tablets	B. Monsanto tester
(iii)	Particle size in suspension	C. Ultrasonifier
(iv)	Homogenization of emulsion	D. Viscometer

(v) For consistency and hardness of relatively rigid   E. Zetameter
      semisolids
(vi) Dissolution of granules and tablets   F. Glass electrode
(vii) pH indicating electrode   G. Hansen-paddle equipment
                                                              H. Penetrometer

39. Given below are equipment used in the manufacturer of following products A to E match
     them correctly.

(i)   Zanasi   A. Tablet granules
(ii)   HEPA filter   B. Tablet coating
(iii) Chilsonator   C. Emulsion
(iv)   Accelacota   D. Injectable
                       E. Capsules

40. Match the ingredients listed into A to E with the purpose for which they are used in the
     formulations.

(i)   Film coating   A. Sodium benzoate
(ii)   Syrups   B. Ethyl cellulose
(iii) Emulsification   C. Eudrajit
(iv)   Enteric coating D. Sucrose
                        E. Sodium oleate

ANSWERS

1. B; 2. B (Titanium dioxide is also a very good sunscreening agent); 3. D (Presence of about 30%
water is essential for maximum germicidal activity); 4. C; 5. C (Calamine contains about 98% zinc
oxide and 2% ferric oxide); 6. C (Carbowax is a polymer); 7. A; 8. A (The pH of the lacrimal fluid
is approximately 7.4. The eye can tolerate a pH from 6 to 8 with a minimum of discomfort); 9. B
(Used to reduce free alkali); 10. D; 11. E; 12. E; 13. D (When expiration dates are expressed only
in terms of month and year the intended expiration date is the last day of the stated month or year
respectively); 14. E (Most drug products are considered useable until approximately 10% loss of
drug or drug activity has occurred. However, some monographs specify other ranges. For example,
digoxin tablets must assay between 92 and 108% of label claim); 15. C [The NBS usually uses
20°C as a standard temperature. A temperature of 15.56°C (60°F) is used for determining alcohol
volumes]; 16. E (The solution is caustic and the vapour is irritating); 17. E (It is an isotonic
electrolyte solution containing Na^+, K^+, Ca^{++} and Cl^- in a balanced physiological proportion); 18.
C (They are both aqueous solution containing 6 g of sodium phosphate and 16 g of sodium
bi-phosphate per 100 ml.); 19.B (The rectal thermometer bulb has a strong, blunt shape which
facilitates insertion into the rectum and retention by sphincter muscles. The oral bulb is cylindrical,
elongated and thin-walled for quick registration of temperature. Rectal thermometers can be used
orally. The oral bulb is too easily broken and is not suitable for rectal use); 20. A (This thermometer
is used to determine the time of ovulation which roughly corresponds with the body temperature

rise. The basal thermometer scale ranges only from 96°F to 100°F and is graduated to 0.1°F); 21. C (If the height in inches is an odd number, substract 17 to get the crutch length, if even, subtract 16); 22. B; 23.C; 24. A (The burn area should be kept in cold water until no further pain is experienced whether in or out of the water); 25. B (Inflammation of the eyelid is **blepharitis,** inflammation of the tongue is **glossitis,** inflammation of the stomach wall is **gastritis**); 26. B (Each gram of carbohydrate supplies 4 calories. Therefore, 50 g dextrose mathematically supply 200 calories); 27. D (The dose will assist in maintaining normal serum levels and provide 3.5 : 1 ratio of potassium to nitrogen necessary for protein synthesis); 28. C (It is better to induce vomiting first with ipecac syrup and then administered activated charcoal. Simultaneous administration is not recommended as the alkaloids present in the ipecac syrup would be adsorbed and inactivated by activated charcol); 29. D; 30 C; 31. i - D; ii - B; iii - A; iv - E; v - C; 32. i - C; ii - B; iii - A; iv - E; v - D; vi - G; vii - F; viii - H; 33. i - C; ii - D; iii - B; iv - E; v - A; 34. i - I; ii - F; iii - E; iv - G; v - D; vi - A; vii - B; viii - C; ix- H; x - J; 35. i - E; ii - C; iii - D; iv - B; v - A; 36. i - C; ii - A; iii - B; iv - E; 37. i - E; ii - E; iii - B; iv - A; 38. i - D; ii - B; iii - A; iv - C; v - H; vi - G; vii - F; 39. i - E; ii - D; iii - A; iv - B; 40. i - B; ii - D; iii - E; iv - C.

Pharmacognosy

CHAPTER 27

History and Scope of Pharmacognosy

- Definition and History of Pharmacognosy
- Various Systems of Classification of Drugs of Natural Origin.

CHARAKA made fifty groups of ten herbs each of which according to him would suffice an ordinary physician's need. Similarly, SUSHRUTA arranged 760 herbs in 7 distir ct sets based on to some of their common properties. Hippocrates, Galen and Paracelsus contributed a lot in ancient science of life. Galen (131-200 A.D.) was the first pharmacist who used a number of pain-relieving materials, including opium. Paracelsus (1493-1541) used a number of mineral salts as curative agents. Hippocrates is credited for developing Unani System of Medicine. Aristotle Golen made valuable contribution to it. In comparison, other traditional systems of medicine, Homeopathy is a newer one and has been developed in eighteenth century by Samuel Hahnemann—a German physician and chemist. Pharmacognosy may be defined as a branch of bioscience, which treats in detail medicinal and related products of crude or primary type obtained from plant, animal and mineral origins.

Classification of crude drugs

Crude drugs are grouped as (according to whether they contain a regular organized cellular structure or not).

    (i) organized (cellular) or

    (ii) unorganized (acellular)

There are alphabetical classification and taxonomical classification. Besides this the following classifications are very popular.

I. Morphological classification of crude drugs

1.	Seeds	Nux vomica, Stropanthus, Isabgol, castor
2.	Leaves	Senna, Digitalis, Vasaka, Eucalyptus
3.	Barks	Cinchona, Kurchi, Cinnamon, Quaillaia
4.	Woods	Quassia, Sandalwood, Sassafras, Red sanders
5.	Roots	Rauwolfia, Ipecacuanha, Aconite, Jalap
6.	Rhizomes	Turmeric, Ginger, Valerian, Podophyllum, Rhubarb, Glycyrrhiza
7.	Flowers	Clove, Pyrethrum, Artemesia, Saffron
8.	Fruits	Corriander, Colocynth, Fennel, Bael
9.	Entire drugs	Ephedra, Ergot, Cantharides, (*Cantharis vesicatoria* contains cantharidin which is a vesicant and rubefacient and hair growth stimulant), Belladonna
10.	Dried latices	Opium, Gutta-percha, Papain
11.	Bulbs	Urginea, Garlic
12.	Tubers	Dioscorea
13.	Fibres	Cotton
14.	Resins and resin combinations	Balsam of tolu, Myrrh, Asafoetida, Benzoin
15.	Dried juices	Aloes, Kino, Red gum
16.	Gums	Acacia, Tragacanth, Ghatti gum, Guar gum
17.	Dried extracts	Gelatin, Catechu, Agar, Curare

II. Chemical classification

The crude drugs are divided into different groups according to the chemical nature of their most important constituent.

1.	Glycosides	Digitalis, Senna, Cascara, Liquorice
2.	Alkaloids	Nux vomica, Ergot, Cinchona, Datura, Opium
3.	Tannins	Myrobalan, Pale catechu, Ashoka
4.	Volatile oils	Peppermint, Clove, Eucalyptus, Garlic
5.	Lipids	Castor oil, Bees wax, Lanolin, Cod liver oil, Kokum butter
6.	Carbohydrates and derived products	Acacia, Agar, Guar gum, Pectin, Honey, Ispaghula, Starch
7.	Resins and resin combinations	Colophony, Jalap, Balsam of Tolu
8.	Vitamins and hormones	Yeast, Shark liver oil, Oxytocin, Insulin, Amla
9.	Proteins and enzymes	Casein, Gelatin, Papain, Trypsin, Diastase, Yeast

III. Pharmacological (therapeutic) classification

(i) Drugs acting on gastrointestinal tract

1.	Bitters	Gentian, Quassia, Cinchona
2.	Carminatives	Dill, Mentha, Cardamom, Fennel, Ajowan, Ginger, Black pepper, Asafoetida, Nutmeg, Cinnamon, Clove
3.	Emetics	Ipecacuanha
4.	Anti-amoebics/Anti-dysentrics	Kurchi, Ipecacuanha
5.	Bulk laxatives	Agar, Ispaghula, Banana
6.	Purgatives	Senna, Castor oil, Aloes, Rhubarb
7.	Peptic ulcer treatment	Derivatives of 18β-glycyrrhetinic acid (Liquorice), Raw Banana

(ii) Drugs acting on respiratory system

1.	Expectorants	Liquorice, Ipecacuanha, Vasaka
2.	Antiexpectorants	Stramonium leaves (Atropine)
3.	Antitussives	Opium (Codeine, Noscapine), Vasaka, Tolu balsam, Tulsi

(Contd.)

	4. Bronchodilators	Ephedra, Tea (Theophylline)
(iii)	**Drugs acting on cardiovascular system**	
	1. Cardiotonics	Digitalis, Squill, Strophanthus, Arjuna
	2. Cardiac depressants	Cinchona (Quinidine) [Quinine and Quinidine are stereoisomers, the first one is antimalarial but the second one is used in cardiac arrhythmia, tachycardia and arterial fibrillation], Veratrum
	3. Vaso-constrictors and oxytocics	Ergot (Ergometrin maleate is an oxytocic, whereas ergotamine tartarate is used in combination with caffeine in the treatment of migraine). Vasicin from *Adhatoda vasica*
	4. Antihypertensives	Rauwolfia, Forskohlin a labdenone di-terpene from *Coleus forskohlii*
(iv)	**Drugs acting on autonomic nervous system**	
	1. Adrenergics	Ephedra
	2. Cholinergics	Physostigma, Pilocarpus (Pilocarpine nitrate, a life-saving drug useful in glaucoma, extracted from *Pilocarpus jaborandi*
	3. Anticholinergics	Belladonna, Datura
(v)	**Drugs acting on central nervous system**	
	1. Central analgesics	Opium (Morphine)
	2. CNS stimulants	Coffee (Caffeine)
	3. Analeptics	Nux vomica, Lobelia, Camphor
	4. CNS depressants	Hyoscyamus, Belladonna, Opium (Morphine, Codeine)
	5. Hallucinogenics	Cannabis, Poppy latex
(vi)	**Antispasmodics**	
	1. Smooth muscle relaxants	Opium (Papaverine), Datura, Hyoscyamus
	2. Skeletal muscle relaxants	Curare
(vii)	**Anticancer**	Vinca, Podophyllum (Etoposide, Teniposide), Camptotheca, Taxus
(viii)	**Antirheumatics**	Aconite, Colchicum, Guggul
(ix)	**Anthelmintics**	Quassia, Male fern, Vidang
(x)	**Immuno-modulatory agents**	Ashwagandha, Tulsi, Ginseng, Amla
(xi)	**Drugs acting on skin and mucous membrane**	Olive oil, Wool fat, Bees wax, Arachis oil, Sesame oil, Balsam of Tolu, Balsam of Peru
(xii)	**Astringents**	Myrobalan, Black catechu
(xiii)	**Antimalarials**	Cinchona, Artemisia annua (*Artemisinin*)
(xiv)	**Immunising agents**	Vaccines, Sera, Toxoids, Antitoxins
(xv)	**Drugs acting chemotherapeutically**	Antibiotics
(xvi)	**Local anaesthetics**	Coca
(xvii)	**Antileprotics**	Chaulmoogra oil, Asiaticoside is a glycoside useful in leprosy and extracted from *Centella asiatica*
(xviii)	**Antidiabetics**	Pterocarpus, Gymnema, Sylvestro
(xix)	**Diuretics**	Gokhru, Punarnava
(xx)	**Antiseptics and disinfectants**	Benzoin, Myrrh, Nim, Curcuma
(xxi)	**Perfumes and flavouring agents**	Peppermint oil, Lemon oil, Orange oil, Lemon grass oil, Sandalwood oil.
(xxii)	**Pharmaceutical aids**	Honey, Arachis oil, Starch, Kaolin, Pectin, Olive oil, Lanolin, Bees wax, Acacia, Tragacanth, Sodium alginate, Agar, Guar gum, Gelatin.
(xxiii)	**Pesticides**	The ester pesticides obtained from pyrethrum, *Chrysanthemum cinerariifolium* are Pyrethrin I and II
(xxiv)	**Antiplaque**	Sanguinarine an antiplaque alkaloid with both preventive and therapeutic effects on dental plaque

CHAPTER 28

Adulteration and Drug Evaluation

- Drug Adulteration
- Methods of Drug Evaluation
- Identifying Chemical Tests
- Resins
- Fibers, Dressings and Sutures.

Drug adulteration

Adulteration is a practice of substituting original crude drug partially or wholly with other similar looking substances but the later is either free from or inferior in chemical and therapeutic properties. Types of adulterants are as follows :

(i) Substitution with substandard commercial varieties : presence of *Strychnos nux-blanda* or *S. potatorum* in place of *S. nux-vomica*; Indian senna substituted with Arabian senna and dog senna; gentian substituted by Kutki.

(ii) Substitution with superficially similar inferior drugs : Belladonna leaves are substituted with Ailanthus leaves; saffron is admixed with dried flower of *Carthamus tinctorius*.

(iii) Substitution with artificially manufactured substances : Compressed chicory in place of coffee; paraffin wax made yellow coloured and substituted for bees wax.

(iv) Substitution of exhausted drugs : This practice is most common in case of volatile oil containing drugs like fennel, clove, coriander, caraway etc. Sometimes exhausted gentian made bitter with aloes, artificial colouring of exhausted saffron etc.

(v) Use of synthetic chemicals to improve organoleptic characters of the crude drug : Addition of benzyl benzoate to balsam of Peru.

(vi) Presence of vegetative matter from the same plant.

(vii) Harmful adulterants : Pieces of amber coloured glass in colophony, limestones in asafoetida, white oil in coconut oil, cocoa butter mixed with stearin or paraffin.

(viii) Adulteration of powders : Dextrin in ipecacuanha etc.

Methods of drug evaluation

Evaluation of a drug means confirmation of its identity and determination of its quality and purity and detection of nature of adulteration.

1. **Morphological or Organoleptic Evaluation** : It refers to evaluation of drugs by colour, odour, taste, size, shape and special features, like touch, texture etc.

2. **Microscopic Evaluation** : The following 'Leaf Constants' measured with the help of a microscope give some idea about the identification of some crude drugs.

   (i) **Palisade ratio** defined as average number of palisade cells beneath each epiderm cell. It can be determined with powdered drugs.

   (ii) **Vein-islet number** defined as the number of vein-islets per square mm of the leaf surface midway between the midrib and the margin.

   (iii) **Vein-termination number** defined as the number of veinlet terminations per square mm of the leaf surface midway between midrib and margin.

   (iv) **Stomatal number** is average number of stomata per square mm of epidermis of the leaf.

   (v) **Stomatal index** is the percentage which the number of stomata form to the total number of epidermal cells; each stomata being counted as one cell. It is calculated by using the following equation :

   $$S.I. = \frac{S}{E+S} \times 100$$

   where

       S.I. = Stomatal Index

       S = Number of stomata per unit area

       E = Number of epidermal cells in the same unit area.

   The technique of determination of leaf constants can be used for microscopic evaluation of several leaf drugs such as senna, datura, digitalis, buchu, coca, belladonna etc.

   (vi) **Water pores** : Water pores are immovable unlike stomata and they are present on the teeth of the margin.

   (vii) **Trichomes** : Trichomes are the tubular elongated or glandular outgrowth of the epidermal cell. These are another important diagnostic characters helpful in the identification of drugs and detection of adulterants.

   Quantitative Microscopy (Lycopodium spore method) : It is an important analytical technique for powdered drugs, especially when chemical and other methods of evaluation of crude drugs fail as accurate measures of quality. Lycopodium spores are very characteristic in shape and appearance and exceptionally uniform in size (25 μm). On an average, 94,000 spores per mg of powdered lycopodium are present.

3. **Physical Evaluation** :

   (i) **Moisture content** : The moisture content of the volatile oil containing drugs is measured by **toluene** distillation method

   (ii) Viscosity   (iii) Melting point   (iv) Solubility   (v) Optical rotation

   (vi) Refractive index

   (vii) Ash values, extractives and volatile oil content.

       a. Water soluble extractives   b. Alcohol soluble extractives

       c. Ether soluble extractives

   (viii) Foreign Organic Matter

(ix) **Microbiological Limits** : The microbiological limits of some of the items prescribed by the I.P. are given below :

Gum acacia powder	1 g sample of acacia powder is free from *E. coli*.
Guar gum	1 g is free from *E. coli* and Salmonella, and total bacterial count should not be more than 5000 per gram.
Starch	1 g is free from *E. coli* and Salmonella.
Dried yeast	1 g meets the requirement of test for absence of Salmonella and *E. coli*
Gelatin	1 g sample is free from *E. coli*, 10 g is free of Salmonella and total count is not more than 1000 per gram.

4. **Chemical Evaluation** : To detect the different chemical constituents present in the crude drugs.

5. **Biological Evaluation** : When the estimation of potency of crude drug or its preparation is done by means of its effect on living organisms like bacteria, fungal growth or animal tissue or entire animal, it is known as **bioassay**.

Drug substances that either suppress or influence the growth of micro-organisms are generally analyzed by **microbiological assay** method. Antibiotics and a few vitamins fall into this category. The procedure employed in microbial assay of antibiotics may be divided into two broad groups :

(i) Cylinder plate method (cup)   (ii) Turbidimetric method.

Identifying chemical tests

Chemical Tests for Alkaloids

		Name of the reagents	Chemical constituents of the reagents	Observation
COMMON TESTS	i	Mayer's	Potassium mercuric iodide solution	Cream coloured ppt.
	ii	Dragendorff's	Potassium bismuth iodide solution	Reddish brown ppt.
	iii	Wagner's	Iodine-potassium iodide solution	Reddish brown ppt.
	iv	Hager's	Picric acid (saturated solution)	Yellow coloured ppt.
v		Murexide test for purine base (caffeine)	Drug + small amount of $KClO_3$ + a drop of hydrochloric acid → evaporated to dryness and exposed to ammonia vapour	Purple colour
vi		Van Urk's reagent (for ergot alkaloid)	p-dimethylamino benzaldehyde	Blue color.
vii		Vitali's test (Vitali-Morin reaction, for tropane alkaloids)	The tropane alkaloid is treated with fuming nitric acid, followed by evaporation to dryness and addition of methanolic KOH solution to an acetone solution of nitrated residue.	Violet coloration takes place due to tropane alkaloid
viii		Test for indole alkaloids	Sulphuric acid + p-dimethyl – ammonium benzaldehyde	Bluish - violet to red colour
ix		Test for colchicine	Mineral acid	Yellow colour
x		Thalleioquin test for quinine and quinidine	Bromine and ammonia	Colour formation
xi		Marquis Reagent (for opium alkaloid)	Formaldehyde-sulphuric acid	Purple complex

Chemical Tests for Proteins

	Reagents	Constituents	Observation
i	Million's reagent	Mercuric nitrate solution	Red on warming
ii	Iodine test	Iodine solution	Ground substance and crystalloid become yellowish brown and globoids remain unstained
iii	Hager's test	Picric acid	Stains the ground substance and crystalloid yellow

Chemical Tests for Carbohydrates

i	Molisch's test	α - naphthol and conc. H_2SO_4	Purple colour
ii	Reduction of Fehling's solution	Fehling's solution A (cupric sulfate solution) + Fehling's solution B (alkaline sodium potassium tartarate)=potassium cupri-tartarate solution.	Brick red ppt. of cuprous oxide (Cu_2O)
		In case of non-reducing sugar (sucrose, trehalose) boil them with acids to convert to reducing sugar. Then neutralize the acid and perform the test with Fehling's solution.	Do
iii	Osazone formation	Phenylhydrazine hydrochloride + sodium acetate + acetic acid are boiled with sugar solution.	Characteristic sugar derivatives known as Osazones are formed.
iv	Resorcinol test for ketones (fructose, honey or hydrolyzed inulin). This is known as Selivanoff's test	Sample + equivolume conc. HCl + a crystal of resorcinol → Warmed on water bath	A rose colour is produced.
v	Test for pentoses	Sample + equivolume conc. HCl containing a little phloroglucinol → heat	A red colour is produced.
vi	Keller-Kiliani test for deoxy sugars found in cardiac glycosides such as those of digitalis and Strophanthus spp.	The sugar is dissolved in acetic acid containing a trace of ferric chloride and transferred to the surface of conc. H_2SO_4	At the junction of the liquid a reddish-brown colour is produced which gradually becomes blue.
vii	Fiehe's test to detect artificial invert sugar, an adulterant of honey contains furfural	Resorcinol in hydrochloric acid	Gives instant red colour

Chemical Tests for Glycoside

i	Borntrager's test (for anthraquinone glycoside)	The drug is extracted with chloroform, ether, or any other organic solvent. Filtered extract is made alkaline either with caustic soda or ammonia	Aqueous layer shows, after shaking, pink, red or violet colours. Borntrager's test is negative in case of anthranols (reduced form)
ii	Modified Borntrager's test to cleave C-glycoside (casca rosides)	Oxidation with 5% $FeCl_3$ and dilute HCl followed by extraction with organic solvent as in case of Borntrager's test.	Same as in the case of Borntrager's test

iii	General tests for aloes		
	a) Bromine test	1 g aloe powder + 10 ml. water → boiled & filtered. To it added a freshly prepared bromine solution	A pale yellow precipitate of tetrabromalin
	b) Schoenteten's reaction (Borax test)	Little quantity of borax is dissolved in the above filtrate. A few drops of the solution are added to a test tube nearly filled with water	A green fluorescence.
iv	Keller-Kiliani test for digitoxose	Same as before	
v	Legal test for digitalis glycoside	The extract is dissolved in pyridine, sodium nitroprusside solution is added to it and made alkaline	Pink or red colour is produced.
vi	Baljet test for digitalis glycoside	To a section of digitalis, sodium picrate solution is added	Yellow to orange colour is produced.

- The solution of Ruthenium red is used to stain the mucilage.
- Halphen's test is used for cotton seed oil.

Resins

Resins are amorphous acellular/unorganized products of complex chemical nature. Depending upon the type of the constituents of the resin, they are further classified as :

1. Acid resins   Colophony (abietic acid), copaiba (capaivic and oxicopaivic acids), sandrac (sandracolic acid), myrrh (commiphoric acid) and shellac (alleuritic acid).

2. Ester resins   Benzoin (coniferyl benzoate) and storax (cinnamyl cinnamate).

3. Resin alcohols   Balsam of peru (with peruresinotannol), gurjan balsam (with gurjuresinol) and guaiacum resin (with guaic-resinol).

Besides these there are :

- *Oleoresins* are homogenous mixture of resins and oils, e.g. copaiba, Canada balsam, capsicum, etc.
- *Oleo-gum resins* are the homogenous mixture of volatile oil, gum and resin, e.g., myrrh, guggul, asafoetida, etc.
- *Glycoresins* are made up of resins and sugars and are present in jalap and ipomoea.
- *Balsam :* If the resin contains benzoic acid and/or cinnamic acid, it is called as a balsam, e.g., balsam of peru, balsam of tolu, storax etc.
- *Resenes :* These are the complex natural substances without any specific chemical properties. They are chemically inert, neither form any salt nor they get hydrolysed. Examples of the drug containing resenes are gum copal, gutta percha, asafoetida, colophony and dammar.

Fibres, Dressings and Sutures

Fibres from various sources may be categorised as follows :

   (i) Plant fibres : Jute, flax, banana, cotton, hemp.

  (ii) Animal fibres : Silk, wool.

 (iii) Mineral fibres : Glass, asbestos.

 (iv) Synthetic fibres :

     a. Fibres regenerated from carbohydrate materials—alginate yarn, artificial silk or rayon or regenerated cellulose.

     b. Fibres regenerated from protein materials—aridil from groundnut protein and fibrolin from milk casein.

     c. Synthetic—nylon (polyamide), terylene, orlean, etc.

Surgical dressings are classified as :

I. **Fibres :**

   (i) Non-mediated fibres—absorbent cotton, wool, rayon, silk etc.

  (ii) Medicated fibres—boric acid wool, capsicum wool etc.

II. **Fabric :** Absorbent lint, absorbent ribbon gauze, boric acid lint, absorbent gauze, X-ray detectable.

III. **Bandages :**

   (i) Non-medicated—crepe, domette, calico, cotton, rubber, elastic bandage, etc.

  (ii) Medicated—plaster of paris, zinc paste, zinc pastel chthamol.

IV. **Rubber and Oil Impregnated Materials :** Belladonna self-adhesive plaster, zinc oxide self adhesive plaster, etc.

Sutures

These are the sterile threads, strings and strands specially prepared for use in surgery meant for sewing tissues together. They must be sterile and non-irritant. Sutures may be of the following types :

1. **Absorbable Sutures :**

   (a) Sterile catgut (muscular layer of small intestine of sheep, ox and appendix of deer).

   (b) Sterile reconstituted collagen suture.

2. **Non-absorbable Sutures :**

   (a) Sterile non-absorbable sutures (silk and cotton)

   (b) Sterile linen sutures

   (c) Sterile polyamide sutures (nylon)

   (d) Sterile polyester sutures (terylene)

   (e) Sterile braided sutures

   (f) Sterile stainless steel and silver sutures.

3. **Haemostatics :**

   (a) Oxidized cellulose

   (b) Absorbable gelatin sponge.

Chemical Tests for Cotton

1. Soak cotton fibres in aqueous iodine solution and dry. Add few ml of 80% H_2SO_4, trichomes assume purplish-blue or bluish green colour → distinction from hemp, wool, silk, jute, nylon, alginate yarn and acetate rayon.

2. Cuoxam-reagent (ammoniacal copper oxide solution) dissolves raw cotton fibres with the formation of balloons, while absorbent cotton dissolves completely with uniform swelling.

3. Cotton is insoluble in dilute sodium hydroxide solution and hydrochloric acid (distinction from silk). It is soluble in 66% of H_2SO_4.

CHAPTER 29

Synonyms, Biological Source, Family, Chemical Constituents, Uses and Chemical Category

Category	Members	Synonyms	Biological Source	Family	Chemical Constituents	Uses	Chemical Category	Any other
1	2	3	4	5	6	7	8	9
LAXATIVES	Aloes	Musabbar, Kumari	Dried juice of leaves of *Aloe vera* *A. barbadensis* *A. ferox*	Liliaceae	Anthracin glycosides – barbaloin, aloe-emodin	Purgative	Anthracin glycoside	
	Rhuburb	Radix rhei, Rheum, Revandchini	Dried rhizome of *Rheum palmatum* *R. emodi* *R. Webbianum*	Polygonaceae	rhein, aloe-emodin	Purgative, bitter, stomachic	Do	
	Castor oil	Ricinus oil	Castor oil is the fixed oil obtained from the seeds of *Ricinus communis*	Euphorbiaceae	Triglyceride of ricinoleic acid (80%), isoricinoleic acid, linoleic acid, stearic acid and isostearic acid.	Cathartic in the preparation of soap, as an emollient in preparation of lipsticks, ointments, creams and polishing. Castor oil does not freeze at lower temperature and hence, is valuable as lubricant	Ester (triglyceride)	The cathartic property of the castor oil is due to irritant action of **ricinoleic acid.**
	Ispaghula	Isapgol, Isabgol, Isabgul, Indian Psyllium.	Dried seeds of *Plantago ovata*	Plantaginaceae	Mucilage consists of pentosan and aldobionic acid; fixed oils and proteins.	Demulcent laxative, emollient, in constipation, amoebic and bacillary dysentery, crusted seeds are used in the form of poultice for rheumatic pain. Mucilage has other application in ice-cream industry, tablet formulation etc.	Carbohydrate	Both seed and seed coats known as Isapgol husk is used
	Senna	Senna leaf (Indian Senna)	Dried leaflets of *Cassia angustifolia*	Leguminosae	Sennosides A & B	Purgative	Anthracin glycoside	

2	3	4	5	6	7	8	9
	Senna leaf (Alexandrian Senna)	Dried leaflets of *C. acuifolia*	Do	Do	Do	Do	
	Seena pods	Dried nearly ripe fruits of *C. acuifolia and C angustifolia*	Do	Do	Do	Do	
Digitalis	Digitalis leaves, Fox glove leaves	Dried leaves of *Digitalis purpurea*	Scrophulariaceae	Purpurea glycoside A on enzymatic hydrolysis yields Digitoxin and glucose, which on further hydrolysis yields digitoxigenin & 3-digitoxose. Purpurea glycoside B on enzymatic hydrolysis yields Gitoxin & glucose which on further hydrolysis yields Gitcxigenin & 3- digitoxose. It also contains 2 saponin glycosides viz. digitonin and gitoxin.	In the treatment of congestive heart failure. Digitalis blocks the sodium -potassium ATP-ase pump of the cardiac muscle so that intracellular concentration of sodium increased. This leads to increase in calcium ions, released from sarcolemma and thereby, brushing action of proteins viz. actin and myosin is enhanced. This is exhibited as more forceful contraction of myocardium, greater output per beat and complete emptying of heart.	Glycoside	Leaves after collection dried immediately at a temperature below 60°C.
	Austrial Digitalis, woolly fox glove leaf	*Digitalis lanata*	Do	Primary glycosides such as lanatosides A, B, C, D & E. The aglycones viz. digoxigenin and diginatigenin are specific to *D lanata* while others are present in *D. purpurca* also.	Do Digoxin is preferred because of less cumulative effects	Do	Do
	Straw Foxglove	*Digitalis lutea*	Do	The drug is as potent as *D. purpurea*	Do	Do	Used as a common substitute of official drug.
	Spanish Foxglove	*D. thapsi*	Do	The drug is 1.25 to 3 times more potent than *D. Purpurea*	Do	Do	

1	2	3	4	5	6	7	8	9
	Arjuna	Arjuna bark	Dried stem bark of the plant *Terminalia arjuna*	Combretaceae	Tannins, triterpenoid saponin, arjunolic acid (diuretic activity) β-sitosterol, ellagic acid and arjunic acid, arjunine and arjunetine	Cardiotonic antidysenteric, diuretic and tonic properties, hypotensive action with vasodilation and decreased heart rate, used in tanneries.	Miscellaneous (tannins)	
	Urginea	Jangli pyaj, Sea onion, Scilla, Indian squill	Dried slices of the bulbs of *Urginea indica*	Liliaceae	Cardiac glycosides (Scillaren A & B) glucoscillaven A and an enzyme scillarenase.	Cardiotonic, expectorant, diuretic in small doses, emetic and cathartic in large doses. It is less cumulative and acts rapidly than digitalis).	Glycoside	
		European squill, white squill	Dried slices of the bulbs of *U. mariiima*	Do	Do (bufadienolide type cardiac glycoside)	Do	Do	
		Red squill	It is a red variety of European squill i.e., *U. mariiima*	Do	Glycoside called scilliroside and scillirubroside, anthocyanin, pigment is responsible for its red colour	As rat poison.	Do	
	Coriander	Coriander fruits	Dried ripe fruits of *Coriandrum sativum*	Umbelliferae	Volatile oil 0.3 to 1%, Fixed oil 13%, Protein 20%. 90% of the volatile oil is D-linalool (coriandrol) and coriandryl acetate	aromatic, carminative, stimulant and flavouring agent having antigripping action in intestine.	Volatile oil.	
	Fennel	Fructus Foeniculum	Dried ripe fruits of *Foeniculum vulgare*	Do	Volatile oil (3 to 7%)about 20% each of proteins and fixed oil. Chief constituents of the volatile oil is fenchone (pungent and aromatic) and anethole (sweet in odour and taste)	carminative, aromatic and stimulant, expectorant, flavouring agent	Volatile oil	

CARMINATIVES AND GI REGULATORS

2	3	4	5	6	7	8	9
Cardamom	Cardamom fruits Cardamom seeds	Dried ripe fruits of *Elettaria cardamomum*	Zingiberaceae	2 to 8% volatile oil which contains cineol along with other aromatic compounds (terpineol and borneol), fixed oil, starch and protein	Aromatic, carminative stimulant and flavouring agent. It is used in the form of compound tincture	Volatile oil	
Ajowan	Trachyspermum copticum, Carum copticum Hieren	Dried ripe fruits of *Trachyspermum ammi*	Umbelliferae	2 to 4% volatile oil which contains 35-60% thymol, 50-55% p-cymene, 30-35% terpinene, pinene etc., fat (21%) proteins (17%) and carbohydrates (25%)	Antispasmodic, stimulant and carminative, antiseptic, antifungal, insecticide, anthelmintic, and deodorant	Volatile Oil	
Clove	Caryophyllum, clove flower, clove buds	Dried flower buds of *Eugenia caryophyllus*	Myrtaceae	15-20% volatile oil which contains eugenol (70-90%), eugenol acetate, caryophyllenes etc., 10-13% of tannin (gallotannic acid) resin, chromone, eugenin etc.	as dental analgesic, carminative, stimulant, flavouring agent, aromatic and antiseptic. In the manufacture of cigarettes and vanillin	Volatile oil	
Nutmeg	Myristica, Nux Moschata	Dried Kernels of the seeds of *Myristica fragrans*	Myristicaceae	5-16% volatile oil which contains 4-8% myristicin, elimicin and safrole; 30% of fat which contains about 60% myristic acid	aromatic, stimulant, carminative. The fat and volatile oil of nutmeg are used in the treatment of rheumatism	Volatile Oil	
Cinnamon	Cinnamon bark, Kalmi-Dalchini, Ceylon Cinnamon	Dried inner bark of the shoots of *Cinnamomum zeylanicum*	Lauraceae	Volatile oil (0.5-1.0%) tannis (phlobatannins) – 1.2%, mannitol (sweet taste). Cinnamon oil contains 60-70% cinnamaldehyde, 5-10% eugenol, benzaldehyde, cuminaldehyde, phellandrene, cymene, pinene etc.	Carminative, stomachic, mild astringent, flavouring agent, stimulant, antiseptic & aromatic. In the preparation of candy dentifrices and perfumes.	Volatile oil	Substituents & Adulterants :- Jungle Cinnamo, cinnamon chips, Saigon cinnamon, Java Cinnamon
Cassia Cinnamon	Cassia bark, Chinese cinnamon	Dried stem bark of *Cinnamomum cassia*	Do	Volatile oil (cassia oil) – 1 to 2% constituents of which is more or less same.	carminative, stimulant, flavouring agent, aromatic and used in spices	Volatile oil	

2	3	4	5	6	7	8	9
Ginger	Zingiber, Zingiberis	Rhizomes of *Zingiber officinale*	Zingiberaceae	Volatile oil (1-4%) starch (40-60%) fat (10%), protein (10%) etc., resinous matter (5-8%). Ginger oil contains monoterpene and sesquiterpene hydrocarbon, phenyl propanoids. Sesquiterpene hydrocarbon includes α - zingiberene, β- bisabolene, α - farnesene etc.	Stomachic, aromatic, carminative, stimulant etc., in the preparation of mouth wash, beverages, liquors etc.	Volatile oil	
Black pepper		Dried unripe fruit of *Piper anagram*	Piperaceae	Alkaloid piperine (5-9%), volatile oil (1-2.5%), pungent resin (6%), piperidine. Volatile oil contains l- phellandrene & caryophyllene.	Aromatic, stimulant, stomachic and carminative and also as spices	Alkaloid and volatile oil	Substitute: *P. attenuatum* *P. brachystach-yum* *P. longum* Adulterants → Gum arabic, rosin, gypsum, red clay, chalk, barley, wheat flour.
Asafoetida	Devils dung, Gum Asafoetida	Oleo-gum resin obtained by incision from the rhizomes and roots of *Ferula foetida, F. rubricaulis* and other species of Ferula	Umbelliferae	Resin (40-65%), gum (20-25%) volatile oil (4-20%). Resin consist of as a resinotannol in the free or combined form with ferulic acid. The chief constituent of oil is secondary butyl propanyl disulphide	Carminative, nervine stimulant, intestinal flatulence and as flavouring agent for curries, sauces and pickles and in veterinary medicine.	Oleo-gum resin	
Brahmi	Mandukpami	The herbs of *Centella asiatica* or *Hydrocotyl asiatica*	Do	Saponins in the form of α - amyrin derivatives called asiaticoside and madecassoside. They yield asiatic and madecasic acid respectively on hydrolysis. Madras & Lucknow varieties from India also contain brahmoside and bramhinoside	Nervine tonic, sedative. spasmolytic and anti-stress action. Also used in skin disease, leprosy and syphilis	Glycosides	

2	3	4	5	6	7	8	9
Visnaga	Khella, Picktooth fruit	Dried ripe fruits of *Ammi visnaga*	Do	Khellin, visnagin khelloside	Smooth muscle relaxant, used as coronary vasodilator in angina pectoris, renal and uterine colic, bronchial asthma and whooping cough	Miscellaneous	
Ammi		Fruits of *Ammi majus*	Do	Xanthotoxin, bergapten isopimpilin etc.	Xanthotoxin in the active constituents of Methoxsalen USP, used to increase the formation of melanin pigment in the skin	Miscellaneous	The drug, 8-methoxy psoralen, used in the treatment of leucoderma is extracted commercially from the inflorescence of Ammi majus`
Caraway	Carum, Caraway seed	Dried ripe fruits of *Carum carvi*	Umbelliferae	Volatile oil (2.5-8%), fixed oil (10%), proteins and resin (15%). Volatile oil contains 45 to 65% of carvone, limonene, dihydro-carvone and trace of carvacrol	Aromatic, stimulant and carminative. As a spice and flavouring the bread, biscuits, cheese and cakes.	Volatile oil	
Dill	Dill fruits, Anethum, European Dill	Dried ripe fruits of *Anethum graveolens*	Do	Volatile oil (2.4 - 4%), fixed oil (20%), proteins (20%). Chief constituents of volatile oil is carvone (43-63%). It also contains dihydro-carvone, D-limonene, phellandrene and other terpene.	Aromatic, stimulant and carminative. The oil is used in the preparation of dill water, gripe water and also as flavouring agent.	Volatile oil	
Anise	Anise fruit, Aniseed	Dried ripe fruits of *Pimpinella anisum*	Do	1.5-3.5% volatile oil, 10% of fixed oil, proteins, mucilage and starch. The volatile oil mainly contains anethol (90%), methylchavicol (13-15%) and anisaldehyde.	Stimulant, carminative, expectorant, condiment and flavour in foods or beverages and also in the manufacture of dentifrices.	Do	

2	3	4	5	6	7	8	9
Cummin	Jira	Dried ripe fruits of *Cuminum cyminum*	Do	2.5-4% volatile oil which mainly contains cuminaldehyde. 10% of fixed oil and proteins	Stimulant and carminative, in diarrhoea and dyspepsia	Do	
Celery	Celery seed, Apium	Dried ripe fruits of *Apium graveolens*	Do	1.5-3% volatile oil, 15-17% of fixed oil, resin and bitter extractives, volatile oil contains d-limonene (60%), sedanoic acid (0.5%), sedanolide (2.5 to 3) and d-selinine (10%)	Stimulant, carminative, nervine sedative and tonic, in the treatment of rheumatism and as a flavour for soft drink and medicaments	Do	
Black Catechu	Cutch	Dried aqueous extract of heartwood of *Acacia catechu*	Leguminosae	Acacatechin, quercetin	astringent for boils, skin eruptions, mainly used for commercial purposes	Condensed tannins	
Pale Catechu	Gambier	Dried aqueous extract of leaves of young shoots of *Unicaria gambier*	Rubiaceae	Catechin, catechutannic acid	Astringent for treatment of diarrhoea	Do	
Hyoscyamus	Henbane, Hyoscyamus herb and leaves	Dried leaves, or leaves of flowering tops of *Hyoscyamus niger*	Solanaceae	The principal alkaloid is hyoscyamine along with atropine and hyoscine. Hyoscyamine is an ester of tropic acid and tropine, and is more active than the racemic form, i.e., atropine. During the extraction, it is racemized to atropine.	To counteract gripping due to purgative, antispasmodic and to relieve spasms of urinary tract, sedative and used to check salivary secretion, expectorant etc.	Alkaloid (tropane)	
Belladonna herb	Belladonna leaf, Deadly night shade leaf, Belladonna Folium	Dried leaves or the leaves and other aerial parts of *Atropa belladonna* (European), or *A. acuminate* (Indian)	Do	The main alkaloids are l – hyoscyamine and its racemic form atropine. The drug also contains belladonine, scopoletin, hyoscine, pyridine and N-methyl pyrroline	Parasympatholytic with anticholinergic properties to reduce the secretion of sweat, saliva and gastric juice and to reduce spasm due to strong purgative. Also as an antidote in opium and chloral hydrate poisoning.	Do	Adulterants and substituents - leaves of *Phytolacca americana*, *Solanum nigrum* and *Ailanthus glandulosa*

1	2	3	4	5	6	7	8	9
	Aconite	Aconite root, Bachnag, Monkshood	Dried root of *Aconitum napellus*	Ranun-culaceae	The main alkaloid is aconitine along with hypaconitine, neopelline, neoline etc.,	It is a highly poisonous drug. Liniment form is used externally only in the treatment of neuralgia, sciatica, rheumatisms and inflammation. Analgesic and cardiac depressant. Its use is restricted to homeopathic medicine.	Diterpene alkaloid	
	Ashwagandha	Withania root, Asgandh	Dried roots and stem of *Withania somnifera*	Solanaceae	The main constituents are alkaloids and steroidal lactones. The main alkaloid is withanine along with somniferine, somnine, somniferinine, withananine, tropine and pseudotropine etc. Steroid lactones are called as "Withanolides"	Sedative, hypnotic, hypotensive, respiratory stimulant and as immunomodulatory agent. In the treatment of rheumatism, gout, hypertension, nervine and skin disease and also as sex-stimulant.	Alkaloid	
	Ephedra	Ma-Huang	Dried young stems of *Ephedra gerardiana* and *E.nebrodensis*	Gnetaceae	Amino alkaloids such as ephedrine, norephedrine, n-methyl ephedrine pseudo-ephedrine etc.	Sympathomimetic, as a bronchodilator in asthma. In the treatment of allergic hay-fever. Ephedrine through peripheral vaso-constriction action corrects the low blood pressure, whereas ephedradines show hypotensive effect.	Alkaloid	
	Opium	Raw opium	Dried latex obtained by incision from the unripe fruits (capsules) of *Papaver somniferum*. Milky latex comes out from the unripe fruits contains the precursors of opium alkaloids. This latex is dried before collection over	Papaveraceae	Benzylisoquinoline type alkaloids such as Narcotine (noscapine). narceine and papaverine and phenanthrene type alkaloids such as morphine, codeine and thebaine. The opium alkaloids are present as salts of *meconic acid*. The minor alkaloids of opium	Morphine is a potent centrally acting analgesic. It has sedation, nausea, vomiting, respiratory depression and constipation action. Codeine has antitussive effect through minimization of local irritation in the bronchial tract. It has mild analgesic	Alkaloid	Codeine is 3- methyl morphine and Heroin is 3,6-diacetyl morphine

1	2	3	4	5	6	7	8	9
			the fruits in expose to air which turns the milky latex brown which is known as raw opium.		are protopine and hydrocotarnine	action Papaverine has relaxant effect on smooth muscles of blood vessels, intestine and bronchial tract. Narcotine has specific depressant action on cough reflex.		
	Cannabis	Cannabis indica, Indian hemp, Ganja, Mari J(h) uana	Dried flowering tops of the female plants of *Cannabis sativa*	Mouraceae (Cannabinaceae)	Resin (15-20%) containing euphoric principle, 1,3,4-transtetra hydrocannabinol. The other constituents of resin is cannabinol, cannabidiol, cannabidiolic acid, cannabichromene and cannabigerol, volatile oil trigonelline and choline	Narcotic, sedative and analgesic. It's psychotropic properties is mainly due to tetrahydro-cannabinol. It causes euphoria, intoxication and mental disturbances.	Resin	
Do	Nux-vomica	Crow-fig., Semen strychni, Nux vomica seed	Dried ripe seeds of *Strychnos nuxvomica*	Loganiaceae	Strychnine, brucine along with small amount of vomicine, α - colubrine, pseudostrychnine etc. Loganin, a glycoside, also present in Nux-vomica	Bitter tonic and stomachic, stimulate CNS, respiratory and cardio-vascular system, increases blood pressure. Strychnine is more potent than Brucine. Brucine is used for denaturing alcohol, arrow-poison etc.	Indole alkaloids	
ANTI-HYPERTENSIVE	Rauwolfia	Sarpagandha, Chootachand, Serpentine root, Rauwolfia root	Dried roots of *Rauwolfia serpentina*	Apocynaceae	Main alkaloids are reserpine and rescinnamine, along with other alkaloids such as ajmaline, ajmalicine, rauwolfinine, reserpinine, Yohimbine, serpentine etc.	Antihypertensive and mild tranquiliser. Reserpine, rescinnamine and ajmalicine are clinically important	Alkaloid	
ANTI-TUSSIVES	Vasaka	Adulsa, Adhatoda	Dried, as well as fresh leaves of *Adhatoda vasica*	Acanthaceae	Vasicine, vasicinone and 6-hydroxy vasicine along with volatile oil, betain, vasakin and adhatodic acid. After biochemical conversion vasicine is	Expectorant and bronchodilator. Vasicine has oxytocic action and abortificient. Its synthetic derivative is bromohexine hydrochloride	Quinazoline alkaloid	

1	2	3	4	5	6	7	8	9
ANTI-RHEUMATICS	Tolu Balsam	Balsam of Tolu	Solid or semi-solid balsam obtained from the trunk region of the tree *Myroxylon balsamum*	Leguminosae	converted to vasicinone which has bronchodilation effect. Cinnamic acid (12-16%). Benzoic acid (8%) and 7.6% oily liquid containing cinnamicin, benzyl benzoate and benzyl cinnamate. Small amount of toluresinotanol, vanillin and styrol are also present	expectorant and flavouring agent in the preparation of perfumery, chewing gums etc., and also has antiseptic action	Resins and resin combination	
	Tulsi	Holy basil, Sacred basil	Dried and fresh leaves of *Ocimum sanctum*	Labiatae	Volatile oil containing eugenol, carvacrol, eugenol-methyl ether, carryophyllin along with small amount of alkaloids, saponin, tannin, vit. C, maleic acid, tartaric and citric acid	antitussive, antibacterial, stimulant, aromatic, spasmolytic, immuno-modulatory and diaphoretic	Volatile oil	
	Guggul	Scented Bdellium	Oleo-gum-resin obtained by deep incisions of stem bark of *Commiphora weightii*	Burseraceae	Steroids, diterpenoids, carbohydrate and aliphatic esters, guggulosterone and guggulosterol is important	Anti-inflammatory, anti-rheumatic, hypolipidemic and hypocholesteremic	Oleo-gum-resin	
ANTI-TUMOUR	Colchicum	Autumn crocus, Meadow saffron seeds	Dried ripe seeds of *Colchicum luteum and C. autumnale*	Liliaceae	Two main alkaloids – Colchicine and demecolcine	For the treatment of gout and rheumatism. Having anti-tumour activity and used in horticulture as a chemical agent for inducing polyploidy (increase in number of chromosome)	Aminoalkaloids	
	Vinca	Periwinkle, Catharanthus	Dried whole plant of *Catharanthus roseus*	Apocynaceae	Two main alkaloids – Vincristine and vinblastine along with other alkaloids such as ajmalicine, locherine, serpentine and tetra hydroalstonine	Antineoplastic (oncolytic) activity. In the treatment of hodgkin's disease. It is also hypotensive and anti diabetic	Alkaloid	

1	2	3	4	5	6	7	8	9
	Chaulmoogra oil	Hydnocarpus oil Gynocardia oil	Fixed oil obtained from ripe seeds of *Taraktogenos kurzii,Hydnocarpus anthelmintic, H. heterophylla* and other species	Flacourtiaceae	Ester (glycerides) of chaulmoogric acid, hydnocarpic acid and palmitic acid	In the treatment of T.B.. leprosy and psoriasis. It is intended for external use only	Fixed oil	Fatty acids of chaulmoogra oil possess strong bactericidal effect against acid fast organisms *Mycobacterium leprae and M. tuberculosis*
	Pterocarpus	Bijasal, Indian kino tree, Malbar Kino	Juice of the plant *Pterocarpus marsupium*, obtained by making vertical incisions of the stem bark.	Leguminosae	Kinotannic acid, kino-red, kino-pyrocatechin (catechol), resin and gallic acid.	It is a powerful astringent, used in the treatment of diabetes, diarrhoea, dysentery, haemorrhage toothache, dyeing and tanning. Aqueous infusion of the wood is used in diabetes	Tannins	
	Gymnema		Leaves of *Gymnema sylvestre*	Ascelpiadaceae	Pentriacontane, hentriacontane, phytin, resin, gymnemic acid, anthraquinone derivatives etc.	Antidiabetic, stimulant, stomachic, laxative and diuretic	Glycoside	
	Gokhru	Punchuvine	Dried fully riped fruits of plant *Tribulus terrestris*	Zygophyllaceae	Alkaloids (harman and harmine), fixed oil, resin, essential oil, saponins which on hydrolysis give steroidal sapogenins like diosgenin, gitogenin, chlorogenin and ruscogenin, flavonoid, kaempferol etc.	Diuretic, demulcent, aphrodisiac (arousing sexual desire), primary nephritis and kidney stone.	Alkaloid and glycoside	
	Punarnava	Hog weed, Rakta Punarnava	Fresh as well as dried plants known as *Boerthanvia diffuss*	Nyctaginaceae	An alkaloid- punarnavine, potassium nitrate and other potassium salts, ursolic acid, β - sitosterol	As diuretic and in chronic edema, expectorant, stomachic, anti-inflammatory. In treatment of jaundice, enlargement of spleen, improves digestive power	Alkaloid	

1	2	3	4	5	6	7	8	9
ANTI-DYSENTRICS	Ipecacuanha	Ipecac	Dried root and rhizome of *Cephaelis ipecacuanha* and *C. acuminata*	Rubiaceae	The principal alkaloids are emetine, cephaeline, psychotrine, o-methyl psychotrine and emetamine, along with ipecacuanhic acid and a glycoside ipecacuanhin.	Expectorant in small doses and emetic in higher doses. Cephaeline has more emetic and less expectorant action than emetine. Emetine hydrochloride has strong action against *Entamoeba histolytica* and used parenterally to treat amoebic dysentery.	Iso-quinoline alkaloid	
ANTISEPTICS AND DISINFECTANTS	Benzoin	Sumatra Benzoin	Balsamic resin obtained from *Styrax benzoin or S. paralleloneurus* or other species of styrax, or *S. tonkinesis* (Siam benzoin)	Styraceae	Sumatra benzoin contains balsamic acids (benzoic, cinnamic) and their esters, triterpenoid acids (sumaresinolic acid and siaresinolic acid). Siam benzoin contains coniferyl benzoate, styrol, vanillin and cinnamate.	Benzoin is an irritating expectorant, carminative and diuretic, used externally as an antiseptic and protective, as perfumes and to mask the unpleasant taste of pharmaceutical preparation.	Balsamic resin	
	Myrrh	Gum Myrrh, Bol	Oleo-gum-resin obtained from *Commiphora molmol*, and also from other species of commiphora	Burseraceae	Volatile oil, gum, resin and bitter principle, α, β and γ commophoric acids, α,β - heerabomyrrholic acids, terpenes, cuminic aldehyde, eugenol etc.	Stimulant, antiseptic and protective. Tincture is used as astringent in mouth washes and gargles.	Oleo-gum resin	
	Neem		*Azadirachta indica*	Meliaceae	Azadirachtin (from leaves and seed), → Meliantriol and Salanin→ (from leaves), Nimbin and Nimbidin → (from seed and bark). Nimbosterol, Myricitin,→ Kaempferol Deacetylazadirachtinol → (fruit) Seed oil ↑	Insect repellant Antifeedant Antiviral Insecticidal paralyzes insects, spermicidal activity. Bark and root has also antibacterial and anti-fungal activity.	Natural pesticide	

1	2	3	4	5	6	7	8	9
ANTI-MALARIAL	Turmeric	Curcuma, Indian saffron	Dried and fresh rhizomes of *Curcuma longa* and other species of Curcuma	Zingiberaceae	Volatile oil, resins, starch, yellow colouring substance (curcuminoids), the chief constituent of which is curcumin. Volatile oil contains α- and β pinene, α-phellandrene, camphor, camphene, zingiberene etc.	As a condiment or spice and colouring agent, anti-inflammatory and anti-arthritic etc.	Resin and Resin combination	
	Cinchona	Peruvian bark, Jesuit's bark	Dried bark of *Cinchona calisaya*, *C. ledgeriana*, *C. officinalis* *C. succirubra* or a suitable hybrid	Rubiaceae	Important alkaloids are quinine, quinidine, cinchonine, cinchonidine along with quinicine, cinchonicine, hydroquinine, hydrocinchonidine, homocinchonidine etc. Cinchona alkaloids are present as salt of Quinic acid and cinchotanic acid. Quinovin, a glycoside, also present in cinchona	Anti-malarial, active against protozoa like *Plasmodium vivax*, *P. falciparum* (malignant malaria), *P. malarie and P. fatal*. It is also used as bitter stomachics, antipyretic	Quinoline alkaloids	Quinine and quinidine are stereoisomers. The former is anti-malarial but the later is anti-arrhythmic used in cardiac arrhythmia as cardiac depressant.
OXYTOCIC	Ergot		Dried sclerotium of a Fungus, *Claviceps purpurea*, developed in ovary of rye plant	Clavicipitaceae or Hypocreaceae	Potent indole alkaloids, which are derivatives of lysergic acid, also called as peptide alkaloids. Only levoforms are medicinally active but dextro forms are inactive	Ergometrine (also known as ergonovine) maleate is used as oxytocic to enhance the labour pains during delivery and also to prevent post-partum haemorrhage. Ergotamine tartarate is used as specific analgesic in treatment of migraine. Lysergic acid diethylamide (LDS) is a	Indole alkaloid	Rye plant is host and ergot is a parasite

1	2	3	4	5	6	7	8	9
					Levo-form **Dextro-form** Ergometrine Ergometrinine Ergotamine Ergotaminine Ergosine Ergosinine Ergocristine Ergocristinine Ergocryptine Ergocryptinine Ergocornine Ergocorninine	semisynthetic derivative, possesses psychotomimetic action and used in psychiatry. Because of its abuse it is narcotic drug. Ergot derivatives such as methyl ergometrine in small doses are used after delivery to control bleeding and maintain uterine firmness.		
VITAMINS — Shark liver oil	Oleum selachoids	Fixed oil obtained from the liver of various species of the shark, mainly *Hypoprion brevirostris and Galeorhinus zyopterus.*		Vitamin A, Glycerides of the saturated and unsaturated fatty acids.	In Vitamin A deficiency as anti-xerophthalmic factor.	Vitamin	I g of oil should contains not less than 6000 I.U. of Vitamin A.
Amla	Indian Goose berry, Emblica	Dried as well as fresh fruits of *Emblica officinalis.*	Euphorbiaceae	It is a rich source of Vitamin C (600 to 750 mg per 100 g of the fresh pulp), minerals (such as phosphorus, iron and calcium), fat, phyllemblin and tannin	used as an acrid, diuretic and laxative. Dried fruits are used in diarrhoea, dysentery, jaundice and anaemia (along with iron compound), also used to prepare inks, hair oil, shampoo etc. Seeds are used in the treatment of bronchial asthma. Fixed oil of fruits possesses the property of promoting hair growth.	Vitamin	
ENZYMES — Papain		It is a mixture of proteolytic enzymes derived from the latex of unripe fruit of melon tree, *Carica papaya*	Caricaceae	Proteolytic enzymes – papain, chymopapain	As enzyme, clarification of beverages, as a meat tenderiser, in cheese manufacturing as a substitute of rennin, degumming of silk fabrics in textile industry, as an anti-inflammatory agent.	Enzyme	
Diastase	Amylase	Amylotic enzyme present in saliva i.e.,		Amylotic enzyme. Also used in fermentation and	As digestant	Enzyme	Zymase, maltase,

1	2	3	4	5	6	7	8	9
			salivary diastase or ptyalin and pancreatic diastase or amylopsin are obtained from animal. It is also formed during the germination of barley grain, known as Malt-diastase.		brewing industry to convert starch to fermentable sugar.			sucrase, cellulase, invertase, hyaluronidase, lysozyme are some important amylolytic enzymes.
	Yeast		It consist of unicellular fungal micro-organisms *Saccharomyces cerevisiae*	Saccharo-mycetaceae	The enzymes invertase, diastase, zymase, and maltase along with traces of thiamine, riboflavin, nicotinic acid, pantothenic acid, folic acid, biotin etc.	In the manufacture of alcohol, beer, various wines and bread, glutathion and invertase are also manufactured from yeast. As a source of vitamin D.	Enzyme	Wine yeast, baker's yeast, brewers yeast, distillers yeast are some common examples of various types of yeast.
PERFUMES AND FLAVOURING AGENTS	Peppermint oil	Mentha oil, Colpermin, Oleum Mentha piperita	The oil obtained by steam distillation of the fresh flowering tops of *Mentha piperita*.	Labiatae	The chief constituent is menthol. Other constituents are menthone, mentho furan, jasmone, menthyl isovalerate, menthyl acetate, terpene derivatives such as limonene, isopulegone, cineole, pinene, camphene etc. Jasmone and esters are responsible for pleasant flavour.	As carminative, stimulant and flavouring agent. In the preparation of tooth-paste, tooth powders, shaving creams, different pharmaceutical dosage forms, chewing gums, candies, jellies, perfumes etc. As antiseptic, muscle relaxant, steam inhalant etc.	Volatile oil	
	Lemongrass oil	Indian Melissa oil, East Indian Lemon-grass oil	Volatile oil obtained by steam distillation from the leaves and aerial parts of *Cymbopogon flexuousus and C. citratus* etc.	Graminae	Citral along with methyl heptenol, nerol, citronellal, dipentene and geraniol.	As a flavouring agent. Citral is used to prepare β-ionine, which is a starting material for the synthesis of vitamin A.	Do	

2	3	4	5	6	7	8	9
Oil of Sandal wood	Oil of sandal Wood. East Indian Sandal Wood Oil	Obtained by distillation from the heart-wood of *Santalum album*	Santalaceae	Two isomeric sesquiterpene alcohols, α-santalol and β-santalol; an aldehyde santalal; santene, santenone, teresantol, santalone and santalene	In the symptomatic treatment of dysurea (painful or difficult urination), in diminishing the frequency of micturition. As a perfume	Volatile oil	
Orange Oil		Volatile oil obtained by expression from the fresh peel of the ripe fruit of *Citrus sinensis*	Rutaceae	Volatile oil containing 1-2% decanal, more than 90% limonene	Flavouring agent	Volatile oil	Some volatile oils cannot be distilled without decomposition and are usually obtained by expression (lemon oil, orange oil)
Lemon Oil		Volatile oil obtained by expression, from the fresh peel of the fruit of *Citrus limon*	Rutaceae	Terpenes chiefly of (+)-limonene, monoterpene hydrocarbons such as β-pinene and γ - terpinene. Lemon oil flavour is mainly due to neral and geranial (together called citral)	As flavouring agent (food, cosmetics and liquid cleansers), stimulant, carminative and stomachic	Volatile oil	
Honey	Madhu, Honey Purified Mel	Sugar secretion deposited in honey comb by the bees, *Apis mellifera* *A. dorsata* and other species of Apis.	Apidae	Glucose, fructose, sucrose, maltose, gum traces of succinic acid, acetic acid, dextrin, formic acid, colouring matter, vitamins and enzymes (invertase, diastase, inulase)	As demulcent and sweetening agent, nutrient, mild antiseptic, as vehicle in the preparation of cough mixture, cough drops, creams lotions, soft drinks, candies etc.	Carbohydrate	Artificial invert sugar, an adulterant of honey contains furfural, which is detected by Fiehe's test. It gives instant red colour with resorcinol in hydrochloric acid

2	3	4	5	6	7	8	9
Arachis oil	Ground nut oil, Peanut oil	Fixed oil expresses from the seed kernels of *Arachis hypogaea*	Leguminosae	Triglycerides of fatty acids, chiefly oleic, linoleic, stearic and arachidic acid. Other acids are lignoceric and palmitic acids. The polyunsaturated fatty acid content of this oil is about 31%.	As edible oil, non-aqueous solvent for intramuscular injection, in the preparation of liniments, plasters, soap and as lubricant. In the preparation of non-staining iodine ointment	Triglycerides (fixed oil)	Raw oil may contain aflatoxin (a carcinogenic substance produced by the fungal growth), which needs refining.
Starch	Amylum	Polysaccharide granules obtained from the grains of *Zea mays* (maize), *Oryza sativa* (rice), *Triticum aestiuum* (wheat)	Gramineae	Two polysaccharides – amylose (β - amylose) and amylopectin (α-amylose), in the proportion of 1:2. Amylose is water-soluble and gives blue colour with iodine. Amylopectin is water insoluble, but swells in water and responsible for gelatinising properties and gives bluish black colour with iodine.	As nutritive, demulcent, protective and absorbent, used in the preparation of glucose, dextrose and dextrin. As tablet disintegrating agent paste is used as binder. It is also used as diluent in dry extract of crude drug, as antidote in iodine poisoning, sizing of paper and cloth, as a component of dusting powder.	Carbohydrate	
		or from the tubers of *Solanum tuberosum* (potato)	Solanaceae				
Kaolin	China-clay, porcelain clay	Powdering of native kaolin, elutriating and collecting the fraction, which complies with the requirements of particle size		Hydrated aluminium silicate	Adsorbent, as filter aid, excipient in poultices, dusting powder. As filler in paper, rubber, paint etc. It is believe that light Kaolin with very high surface area adsorb toxin from the G.I tract and used in the treatment of enteritis, dysentery and in alkaloidal and food poisoning.	Clay	Light kaolin and Heavy kaolin chemically are same. The former is very light having low bulk density due to low particle size

2	3	4	5	6	7	8	9
Pectin		Lemon peel, orange peel, apple pomace, carrots, sunflower heads etc. are the source of pectin *Citrus-limon, C. aurantium.*	Different, mainly Rutaceae	Pectins are polyuronides which on hydrolysis yields D-galacturonic acid, methyl alcohol, small amount of galactose and arabinose; pectic acid.	As a sorbent in the treatment of diarrhoea, as a haemostatic for internal and external haemorrhage, as emulsifying agent, gelling agent in acid medium & as a plasma substitute. In food industry as thickening agent for sauces, jams, ketchup etc., in cosmetic preparations. Pectin in combination with gelatin has been suggested to be used as an encapsulating agent in pharmaceutical formulations to promote sustained release.	Carbohydrate	
Olive oil	Oleum Olivae	Fixed oil expressed from the ripe fruit of *Olea europoea*	Oleaceae	Triglycerides (ester of glycerol with fatty acids) mainly in the form of olein, palmitin and linolein.	Externally, it is an emollient and soothing agent. Internally it is used as nutrient, demulcent and also, as mild laxative. It is used as a vehicle for oily suspensions for injection.	Triglyceride	
Lanolin	Hydrous wool fat, Adeps Lanae	Purified fat like substance obtained from the wool of the sheeps, *Ovis aries.* It contains 25-30% water and therefore is commonly called hydrous wool fat. Anhydrous Lanolin (water content not more than 0.25%) is usually referred to as wool fat.	Bovidae	Esters and polyesters of 33 high molecular weight alcohols and 36 fatty acids. Mainly esters of cholesterol and isocholesterol with caranubic, oleic, myristic, palmitic, lanoceric and lanopalmitic acids.	As water absorbable ointment base. It is a common ingredient and base for several water soluble creams and cosmetic preparations	Ester	In very few cases lanolin can be allergic also.

2	3	4	5	6	7	8	9
Bees wax	Yellow Bees wax, Cera-flava	Purified wax obtained from the honey comb of the bees *Apis mellifera* & other species of Apis.	Apidae	Ester of straight-chain monohydric alcohol with straight chain acids. The chief constituent of the bees wax is myricin i.e., myricyl palmitate; free cerotic acid, aromatic substance cerolein etc.	As an ingredient of ointment base as hardening (stiffening) agent, plasters, polishes, candles, dental preparation, lipsticks, face creams etc. It is an ingredient of Paraffin Ointment I.P.	Ester	White bees wax obtained by bleaching yellow bees wax and should not be used for ophthalmic purpose due to the presence of residual amount of toxic bleaching agent.
Acacia	Indian gum, Gum acacia, Gum arabic	Dried gummy exudation obtained from the stem and branches of *Acacia arabica*	Leguminosae	Arabin (a complex mixture of calcium, magnesium and potassium salts of arabic acid). It also contains enzyme oxidase, and peroxides	Acacia is a demulcent. As suspending agent, emulsifying agent. It is a very good binding agent and used in the preparation of compressed tablets, lozenges, pastilles. In combination with gelatin, it is used to form coaservate for microencapsulation of drug.	Carbohydrate	
Tragacanth	Gum Tragacanth	Dried gummy exudation obtained by incision from steams and branches of *Astragalus gummifer* and other species of Astragalus	Leguminosae	Tragacanth in (water-soluble portion of Tragacanth) and bassorin (water insoluble portion of Tragacanth), tragacanthic acid. Methoxy group present (about 15%) is responsible for its high viscosity.	As demulcent, emollient suspending agent, emulsifying agent. In combination with acacia used as suspending agent. Mucilage is used as a binding agent in the tablet and also as an excipient in the pills; as an adhesive, in lotions, spermicidal jellies, and ice-cream.	Carbohydrate	

1	2	3	4	5	6	7	8	9
	Sodium alginate	Algin, Sodium polymannur-onate.	It is the sodium salt of alginic acid (polyuronic acid composed of reduced mannuronic and glucoronic acids) obtained from the brown seaweed (algae). The common species are *Macrocystis pyrifera*, *Laminaria hyperborea*, *Laminaria digitata*, & *Ascobyllum nodosum*	Phaeophyceae	Alginic acid which is polyuronic acid composed of reduced mannuronic and glucoronic acids.	In the preparation of paste, cream, jellies, ice-cream etc. As thickening, suspending agent, stabilizing emulsion, as binding and disintegrating agent. It can be sterilized by autoclave and is preserved by the addition of 0.1% of chloroxylenol, chlorocresol, benzoic acid or parabens.	Carbohydrate	
	Agar	Agar-agar, Japanese-Isinglass, vegetable gelatin.	Dried gelatinous substance obtained from *Gelidium amansii* and several other species.	Gelidaceae and Gracilariaceae	Two polysaccharides known as agarose (responsible for gel strength of agar) and agaropectin (responsible for the viscosity of agar solution)	Mainly used for the preparation of bacteriological culture medium, also used as emulsifying agent, bulk laxative, in the preparation of jellies etc.	Sulphonated polysaccharide	
	Guar Gum	Guar flour, Jaguar gum	Powder of the endosperm of the seeds of *Cyamopsis tetragonolobus*	Leguminosae	The chief water soluble constituent is Guaran, a high molecular weight hydrocolloidal polysaccharide.	As protective colloid, binding disintegrating and emulsifying agent, bulk laxative, appetite depressant, in peptic ulcer therapy, textile, cosmetic and food industry	Polysaccharide	
	Gelatin		Gelatin is extracted from the collagenous tissue like skins, tendons ligaments and bones of animal		Gelatin is a protein, naturally contains different amino acids mainly lysine. Gelatin is mainly composed of glutin protein.	In manufacture of hard and flexible capsule shells, pessaries, suppositories etc. In the preparation of bacteriological culture media, microcapsules. Absorbable gelatin sponge is used as haemostatic. As a vehicle for certain injection, like hepari.. in the form of	Protein	The quality of gelatin is expressed as "bloom strength". It is the weight in gram which when applied to a plunger, 12.7 mm in

1	2	3	4	5	6	7	8	9
								diameter under controlled conditions shall
	Liquorice	Glycerrhiza, Glycerrhiza radix, Liquorice root, Mulethi	Dried root and stolon of *Glycyrrhiza glabra* and other species of Glycyrrhiza	Leguminosae	The chief constituent of liquorice is a triterpenoid saponin known as glycyrrhizin, which is a potassium and calcium salt of glycyrrhizinic acid. Glycyrrhizinic acid is a glycoside. Liquorice also contains flavonoids (liquiritin and isoliquiritin) useful in peptic ulcer treatment.	As an expectorant, demulcent flavouring agent for tobacco, pharmaceutical preparation etc, in cough mixture. Antigastric effect (due to flavonoid). It has also antispasmodic effect due to flavonoid glycoside isoliquiritin. It is also used as sweetening agent.	Glycoside	produce a depression exactly 4 mm deep in a jelly matured at 10°C & containing 6.66% w/w gelatin in water.
	Garlic	Allium	bulbs of *Allium sativum*	Liliaceae	Carbohydrates, proteins, fat, mucilage and volatile oil along with phosphorus, iron and copper. Chief active constituent is volatile oil, which contains allyl propyl disulphide, diallyl disulphide, alliin and allicin.	As carminative, aphrodisiac (arousing sexual desire), expectorant, stimulant, disinfectant, anthelmintic, rubefacient. Garlic oil is useful in high blood pressure and atherosclerosis.	Volatile oil	
	Picrorrhiza	Indian gentian, Kutki	Dried rhizomes of the plant *Picrorrhiza kurroa*	Scrophulariaceae	Picroside I & II & Kutkoside	As bitter tonic, antiperiodic, febrifuge (dispelling fever) and stomachic, laxative in large doses and to treat jaundice	Glycoside	
	Dioscorea	Yam, Rheumatism root	Dried tubers of *Dioscorea deltoidea, D. composita* and other species of Dioscorea	Dioscoreaceae	The chief constituent of dioscorea is diosgenin a steroidal sapogenin. Rhizomes are also found to contain an enzyme sapogenase. Tubers are	Diosgenin being steroidal in structure is used as precursor for synthesis of several cortisco-steroids, sex hormones, oral-contraceptives etc.	Steroid	

MISCELLANEOUS

1	2	3	4	5	6	7	8	9
					also rich in glycosides, phenolic compounds etc. Diosgenin is the hydrolytic product of saponin-dioscin.	Dioscorea is also used in the treatment of rheumatic arthritis.		
	Linseed oil		Fixed oil obtained from the dried fully ripe seeds of *Linum usitatissimum*	Linaceae	Glycerides of palmitic, stearic, oleic, linolic and linolenic acids. It also contains sterols, tocopherol, squalene, cyanogenetic glycoside linamarin and mucilage.	In the preparation of lotions, liniments, paints, varnishes, soap, plasticisers, greases etc. It has high iodine value and used in the preparation of non-staining iodine ointment and also in the preparation of cresol with soap solution.	Triglycerides	
	Shatavari	Shatmuli	Dried roots and leaves of the plant known as *Asparagus racemosus*	Lilliaceae	Shatavari contains 4 steroid saponins shatavarin I, II, III & IV. In shatavarin I glycoside 3 glucose and one rhamnose moieties are attached with sarsapogenin, where as in shatavarin IV two glucose and one rhamnose moieties are attached.	As galactogogue, tonic and diuretic. It has anti-oxytocic property and used in threatened abortion and safe delivery by uterine blocking activity in the treatment of rheumatism and nervine disorders.	Glycoside	
	Pyrethrum	Insect flowers, Dalmation Insect Flowers	Expanded flower heads of *Chrysanthemum cinerariaefolium*	Compositae	Insecticidal principles such as pyrethrin I & II, cinerin I & II and Jasmoline I & II. Pyrethrum also contains pyrethrosin, pyrethrol and sesquiterpene lactones	Naturally occurring insecticides and pesticides	Esters	
	Tobacco	Nicotine	Volatile liquid alkaloid obtained from the dried leaves of the tobacco, i.e., *Nicotiana tabacum*	Solanaceae	Nicotine	Insecticide and pesticides		
	Shankha pushpi	Shankhud, Shankhphull	Aerial parts of the plant *Conscoradecussata schunt*	Gentianceae	Bitter principle, oleo resin, triterpenes, alkaloids and xanthones	Bitter, nervine tonic, entire plant and fresh juice are used in insanity, epilepsy, nervous disability and as antiviral		

	2	3	4	5	6	7	8	9
LOCAL ANAESTHETICS	Coca leaves	Coca	Dried leaves of *Erythroxylon coca and E. truxillense*	Erythroxylaceae	Derived tropane alkaloids such as cocaine cinamyl cocaine, α- truxilline, cinnamoylecgonine, tropocaine benzoyltropine, dihydroxy-tropane, benzoylecgonine etc.	Cocaine is local anaesthetic; as stimulant, restorative and also in convulsions; CNS stimulating action and reduces the sedative and respiratory depressant effects of morphine and allied drugs. It has hallucinogenic and addictive effect.	Topane alkaloid.	

CHAPTER 30

Model Questions
of Pharmacognosy

- Model Questions of Pharmacognosy

---

1. The evaluation of a crude drug is necessary because
   A. biochemical variation in the drug
   B. deterioration of active principle due to treatment and during storage
   C. substitution and adulteration deliberately or as a result of carelessness or ignorance
   D. all of the above.
2. The term "Organoleptic evaluation" refers to
   A. evaluation of organic matter present in the crude drug
   B. evaluation with the help of sensory organs
   C. evaluation based on organic reactions
   D. none of the above.
3. The term "Chemomicroscopy" refers to
   A. the use of a compound microscope fitted with eye-piece micrometer
   B. the microscope whose mechanism of action is based on chemical reaction
   C. the study of constituents by application of chemical methods to small quantities of crude drugs
   D. none of the above.
4. The number of stomata per unit area of a leafy drug is 80 and the number of epidermal cells in the area is 12. The Stomatal index would be
   A. 86.96   B. 80.0   C. 12.0   D. 92.0
5. Clove is classed as a flower. It contains
   A. Safrole   B. Eugenol   C. Anethol   D. Cineole

6. All the volatile oils mentioned below are separated and collected by way of steam distillation. The exception is
   - A. sandal wood oil
   - B. lemon oil and orange oil
   - C. lemon grass oil
   - D. rose oil
   - E. peppermint oil

7. The opium alkaloids are present as
   - A. free bases
   - B. free acids
   - C. salts of meconic acid
   - D. salts of tartaric acid
   - E. none of the above

8. Codeine is
   - A. 3,6-dimethyl morphine
   - B. 6-methyl morphine
   - C. ethyl morphine
   - D. 3-methyl morphine
   - E. none of the above

9. Heroin is
   - A. 3,6-diacetyl morphine
   - B. brown sugar
   - C. addictive
   - D. all of the above
   - E. none of the above

10. A glycoside present in nux-vomica seed is
    - A. loganin
    - B. strychnine
    - C. brucine
    - D. vomicine
    - E. all of the above

11. All the following statements regarding rescinnamine are true except
    - A. it is an alkaloid
    - B. it is a stereoisomer of reserpine
    - C. it is obtained from the root of *Rauwolfia serpentina*
    - D. it is an inactive form of reserpine
    - E. it is an anti-hypertensive

12. A glycoside present in ipecacuanha is
    - A. emetine
    - B. cephaeline
    - C. ipecacuanhin
    - D. psychotrine
    - E. all of the above

13. A glycoside present in cinchona is
    - A. quinovin
    - B. quinine
    - C. quinidine
    - D. cinchonine
    - E. all of the above

14. Quinidine is
    - A. a stereo isomer of quinine
    - B. an anti-arrhythmic used in cardiac arrhythmia
    - C. obtained from cinchona
    - D. a cardiac depressant
    - E. all of the above

15. Cinchona alkaloids are present as
    - A. free bases
    - B. free acids
    - C. salts of meconic acid
    - D. salts of quinic and cinchotanic acid
    - E. none of the above

16. Terpenes are characterized by the presence of repeat unit of
    - A. isoprene
    - B. ethylene
    - C. acetyl groups
    - D. butene

17. The cathartic action of the castor oil is due to the irritant action of
    A. palmitic acid   B. stearic acid   C. oleic acid
    D. anthraquinone glycoside   E. ricinoleic acid
18. Fresh leaves of digitalis after collection should be dried
    A. immediately at a temperature below 60°C
    B. immediately at a temperature below 0°C (freeze drying)
    C. immediately above 100°C for quick evaporation of moisture
    D. under shade
    E. none of the above
19. The most preferred digitalis cardiac glycoside due to its less cumulative effect is
    A. digitoxin   B. gitoxin   C. digitonin   D. digoxin   E. lanatoside B
20. Sweetish odour and taste of fennel is mainly due to
    A. fenchone present in volatile oil fraction
    B. anethole present in volatile oil fraction
    C. the fixed oil present
    D. the presence of protein
    E. none of the above
21. All the statements about xanthotoxin are true except
    A. it is obtained from a plant source *Ammi majus*
    B. it is extracted from fruits
    C. it is an active constituents of Methoxsalen USP
    D. it is oxytocic in nature
    E. it increases the formation of melanin pigment in the skin
22. Cineole is a terpene belonging to the class of
    A. sesquiterpene B. monoterpene C. diterpene   D. triterpene
23. All the statements regarding 'hyoscyamine' are correct except
    A. it is an ester of tropic acid and tropine
    B. it is more active than atropine
    C. it is a racemic form of atropine
    D. during extraction it is recemized to atropine
    E. it is an indole alkaloid
24. An alkaloid present in opium and having smooth muscle relaxant effect is
    A. morphine   B. papaverine   C. codeine   D. narcotine   E. narceine
25. The euphoric action of cannabis is due to the presence of
    A. 1,3,4-transtetrahydrocannabinol   B. cannabidiol
    C. cannabichromene   D. cannabigerol   E. volatile oil
26. The synonym(s) of cannabis is
    A. cannabis indica   B. Indian hemp   C. ganja
    D. mari-j(h)uana   E. all of the above
27. The pleasant flavour of peppermint oil is due to the presence of
    A. menthol   B. menthone   C. jasmone and esters
    D. menthofuran   E. none of the above

28. The flavour of the lemon oil is mainly due to the presence of
    A. limonene   B. β-pinene   C. γ-terpinene
    D. neral and geranial (citral)   E. all of the above

29. Following are the drugs of mineral origin except
    A. bentonite   B. veegum   C. calamine   D. kaolin   E. talc
    F. pectin   G. kieselguhr

30. Which one of the following is derived from the plant source?
    A. Olive oil   B. Gelatin   C. Veegum   D. Lanolin   E. Kaolin

31. Which of the following pharmaceutical aid is also known as "vegetable gelatin"?
    A. Acacia   B. Tragacanth   C. Sodium alginate
    D. Agar   E. Guar gum

32. Which of the following gummy material is derived from the endosperm of seed?
    A. Acacia   B. Tragacanth   C. Sodium alginate
    D. Agar   E. Guar gum

33. "Pitkin's menstruum" for heparin injection contains which of the following ingredients along with dextrose, acetic acid and water?
    A. Gelatin   B. L-lysine mono hydrochloride
    C. Ferric chloride   D. Alcohol   E. None of the above

34. Which is the isomeric pair?
    A. Thymol-carvacrol   B. Anethole-safrole   C. Citral-geraniol
    D. Menthol-eugenol

35. Reserpine and Rescinnamine differ from each other in respect of
    A. methylation at C-10   B. acetyl group at C-16   C. methylation at C-17
    D. acetyl group at C-18

36. Most alkaloids occur in nature as
    A. free bases
    B. water soluble salts
    C. alcohol soluble salts of organic acids
    D. insoluble salts of organic acids

37. Liebermann Burchard test is performed for detecting
    A. hormonal steroids   B. phytosterols   C. cardenolide aglycones
    D. desoxysugars of glycosides

38. Tropane alkaloids show their pharmacological activity by
    A. blocking phosphodiesterase in the muscles
    B. sympathetic ganglionic blocking
    C. parasympathetic ganglionic blocking
    D. cholinergic receptor blocking

39. Among the purine alkaloids which compound has the highest diuretic activity?
    A. 3,7-Dimethyl xanthine   B. 1,3,7-Trimethyl xanthine
    C. 1,7-Dimethyl xanthine   D. 1,3-Dimethyl xanthine

40. Morphine is present in

    A. *Atropa belladonna*   B. *Solanum nigrum*   C. *Ricinus communis*

    D. *Papaver somniferum*

41. Morphine and heroin differ from each other in respect of

    A. methyl group on nitrogen

    B. acetyl groups at C_3 and C_6

    C. absence of double bond between C_5 and C_6

    D. absence of 'D' ring

42. A rhamno-glucoside on complete hydrolysis will give

    A. aglycone + fructose + rhamnose

    B. aglycone + ribose + rhamnose

    C. aglycone + rhamnose + glucose

    D. rhamnose + fructose

43. Indian (Tinnevelly) and African senna leaves differ from each other with respect to

    A. vein-islet number   B. stomatal index   C. colour

    D. all of the above

44. Salicin, a phenolic glycoside, on hydrolysis yields

    A. salicylic acid + glucose

    B. phenol + glucose

    C. salicyl alcohol + glucose

    D. salicyl aldehyde + glucose

45. Wagner's test is used to detect the presence of

    A. steroids   B. alkaloids   C. glycosides   D. terpenes

46. Atropine on hydrolysis with barium hydroxide gives

    A. tropanol and tropic acid

    B. ecgonine and benzoic acid

    C. benzyl ecgonine and methanol

    D. scopine and tropic acid

47. *Claviceps purpurea* yields after infecting overies of graminaceous plants :

    A. reserpine   B. polypeptides   C. lysergic acid derivatives

    D. digitoxin

48. Idioblasts of crystal layer of calcium oxalate is a diagnostic feature of :

    A. *Hyoscyamus niger* leaves

    B. deadly night shade leaves

    C. cinchona bark

    D. senna leaves

49. Anamocytic type of stomata are found in the leaves of

    A. *Urginea maritima*

    B. *Atropa belladonna*

    C. Fox glove

    D. *Cassia acutifolia*

50. Peroxidase enzyme present in acacia is identified by
    A. oxidation and treatment with benzidine
    B. oxidation and extraction in benzene
    C. Molisch's test
    D. Borntrager's test

51. More of earthy matter in a rhizome is determined by
    A. total ash value
    B. the earthy material is separated and then weighed
    C. acid insoluble ash value
    D. the rhizome is washed in water and then in hydrochloric acid finally it is weighed

52. The gummy nature of *Astragalus gummifer* is dependent on
    A. the carbohydrate content
    B. more of hydroxyl groups of the sugar moiety
    C. more of protein content of the drug
    D. more of methoxyl groups of bassorin

53. The sugar moiety of *Digitalis purpurea* is
    A. 2 : 6 deoxy allose
    B. 2 : 6 deoxy glucose
    C. 2 deoxy rhamnose
    D. 2 : 6 deoxy galactose

54. Reserpine on hydrolysis gives
    A. reserpic acid + methyl alcohol + trimethoxy cinnamic acid
    B. reserpic acid + methyl alcohol + trimethoxy benzoic acid
    C. reserpic acid + acetic acid + trimethoxy benzaldehyde
    D. reserpic acid + methyl alcohol + trimethoxy cinnamaldehyde

55. Powdered ergot when treated with sodium hydroxide solution develops
    A. a strong odour of ammonia
    B. a strong odour of trimethylamine
    C. a strong odour of indole
    D. a strong odour of urea

56. Powdered digitalis is dried at a temperature
    A. not exceeding 60°C   B. 65°C
    C. 75°C   D. 100°C

57. Alkaloids in cinchona bark are detected by
    A. Iodine test
    B. Thalleioquin test
    C. Leibermann-Burchard test
    D. Nessler's test

58. Strychnine produces which of the following colors in the presence of sulfuric acid and potassium dichromate?
    A. Reddish-orange   B. Black   C. Yellow green
    D. Blue violet   E. Brown

59. Aloes are used to treat
    A. burns   B. gastritis   C. blood dyscrasias
    D. carcinomas   E. vertigo

60. Most volatile oils are rich in
    A. sulfur-containing compound
    B. fluorinated hydrocarbons
    C. purines and pyrimidines
    D. glucocorticoids
    E. terpenes and sesquiterpenes

61. Opium is obtained by
    A. levigation followed by extraction
    B. chemical synthesis
    C. incision of unripe capsules of a plant
    D. extraction from leaves of a plant
    E. repeated maceration of unorganised drug

62. Which of the following alkaloids has steroidal structure?
    A. Conessine   B. Morphine   C. Atropine   D. Caffeine

63. Which of the following crude drug contains higher concentration of eugenol?
    A. Tulsi   B. Clove   C. Fennel   D. Coriander

64. Keller-Kiliani Test is performed to identify the following drug.
    A. Cocaine   B. Senna   C. Atropine   D. Digoxin

65. Wool wax alcohol is
    A. cholesterol   B. cetyl alcohol   C. stearyl alcohol
    D. myricyl alcohol   E. phytosterol

66. Which of the following is insoluble in alcohol?
    A. Resins   B. Volatile oils   C. Gums   D. Ether   E. Esters

67. The emetic action of morphine is due to
    A. irritation of gastrointestinal tract
    B. stimulation of emetic chemoreceptor trigger zone
    C. stimulation of medullary vomiting center
    D. stimulation of cerebral cortex
    E. none of the above

68. Colchicine is used mainly to treat
    A. high blood pressure   B. diabetes   C. cancer
    D. arthritis   E. gout

69. One procedure in the treatment of digitalis intoxication is to
    A. administer diuretics to the patient
    B. administer quinidine
    C. stop the administration of the drug
    D. supplement K^+ salts
    E. use permanganate or tannin as antidote

70. The action of quinidine differs from that of digitalis in
    A. decreasing irritability of cardiac muscle
    B. preventing passage of impulses to the ventricle
    C. reducing conductivity
    D. increasing irritability of heart muscle
    E. none of the above
71. Morphine stimulates
    A. propulsive contractions in small intestine of man
    B. biliary and pancreatic secretions
    C. human uterus at full term
    D. propulsive peristaltic waves in colon
    E. non-propulsive rhythmic contractions of small intestine of man.
72. Cardiac glycoside consists of
    A. amino acid and sugar
    B. a steroid combined with sugar residue
    C. a polypeptide and sugar
    D. none of the above
73. Which of the following is useful in severe cases of dysentery?
    A. Sulfamylol   B. Pyrvinium salts   C. Lithium salts
    D. Emetine   E. Praziquantel
74. Oxytocin is used to
    A. raise blood pressure   B. treat hypogonadism   C. induce labor
    D. treat amenorrhea (absence or abnormal stoppage of the menses)
    E. prevent conception
75. A source of anticarcinogenic drugs is
    A. belladonna   B. nux vomica   C. cascara   D. digitalis   E. vinca rosea
76. Capsicum is used in OTC liniments
    A. to promote easy spread
    B. as an analgesic
    C. for its odor
    D. to produce warmth or heat
    E. none of the above
77. Overuse of digitalis may result in
    A. habituation   B. tolerance   C. cumulative poisoning
    D. addiction   E. physical dependence
78. Strychnine deaths in humans usually occur from
    A. fatigue of spinal reflexes
    B. cardiac failure
    C. fatigue of respiratory muscles
    D. kidney failure
    E. exhaustion of the respiratory center

79. Strychnine acts by
    A. stimulating acetylcholine production
    B. stimulating cholinesterase production
    C. inhibiting cholinesterase
    D. stimulating nerve cell metabolism
    E. depressing inhibitory centers in the spinal cord
80. The action of digitalis is enhanced by
    A. magnesium   B. potassium   C. chloride   D. sodium   E. calcium
81. The first toxic symptoms of digitalis poisoning are
    A. undue depression of heart rate
    B. gastrointestinal irritation
    C. flushing of skin
    D. cerebral excitement
    E. colored vision
82. The principal active alkaloid of ipecac is
    A. yohimbine   B. apomorphine   C. caffeine   D. lobeline   E. emetine
83. Which of the following drug is derived from entire plant?
    A. Aconite   B. Digitalis   C. Vasaka   D. Ephedra
84. Codeine acts as a cough sedative by
    A. depressing bronchiolar secretions
    B. depressing cough center
    C. depressing pulmonary action
    D. producing mild nausea
    E. paralyzing sensory nerves of bronchi
85. The greatest threat from morphine poisoning is
    A. renal shutdown
    B. respiratory depression
    C. paralysis of spinal cord
    D. damage of kidney
    E. heart failure
86. A very common side effect of morphine is
    A. allergic response   B. blood dyscrasias   C. constipation
    D. liver damage   E. kidney damage
87. Chemically "Wagner's reagent" is
    A. potassium mercuric iodide solution
    B. potassium bismuth iodide solution
    C. iodine in KI solution
    D. saturated picric acid solution
88. Which of the following symptoms is NOT present in digitalis intoxication?
    A. AV block   B. Visual disturbances   C. Vomiting
    D. Ventricular tachycardia   E. Vagal arrest of the heart

89. A class of plant alkaloids that are widely used to treat migraine is
    A. ergot alkaloids   B. belladonna alkaloids   C. stramonium alkaloids
    D. opium alkaloids   E. vinca alkaloids

90. Ergotamine is indicated to which of the following diseases or conditions?
    A. Hay fever   B. Epilepsy   C. Gout   D. Migraine   E. Insomnia

91. A common side effect of ephedrine is
    A. rashes   B. blood dyscrasias   C. ulcers
    D. drowsiness   E. nervousness

92. The common side effect of reserpine is
    A. postural hypotension   B. constipation   C. respiratory distress
    D. agranulocytosis   E. stomatitis (generalized inflammation of the oral mucosa)

93. Colchicine can give false-positive tests for
    A. glucose   B. uric acid   C. RBC   D. ketones   E. urates

94. Which of the following is classified as a polysaccharide?
    A. Lactose   B. Maltose   C. Saccharin
    D. Starch   E. Cyclamate sodium

95. The cardiac glycoside, due to its high water solubility, most irregularly absorbed from the
    G.I. tract is
    A. digoxin   B. gitalin   C. ouabain (stropanthin)
    D. lanatoside C   E. digitoxin

96. Colchicine is usually administered orally in a dose of
    A. 5 µg   B. 50 µg   C. 500 µg   D. 5 mg   E. 50 mg

97. Which of the following antineoplastics is a plant alkaloid?
    A. 6-Mercaptopurine   B. Vincristine   C. Cytarabine
    D. Busulfan   E. Chlorambucil

98. Vitali Morin test is done for the identification of
    A. atropine   B. pilocarpine   C. morphine   D. reserpine

99. Which of the following is NOT soluble in or miscible with Alcohol USP?
    A. Acacia   B. Methanol   C. Ether   D. Phenol   E. Water
    D. Phenobarbital E. Water

100. Which is NOT true for camphor?
    A. Has a therapeutically useful topical antipruritic action
    B. Dissolves readily in water
    C. Forms eutectic mixture with menthol or thymol or phenol
    D. Can be powdered by rubbing with a small amount of alcohol or ether
    E. Is a ketone

101. Xanthines such as caffeine and theophylline exert all of the following pharmacological
    effects except
    A. cardiac stimulation

    B. peripheral vasoconstriction
    C. central nervous system stimulation
    D. relaxation of smooth muscle
    E. diuresis

102. Papaverine is used primarily for its ability to produce
    A. cough suppression
    B. skeletal muscle relaxation
    C. analgesia
    D. vasodilation
    E. emesis

103. The ergot alkaloids have been found to be useful in the treatment of migraine, headaches and are also used extensively as
    A. oxytocics
    B. skeletal muscle relaxants
    C. antineoplastic
    D. nasal decongestants
    E. local anesthetics

104. Which of the following cardiac glycosides, due to its high lipophilicity, is most completely absorbed after oral administration?
    A. digoxin   B. lanatoside   C. digitoxin   D. ouabain   E. gitalin

105. Which of the following is not an effect of atropine on the human body?
    A. Mydriasis
    B. Reduction of gastrointestinal tone
    C. Stimulation of gastric secretion
    D. Diminished sweating
    E. Cardiac stimulation

106. The constipating component of camphorated tincture of opium is
    A. codeine   B. heroin   C. morphine
    D. oxymorphone   E. hydrocodone.

107. The cardiac glycoside present in digitalis leaf in the largest amount is
    A. gitalin   B. ouabain   C. digoxin   D. lanatoside C   E. digitoxin

108. Ipecac fluid extract was deleted from the official compendia because it
    A. could not be assayed accurately
    B. was too weak to be therapeutically useful
    C. had poor chemical stability
    D. was sometimes confused with ipecac syrup
    E. tended to evaporate

109. Which of the following drugs is derived from bark?
    A. Ipecac   B. Coca   C. Cassia   D. Senna

110. Which of the following is insoluble in 60% H_2SO_4 solution?
    A. Jute   B. Absorbent cotton   C. Rayon
    D. All of the above

111. In cerebral and spinal sedative the natural product belongs to
   A. Solanaceae   B. Labiateae   C. Umbelliferae
   D. Apocynaceae

112. Lanolin has been reported to be a sensitizing agent. The component(s) of lanolin believed to be allergic is/are the
   A. low-molecular-weight esters
   B. aromatic alcohols
   C. minor impurities that may be present
   D. wool wax alcohols
   E. aliphatic fraction of the lanolin acids

113. Which of the following is NOT a pharmacological effect of morphine?
   A. CNS depression   B. Diarrhoea   C. Nausea and vomiting
   D. Respiratory depression E. Constriction of the pupils

114. The major effects of Opium Tincture USP are related to its content of
   A. morphine   B. papaverine   C. codeine
   D. dihydrocodeinone   E. alfentanil

115. The function of papain in a soft contact lens product is to
   A. keep the lens soft
   B. remove proteinaceous residues
   C. remove oil films
   D. disinfect
   E. prevent dehydration of the lens

116. In congestive cardiac failure, digitalis glycosides are used because it increases
   A. the heart rate
   B. the force of myocardial contraction
   C. the venous pressure
   D. the cardiac filling pressure

117. Rancidity of a fat is due to
   A. oxidation   B. saponification   C. hydrolysis
   D. neutralisation

118. Fruits which are derived from the plants umbelliferae are all of the type
   A. cremocarp   B. pericarp   C. epicarp
   D. mesocarp

119. Amygdaline on hydrolysis gives
   A. mandelonitrile + benzaldehyde
   B. mandelonitrile + benzaldehyde + glucose
   C. mandelonitrile + glucose
   D. mandelonitrile + benzaldehyde + rhamnose

120. Digoxin
   A. has its action terminated by metabolism in the liver
   B. has a plasma $t_{1/2}$ of 6 hours

    C. should be given half of its normal dose to hypothyroid patients

    D. provides benefit in atrial fibrillation by increasing the force of contraction

121. Vinca alkaloids are isolated from

    A. *Catharanthus roseus* and contain indole and indoline moieties

    B. *Roseo chromogens* and contain indole and indoline moieties

    C. *Catharanthus roseus* and contain quinoline and quinaldine moieties

    D. *Catharanthus indicus* and contain quinoline and indole moieties.

122. Ergot is the sclerotium of

    A. fungus *Claviceps purpurea*

    B. fungus *Claviceps notatum*

    C. *Strychnos mixpotatorum*

    D. fungus *Penicillum chrysogenum*

123. Cocaine is a monoacid tertiary base, on treatment with hot dilute acids produces

    A. ecgonine, methyl alcohol and scopic acid

    B. ecgonine, methyl alcohol and cinnamic acid

    C. ecgonine, methyl alcohol and benzoic acid

    D. ecgonine, ethyl alcohol and benzoic acid

124. Diosgenin is

    A. an alkaloid obtained from dioscorea

    B. a carbohydrate obtained from dioscorea

    C. a glycoside obtained from dioscorea

    D. none of the above

125. Senna Leaf I.P. consists of

    A. dried leaflets of *Cassia acutifolia* and *Cassia angustifolia*

    B. dried leaflets of *Cassia indica*

    C. dried leaflets of *Cassia carpinifolia*

    D. dried leaflets of *Cassia carpinifolia* and *Cassia acutifolia*

126. Natural camphor is

    A. an optically inactive aldehyde obtained from *Cinnamomum camphora*

    B. a white dextrorotatory ketone obtained from the wood of *Cinnamomum camphora*

    C. a white optically inactive ketone obtained from the bark of *Cinnamomum camphora*

    D. a white volatile aldehyde obtained from the bark of *Cinnamomum camphora*

127. The principal constituent anethole (50-60%) and fenchone (18-20%) is present in the volatile oil obtained from

    A. fruits of *Ammi visnaga* Linn

    B. fruits of *Foeniculum capillaceum* G (*F. vulgare*)

    C. fruits of *Carum carvi* Linn

    D. fruits of *Anethum graveolens* Linn

128. Caffeine on oxidation with $KClO_3/HCl$ gives

    A. trimethyl alloxan and urea

    B. methyl alloxan and dimethyl urea

    C. dimethyl alloxan and methyl urea

    D. none of the above

129. Which one of the following general characteristics is not true for alkaloids?
    A. Nitrogen in the hetrocyclic nucleus
    B. Good solubility in organic solvents
    C. pK_as less than 7
    D. Exhibit optical activity

130. Borntrager's test is performed for identification of
    A. digitoxin   B. reserpine   C. digoxin   D. dianthrone of rhein

131. Choose the correct name for Digitoxigenin.
    A. 3β,14β,16β-trihydroxy cardenolide
    B. 3β,12β,14β-trihydroxy cardenolide
    C. 3β,14β-dihydroxy cardenolide
    D. 1,3,5,11α,14,19β-hexahydroxy cardenolide

132. Ellipsoidal schizolysigenous oils glands are important diagnostic characteristics of
    A. ergot   B. ginseng   C. cinnamon   D. clove

133. Hyoscyamine an alkaloid obtained from *Atropa belladonna*
    A. readily racemises to atropine with ethanolic alkali. Atropine is (±) Hyoscyamine
    B. readily disintegrates into atropine with acid solution. Atropine is (−) Hyoscyamine
    C. readily rearranges into atropine with alkali solution. Atropine is (+) Hyoscyamine
    D. readily racemises to atropine with ethanolic alkali

134. The opium alkaloids in *Papaver somniferum* is present as one of the following. Identify.
    A. Free alkaloids
    B. As salts of citric acid
    C. As salts of meconic acid
    D. None of the above

135. The biological source of cinnamon bark is
    A. dried inner bark of the shoots of coppiced trees of *Cinnamomum zeylanicum*; Family - Lauraceae.
    B. dried inner bark of the shoots of coppiced trees of *Cinnamomum indium*; Family - Lauraceae
    C. dried wood bark of *Cinnamomum camphora*; Family - Lauraceae
    D. dried inner bark of the shoots of coppiced trees of *Cinnamomum loureirii*; Family - Lauraceae.

136. Which of the following is (are) true of the ergot alkaloids? I. Natural source is a fungus; II. Their salts would be compatible with acids; III. Used as oxytocic or antimigraine drugs.
    A. I only   B. III only   C. I and II only
    D. II and III only   E. I, II and III

137. One of the uses given below for opioids (synthetic morphine-like compounds which are non-habit forming, but possess the medicinal activity of morphine) is not correct. Indicate.
    A. Antitussive   B. Analgesic   C. Anti-inflammatory
    D. Antidiarrhoeal

138. Choose the correct characteristic of the epidermal cells and cuticle of *Atropa belladonna* leaf.
    A. Pitted walls with striated cuticle
    B. Wavy walls with striated cuticle
    C. Algal cells walls with smooth cuticle
    D. Striated walls with wavy cuticle
139. Starches from various sources may be characterised by
    A. gelatinisation temperature
    B. carbohydrate content
    C. iodine colour test
    D. NMR spectroscopy.
140. Which one is not related with leaf characteristics?
    A. Vein-islet   B. Palisade ratio   C. Idioblasts
    D. Annular layers.
141. The sound of fracture test is categorised under
    A. organoleptic test   B. physical evaluation
    C. physico-chemical test   D. test for water content.
142. Concentrations of calcium carbonate formed on out growths of the cell wall are termed
    A. otoliths   B. cystoliths   C. rosette   D. idioblast.
143. Covering trichomes may be
    A. either unicellular or pluricellular
    B. always unicellular
    C. always multicellular
    D. none of the above.
144. Cutin by chemical nature is
    A. carbohydrate   B. fatty acids mixture   C. proteins
    D. flavones.
145. Resorcinol test for ketones is known as
    A. Selivanoff's test   B. Molisch's test   C. Mayer's test
    D. Grignard test
146. In α-methyl glycoside the -OCH_3 is
    A. axial   B. equatorial   C. endo   D. exo
147. Indian squill is cut and dried fleshy inner scales of the bulb of
    A. foxglove   B. *Digitalis purpurea*   C. *Pimpenella anisum*
    D. *Urginea maritima.*
148. Lanatoside-E, carbohydrate portion contain
    A. 3-digitoxose, 1-acetyl group, 1-glucose
    B. 3-digitoxose, 1-acetyl group, 1- fructose
    C. 3-digitoxose, 1-glucose
    D. 3-digitoxose, 1-fructose.

149. Flavonol glycoside amongst the following compound is
   A. amygdaline   B. rutin   C. arbutin   D. digoxin

150. Cardenolides contain following ring
   A. unsaturated β-lactone   B. unsaturated α-lactone   C. unsaturated δ-lactone
   D. unsaturated γ-lactone

151. Anthraquinone derivatives in glycosides are
   A. bi-cyclic   B. tri-cyclic - linear type   C. tri-cyclic - angular type
   D. tetracyclic

152. Useful test for detecting anthraquinone glycosides is
   A. Benedict's test   B. Fehling's test   C. Borntrager's test
   D. none of the above

153. Amygdaline on complete hydrolysis gives
   A. benzaldehyde + HCN + sugars
   B. cinnamaldehyde + HCN + sugars
   C. salicylaldehyde + HCN + sugars
   D. none of the above

154. Sinigrin on hydrolysis gives
   A. acrinyl isothiocyanate
   B. β-hydroxybenzyl isothiocyanate
   C. allyl isothiocyanate
   D. benzyl isothiocyanate.

155. The active principle of picrorrhiza is
   A. picrotoxin   B. picrosides   C. endotoxins   D. sennosides

156. Tobacco contains following alkaloid
   A. caffeine   B. anabasine   C. coniine   D. atropine

157. Coca leaf contains alkaloid cocaine which shows the activity
   A. antihypertensive   B. antispasmodic   C. local anaesthetic
   D. diuretic.

158. The arrow poison alkaloid used by South Americans is
   A. curare   B. colchicine   C. lobeline   D. atropine

159. Rauwolfia alkaloid belongs to the chemical class of
   A. quinoline   B. isoquinoline   C. piperidine   D. indole

160. A crude drug containing anticancer properties
   A. *Catharanthus roseus*   B. nux vomica   C. *Rauwolfia serpentina*
   D. *Papaver somniferum*

161. Ergot alkaloid have the pharmacologic action
   A. antipsychotic   B. diuretic   C. hypnotic   D. oxytocic

162. LSD a drug of abuse may be synthesised from
   A. morphine   B. cocaine   C. ergot   D. cannabis

163. The useful test for detection of alkaloids in the crude drug is
    A. Dragandroff's reagent   B. Fehling's test   C. Red dye test
    D. Benedict's test
164. Psychotrine may be converted to emetine by
    A. ethylation and reduction
    B. methylation and reduction
    C. reduction and methylation
    D. none of the above
165. Essential oils are called as essential oils because
    A. they are essential to the plant
    B. they produce essence
    C. they are essential for perfumery
    D. none of the above
166. Lemon peel is rich in terpenes chiefly of
    A. thymol   B. eugenol   C. citral   D. limonene
167. Spearmint contains :
    A. carvone + limonene   B. eugenol + citral   C. cresol + carvone
    D. guaiacol + thymol
168. Drug(s) derived from natural sources is/are I. chloroquine; II. liquorice; III. digitalis; IV. neostigmine.
    A. I only   B. II and III only   C. I, II, III only
    D. all the above
169. Heroin is a
    A. natural product   B. semi-synthetic product   C. synthetic product
    D. none of the above
170. Which of the following alkaloid is liquid in nature?
    A. Morphine   B. Reserpine   C. Atropine   D. Nicotine
171. Which of the following is the drug of choice for acute gout?
    A. Probenecid   B. Allopurinol   C. Indomethacin
    D. Colchicine
172. The anticoagulant heparin is obtained from
    A. sheep's lung   B. dog's kidney   C. rabbit's heart
    D. rat's uterus
173. The principal constituent anethole and fenchone is present in the volatile oil obtained from
    A. *Ammi visnaga*   B. *Foeniculum capillaceum*   C. *Carum carvi*
    D. *Anethum graveolens*
174. Which one of the following is an important plant glycoside used as anticancer agent?
    A. Vincristine   B. Podophyllin
    C. Mitomycin   D. Emetine

175. An antitussive alkaloid obtained from opium
    A. morphine   B. emetine   C. codeine   D. reserpine

176. Quinine is obtained from
    A. tulsi   B. sarpagandha   C. cinchona   D. vasak

177. Which one of the following is obtained from animal source?
    A. Atropine   B. Morphine   C. Physostigmine
    D. Insulin

178. Which part is used for therapeutic activity of digitalis?
    A. Leaves   B. Whole aerial part   C. Seeds
    D. Roots and rhizomes

179. Myristicin is the active constituent of
    A. myrobalan   B. nutmeg   C. mustard   D. mylabris

180. Chebulic acid is obtained from
    A. myrobalan   B. black catechu C. cinchona   D. clove

181. Which of the following alkaloids is not present in opium?
    A. Codeine   B. Thebaine   C. Morphine   D. Papaverine   E. Cyclazocaine

182. Which of the following drug is derived from the seed?
    A. Acacia   B. Castor   C. Saffron   D. Clove

183. Which of the following drugs contains/classified "resinous substance" as phytoconstituents?
    A. Capsicum   B. Wax   C. Catechu   D. Pectin

184. In congestive cardiac failure the natural product used belongs to the family.
    A. Apocynaceae   B. Leguminosae   C. Scrophulariaceae
    D. Solanaceae

185. Which of the following adrenergic drugs occurs in nature in plants?
    A. Adrenaline   B. Salbutamol   C. Noradrenaline
    D. Ephedrine

186. Heparin is
    A. an extract of animal tissue B. a metal   C. an extract of plant
    D. none of the above

187. Which of the following drugs contains/classified, "alkaloid" as phyto-constituents?
    A. Acacia   B. Colchicum   C. Aloe   D. Castor

188. Which of the following drugs contains classified, "steroidal glycoside" as phytoconstituents?
    A. Digitalis   B. Quillia   C. Senna   D. Cascara

189. Marquis reagent in the presence of opium alkaloids gives which of the following colours?
    A. Red   B. Orange   C. Purple   D. Green   E. Yellow

190. Hashish is directly related to
    A. opium   B. heroin   C. marijuana   D. LSD   E. mescaline

191. A natural product is used in Hodgkin's disease, whose family is

    A. Apocynaceae   B. Rubiaceae   C. Labiatae

    D. Leguminosae

192. Which one of the following is true for alkaloidal bases?

    A. Water solubility and organic solvent insolubility

    B. Water insolubility and organic solvent insolubility

    C. Water solubility and organic solvent solubility

    D. Water insolubility and organic solvent solubility

193. Which of the following is not a natural alkaloid?

    A. Papaverine   B. Ergotamine   C. Scopolamine

    D. Lobeline   E. Apomorphine

194. A test solution for alkaloids used to test for completeness of extraction is

    A. hydrogen sulfide   B. silver nitrate   C. mercury potassium iodide

    D. mercuric oxide   E. gold chloride

195. Which of the following statements most correctly describes the solubility of alkaloids?

    A. Sparingly soluble in water, soluble in dilute acid.

    B. Sparingly soluble in water, soluble in nonpolar solvent.

    C. Sparingly soluble in water, insoluble in dilute acid.

    D. Insoluble in water, insoluble in dilute acid.

    E. Insoluble in water, insoluble in nonpolar solvent.

196. Emetine is used in the treatment of

    A. amebiasis   B. tuberculosis   C. malaria

    D. schistosomiasis   E. none of the above

197. Which one of the following is a class I controlled drug?

    A. Morphine   B. Heroin   C. Paregoric

    D. Demerol   E. None of the above

198. The principal use of ephedrine is

    A. diuretic   B. antiarrhythmic   C. treatment of shock

    D. bronchodilator   E. antineoplastic

199. Which one of the following general characteristics is NOT true for alkaloids?

    A. Have poor water solubility

    B. Often exhibit stereoisomerisms

    C. Contain nitrogen in the molecule

    D. Have good alcohol solubility

    E. Have pK_as less than 7

200. Vinblastine and vincristine act by

    A. Interfering with the synthesis of transfer RNA

    B. Inhibiting the fragmentation of DNA

    C. Binding to protein

    D. Incorporating into folic acid metabolism

201. An OTC cough syrup that contains ipecac as the expectorant is

    A. cerose   B. novahistine   C. robitussin   D. triaminic   E. trind

202. Which of the following narcotics may not be used for medicinal purposes in this country?

    A. Diacetylmorphine   B. Ethylmorphine   C. Methylmorphine

    D. Dihydrocodeinone   E. All are permitted

203. Lanolin differs from wool fat in that lanolin

    A. contains more water   B. contains less water   C. has been further purified

    D. is obtained from natural sources

    E. contains a greater quantity of cholesterol

204. Given below in A to L are the list of synonym of drugs. Match them correctly with the common name of the drugs given below.

    (i)   Aloes   A. Radix rhei
    (ii)   Rhubarb   B. Jangli pyaj
    (iii) Digitalis   C. Jira
    (iv)   Urginea   D. Deadly night shade leaf
    (v)   Cinnamon   E. Musabbar
    (vi)   Asafoetida   F. Fox glove
    (vii) Cumin   G. Kalmi-Dalchini
    (viii) Belladonna herb   H. Devil's dung
    (ix)   Ephedra   I. Periwinkle
    (x)   Rauwolfia   J. Indian saffron
    (xi)   Vinca   K. Ma-Huang
                              L. Sarpagandha

205. Given below are the chemical nature of alkaloids (A to G) and the natural drugs of pharmacognostic origin from which they are isolated. Match them correctly.

    (i)   Aconite   A. Tropane alkaloid
    (ii)   Nux vomica/Ergot   B. Quinazoline alkaloid
    (iii) Hyoscyamus/Belladonna/Coca   C. Isoquinoline alkaloid
    (iv)   Vasaka   D. Quinoline alkaloid
    (v)   Colchicum   E. Indole alkaloid
    (vi)   Ipecacuanha   F. Amino alkaloid
    (vii) Cinchona   G. Diterpene alkaloid

206. Given below are the pharmacological actions of the alkaloids listed in A to E. Match them correctly.

    (i)   Alkaloid having strong analgesic action   A. Ephedrine
    (ii)   Alkaloid having bronchodilator action   B. Quinidine
    (iii) Alkaloid having CNS stimulating action   C. Reserpine
    (iv)   Alkaloid having antiarrhythmic action   D. Morphine
                                                        E. Strychnine

207. Choose the most appropriate action from the group (A to E) below to match the drugs.

    (i)   Cocaine   A. Central stimulant
    (ii) Codeine   B. Acetylcholinesterase inhibitor
    (iii) Physostigmine   C. Cardiotonic
    (iv) Atropine   D. Relief of mild pain
                                   E. Mydriatic

208. Choose the most appropriate item (from A to E) below related to the substances listed.

    (i)   Alkaloidal substances occurring in some Solanaceous plants. A. Claviceps purpurea
    (ii) An aglycone with a dianthrone structure. B. Apomorphine
    (iii) Source of lysergic acid derivatives. C. Sennidin
    (iv) Alkaloidal substance not occurring in nature. D. *Thevetia peruviana*
                                   E. Steroidal alkamines

209. Given below are some microscopial diagnostic features of the drugs listed in A to E. Choose the appropriate one.

    (i)   Unlignified seplate fibre A. Rhubarb
    (ii) Raphides of calcium oxalate embedded in mucilage B. Liquorice
    (iii) Anisocytic type of stomata C. Ginger
    (iv) Star spots. D. Squill
                                   E. Solanaceous plants

210. Following are the reactions/test observed in case of drugs listed in A to E. Match them correctly.

    (i)   When fixed oil is exposed to U.V. rays, blue fluorescence is produced. A. *Digoxin*
    (ii) On oxidation with $KMnO_4$, benzaldehyde odour is perceived. B. Benzoin
    (iii) With ammoniacal quaxom characteristic balooned fibre is seen under microscope. C. Cinchona
    (iv) Bark powder exhibits fluorescence with sulphuric acid. D. Palmolein
                                   E. *Gossypium barbadance*

211. Listed in A to E are some of the analytical constants. Match them correctly with the drugs given below.

    (i)   A leafy drug A. Total Ash value
    (ii) A bark B. Cineole content
    (iii) Eucalyptus oil C. Fibre length
    (iv) A fixed oil having more of unsaturated fatty acid glycerides. D. Iodine value
                                   E. Stomatal index

212. Given below in A to E are the list of drugs. Appropriate tests are given below for the drugs. Match them correctly.

    (i)   Alcoholic solution of α-naphthol and sulphuric acid. A. Atropine
    (ii) Murexide test. B. Reserpine

(iii) Para dimethylamino benzaldehyde

(iv) Ninhydrin

C. Caffeine

D. Gelatin

E. *Triticum sativum* powder

213. Match the following

    (i) Amaranth   A. Ointment base

    (ii) Acacia   B. Suspending agent

    (iii) Petrolatum   C. Coloring agent

    (iv) Starch paste   D. Binding agents for tablets

                       E. Flavouring agent

214. Match each drug with the appropriate dosage, dosage range given.

    (i) Digoxin   A. 0.5 to 1.5 mg

    (ii) Codeine   B. 65 mg

                    C. 0.3 to 0.4 μg

                    D. 125-750 mg per day

215. Match the following.

    (i) Weakest of the phenanthrene analgesics   A. Morphine

    (ii) No antagonism by nalorphine   B. Methadone

    (iii) Most abundant alkaloid in opium   C. Codeine

                                        D. Papaverine

216. Match the following oils with the appropriate synonyms given below in A to E.

    (i) Peanut oil   A. Cocoa butter

    (ii) Theobroma oil   B. Teel oil

    (iii) Olive oil   C. Arachis oil

    (iv) Castor oil   D. Oleum ricini

                    E. Sweet oil

217. Given below is a list of medicinal plants. Choose for each one of them appropriate names (from A-E) as they are commonly called.

    (i) *Digitalis purpurea*   A. Periwinkle

    (ii) *Atropa belladonna*   B. Thorn apple

    (iii) *Vinca rosea*   C. Fox glove

    (iv) *Withania somnifera*   D. Deadly night shade

                           E. Ashwagandha

218. Given below are some important drugs. Find out the constituents listed A to E derived from them.

    (i) *Cephaelis ipecacuanha*   A. Cineole

    (ii) *Papaver somniferum*   B. Safrole and myristicin

    (iii) *Cascara sagrada*   C. Morphine

    (iv) *Myristica fragrans*   D. Anthraquinone glycoside

                         E. Emetine

219. Given below are some important drugs. Appropriate tests are listed in A to E. Match them correctly.

     (i)   Cardiac glycoside   A. p-Dimethylamino benzaldehyde
     (ii) Ergot alkaloids   B. Fluorescence test with dil H_2SO_4
     (iii) Quinidine sulphate   C. Liebermann Burchard test
     (iv) Camphor   D. 2,4-Dinitrophenyl hydrazine
                                    E. Benedict's test

220. The sources and constituents of the following umbelliferous fruits are listed in A to E. Match them correctly.

     (i)   Caraway   A. *Foeniculum vulgare* Anethole/Fenchone
     (ii) Fennel   B. *Carum carvi* Carvone
     (iii) Dill   C. *Anethum graveolens* Carvone
     (iv) Coriander   D. *Cuminum cyminum* Cuminic aldehyde
                       E. *Coriandrum sativum* Linalol

221. Given below are some of the microscopical diagnostic features of the drugs listed in A to E. Choose the appropriate one.

     (i)   Cluster crystals of calcium oxalate   A. Stramonium leaves
     (ii) Candelabra trichomes   B. Cinnamon bark
     (iii) Phloem fibres   C. Alexandrian senna
     (iv) Glandular trichomes   D. *Digitalis purpurea*
                                                 E. *Verbascum thapsus*

222. The emulgents and their sources are given below. Match them.

     (i)   Karaya   A. Synthetic
     (ii) Carrageenan   B. Collagen
     (iii) Guar   C. Sea weed
     (iv) Gelatin   D. Gum exudate
                         E. Seed extract

223. Given below a list of medicinal plants. Match them correctly with the list of constituents given in A to E.

     (i)   *Holarrhena antidysenterica*   A. Conessine
     (ii) *Cymbopozan flexuosus*   B. Citral
     (iii) *Urginea indica*   C. Mucilage
     (iv) *Linum usitatissimum*   D. Cocaine
                                          E. Scillarenin

224. Listed are some of the crude drugs which are tested for the active constituents by the tests mentioned in A to E. Match them correctly.

     (i)   Cinchona bark   A. Fluorescence test
     (ii) Nux vomica seeds   B. Keller-Kiliani test
     (iii) Digitalis leaves   C. Borntrager's test

(iv) Senna leaves   D. Mayer's test

                     E. Sham test

225. Listed are some of the common volatile oils. Their active constituents are given in A to E. Match them correctly.

    (i) Peppermint oil   A. (+) Limonene
    (ii) Turpentine oil   B. 1 : 8 Cineole
    (iii) Eucalyptus oil   C. α-Pinene
    (iv) Lemon oil   D. (–) Menthol
                     E. (+) Menthol

226. The following umbelliferous fruits are obtained from the plants mentioned in A to E. Match them.

    (i) Ani seed   A. *Anethum graveolens*
    (ii) Caraway   B. *Foeniculum vulgare*
    (iii) Coriander   C. *Carum carvi*
    (iv) Dill   D. *Pimpinella anisum*
                E. *Coriandrum sativum*

227. Microscopical characters A to E are associated with the plant drugs listed below. Match them.

    (i) *Elettaria cardamomum*   A. Rhytidomes
    (ii) *Quillaia saponaria*   B. Clothing and glandular trichomes
    (iii) *Digitalis purpurea*   C. Thin membranous arillus
    (iv) *Atropa belladonna*   D. Stomata of the anisocytic type
                          E. Concave midrib

228. Pharmacological activity of certain well known plant drugs are listed in A to E. Match them.

    (i) Papaverine   A. Weak analeptic (restorative)
    (ii) Camphor   B. Vasodilator
    (iii) Veratrum alkaloids   C. Antineoplastic
    (iv) Vincristine   D. Central vasoconstrictor
                     E. Anxiolytic

229. Match the following descriptions given in A to F with the products mentioned below

    (i) *Agar*   A. Chief carbohydrate from macrocystic pyrifera
    (ii) Carageenan   B. Dried exudate from *Astragalus gummifer*
    (iii) Tragacanth   C. Closely related hydrocolloids from *Chrondus crispus*
    (iv) Algin   D. Hydrophilic colloid from *Geledum cartilagenum*
                E. Powdered endosperm of the seed of *Cyamopsis tetragonolobus*
                F. Carbohydrates from the Rhizomes of Zingeber sps.

230. Match the following terms with the phytoconstituents mentioned below.

    (i) Opium   A. Tropane alkaloid
    (ii) Ergometrine   B. Cardiac glycosides
    (iii) Scopolamine   C. Latex of poppy capsules

      (iv) Ginsenosides   D. Oxytocic effects

                           E. Adaptogenic and tonic

                           F. Cyanogenetic aglycone

231. The diagnostic features of crude drugs are given in i to iv. Their descriptions are given in A to F. Match them.

    (i)   *Trichome*   A. Two similar cells placed with their long axis parallel and having smaller intercellular space.

    (ii) Cicatrix   B. Epidermal cells which do not have any definite function

    (iii) Stomata   C. An elongated tubular outgrowth of an epidermal cell.

    (iv) Mesophyll   D. Trichomes having fallen or been rubbed off leaving a scar.

                           E. The whole of the parenchymatous ground tissue between two epidermises.

                           F. Flat and has one or more rows of palisade cells

232. Heterocyclic systems (i-iv) and the natural products in which they are present is given in A-F. Match them.

    (i)   Imidazole   A. Reserpine

    (ii) β-Carboline   B. Pilocarpine

    (iii) Hetrosteroidal C. Conessine

    (iv) Isoquinoline D. Ergotamine

                          E. Papaverine

                          F. Scopolamine

233. The following glycosides of Digitalis purpurea gives on hydrolysis the genins and sugars listed in A to D. Match them.

    (i) Purpurea glycoside-A   A. $1,3,5,11\alpha,14,19$-hexahydroxy cardenolide + glucose + digitoxose

    (ii) Purpurea glycoside-B   B. $3\beta,14\beta$-dihydroxy cardenolide + glucose + digitoxose

                                     C. $3\beta,14\beta,16\beta$-trihydroxy cardenolide + glucose + digitoxose

                                     D. $3\beta,12\beta,14\beta$-trihydroxy cardenolide + glucose + digitoxose

234. The following microscopical characteristic is associated with the drugs mentioned in A to D. Match them.

    (i) Rubiaceous type of stomata (Parasitic)   A. *Atropa belladonna* leaves

    (ii) Ranunculaceous type of stomata   B. *Cassia acutifolia* leaves

                                              C. *Cassia auriculata* leaves

                                                    D. *Digitalis purpurea* leaves

235. Following ring systems are present in the alkaloids given in A to D. Match them.

    (i)   Imidazole   A. Pelleterine

    (ii) Isoquinoline B. Nicotine

                           C. Papaverine

                           D. Pilocarpine

236. The ring structure present in the alkaloids listed below are given in A-D. Match them.

(i) Codeine   A. Phenanthrene
(ii) Ergotamine   B. Indole
                      C. Quinoline
                      D. Iso-quinoline.

237. The following terms are used to describe the parts of certain plants listed in A-D. Match them.

(i) Hypanthium   A. *Prunus communis*
(ii) Rhytidoma   B. Cinnamon bark
                      C. Roots of *Rauwolfia serpentina*
                      D. *Eugenia caryophyllus*

238. The chief active constituents of some umbelliferous fruits are listed in A-D. Match them with the correct plant source.

(i) *Foeniculum capillaceum*   A. Anethol
(ii) *Anethum graveolens*   B. Carvone
                                C. Khellin
                                D. Linalol

239. Listed are some of the microscopical characters of bark powder obtained from the plants mentioned in A to D. Match them.

(i) Narrow slender lignified phloem fibres occur singly   A. *Cinchona succirubra*
     or tangential rows of 2-5. Lignified, colourless
     narrow subrectangular parenchyma with small starch
     grains. Less amount of cork
(ii) Wider phloem fibres, larger starch grains, longer   B. *Cinnamomum zeylanicum*
     fibres, abundant cork
                                                            C. *Cinnamomum cassia*
                                                            D. *Holarrhena antidysenterica*

240. Following tests are associated with the drugs mentioned in A to E. Match them correctly.

(i)   Vitali Morin test   A. Digitalis (Digitoxose)
(ii) Borntrager's test   B. Tannin
(iii) Ruthenium Red test   C. Mucilage
(iv) Gold Beater's skin test   D. Anthraquinone glycosides (Senna)
(v)   Keller-Kiliani test   E. Tropane alkaloids (Cocaine, Atropine)

241. Following reagents used for the test of alkaloids are associated with the chemicals listed in A to D. Match them properly.

(i)   Mayer's reagent   A. Saturated picric acid solution
(ii) Dragendroff's reagent   B. Iodine in KI solution
(iii) Wagner's reagent   C. Pot. bismuth iodide solution
(iv) Hager's reagent   D. Pot. mercuric iodide solution

242. Indicate the appropriate drug of pharmacognostic origin from those given (A to H) against their used listed :

    (i)   Seed   A. Clove

    (ii)   Flower   B. Urginea

    (iii) Entire drug   C. Aloes

    (iv) Bulb   D. Ephedra

    (v)   Tuber   E. Agar

    (vi) Dried juices   F. Benzoin

    (vii) Dried extracts G. Dioscorea

                          H. Castor

243. Given below in A to D. are the lists of starch. Biological sources are given below for the starch. Match them correctly.

    (i)   *Zea mays*   A. Potato

    (ii)   *Oryza sativa*   B. Rice

    (iii) *Triticum aestivum* C. Wheat

    (iv) *Solanum tuberosum* D. Maize

244. Indicate from the group A to E the correct compound for the given source

    (i)   *Urginea maritima*   A. Camphene

    (ii)   *Rheum palmatum*   B. Scilliroside

    (iii) *Myristica fragrans*   C. Emodine

    (iv) *Claviceps purpurea* D. Atropine

                             E. Ergometrine

245. Fill in the blanks :

    (i)   Synthetic camphor is optically ...... 1 ...... and is prepared from ...... 2 ...... whereas natural camphor is optically ...... 3 ...... and is obtained from ...... 4 ....

    (ii) Alkaloids of ergot exist in stereoisomeric pairs and they are derived from optically isomeric forms. They are known as ...... 5 ...... and ...... 6 ...... which differ only in configuration at the asymmetric carbon atom which carries ...... 7 ...... group.

    (iii) In quillaia bark, the dark patches often found on the outer surface are known as ...... 8 ....

    (iv) A sample of ginger when boiled with ...... 9 ...... the pungency is lost.

    (v)   Colchicine is an alkaloid obtained from ...... 10 ....

    (vi) The most important property of digitalis glycosides is their positive ...... 11 ....

    (vii) Papain is a ...... 12 ...... enzyme.

  (viii) Dragendorff's reagent used in testing alkaloids is chemically ...... 13 ....

    (ix) Crude drugs are vegetables or animal drugs which consist of natural substances that have undergone no other processes than ...... 14 ...... and ...... 15 ....

    (x)   Tannin containing drugs have more ...... 16 ...... soluble extractives while resin containing drugs have more ...... 17 ...... soluble extractives.

    (xi) The starch-iodine colour (blue) ...... 18 ...... on heating and ...... 19 ...... on cooling.

    (xii) The position and form of the ...... 20 ...... and the presence or absence of well defined ...... 21 ...... are of importance in the characterization of starches.

(xiii) In Molisch's test ...... 22 ...... and sulphuric acid are used.

(xiv) Keller-Kiliani test is used for identification of ...... 23 ...... sugar.

(xv) Mayer's reagent is ...... 24 ...... and useful for identification of ...... 25 ....

(xvi) An elongated tubular outgrowth of an epidermal cell is termed as ...... 26 ....

(xvii) Phenol group glycoside found in Uva-Ursi is ...... 27 ....

(xviii) Rhubarb gives ...... 28 ...... colour when treated with ammonia.

(xix) Rhubarb gives ...... 29 ...... colour with 5% potassium hydroxide.

(xx) Ouabain is a glycoside with aglycone ...... 30 ...... and sugar ...... 31 ....

(xxi) Borntrager's test is used to identify ...... 32 ...... class of glycosides.

(xxii) Squill produces cardioactive glycosides, the principle are being ...... 33 ....

(xxiii) Aloe barbadensis gives glycoside barbaloin and ...... 34 ....

(xxiv) Sinalbin $\xrightarrow[\text{Myrosin}]{\text{H}_2\text{O}}$ 35 ...... + ... 36 ...... + ... 37 ....

(xv) Cochineal consists of the dried female insect ...... 38 ....

(xxvi) Morphine belongs to ...... 39 ...... class of alkaloid.

(xxvii) Black pepper contains crystalline alkaloids ...... 40 ...... and ...... 41 ....

(xxviii) Atropine is recemate of ...... 42 ....

(xxix) Cocaine on hydrolysis gives ...... 43 ...... and ...... 44 ....

(xxx) The colour reaction for quinine and quinidine alkaloids using bromine and ammonia is known as the ...... 45 ...... test.

(xxxi) Lysergic acid and isolysergic acid are found in ...... 46 ...... alkaloids.

(xxxii) Two glycoside sinigrine of mustard oil is hydrolyzed by the enzyme ...... 47 ...... with the production of volatile mustard oil.

(xxxiii) Nutmeg is the dried ripe seed of ...... 48 ....

(xxxiv) The common name for 4-allyl-2-methoxyphenol is ...... 49 ....

(xxxv) The spearmint oil contains about 40-60% of ...... 50 ....

(xxxvi) Lemon oil contains about 90% of terpenes consisting chiefly of ...... 51 ....

(xxxvii) α-pinene on treatment with hydrochloric acid gas at 10° gives ...... 52 ....

(xxxviii) All natural monocyclic monoterpenes are derivatives of ...... 53 ....

(xxxix) ...... 54 ...... is a naturally occurring local anaesthetic.

(xl) ...... 55 ...... is an anti-hypertensive alkaloid.

(xli) Morphine dependence can be treated by ...... 56 ....

(xlii) Clove oil contains about 70-90% of ...... 57 ....

(xliii) Gold Beater Skin Test is used for the identification of ...... 58 ....

(xliv) D-Linalol is the chief constituent of ...... 59 ....

(xlv) Tragacanth gives pink colour with Ruthenium Red due to the presence of ...... 60 ....

(xlvi) The irritant cathartic action of castor oil is due to the presence of ...... 61 ....

(xlvii) Codeine is obtained from ...... 62 ....

(xlviii) The cardiac depressant drug used in cardiac arrythmia, obtained from Cinchona bark is ...... 63 ....

(xlix) Cremocarpus fruit is the characteristic of ...... 64 ....

(l) Starch contains two polysaccharide namely ...... 65 ...... and ...... 66 ....

246. State True or False
    (i) Pharmaceutical pectin differs from commercial pectin because it does not contain sugar or organic acid.
    (ii) Balsams are resinous mixtures that contain large proportions of benzoic acid, cinnamic acid, salicylic acid or esters of these acids.

ANSWERS

1. D; 2. B; 3. C; 4. A; 5. B; 6. B; 7. C; 8. D; 9. D; 10. A; 11. D; 12. C; 13. A; 14. E; 15. D; 16. A; 17. E; 18. A; 19. D; 20. B; 21. D; 22. B; 23. E; 24. B; 25. A; 26. E; 27. C; 28. D; 29. F; 30. A; 31. D; 32. E; 33. A; 34. A; 35. D; 36. B; 37. B; 38. D; 39. D; 40. D; 41. B; 42. C; 43. D; 44. C; 45. B; 46. A; 47. C; 48. B; 49. C; 50. A; 51. C; 52. D; 53. A; 54. B; 55. B; 56. A; 57. B; 58. D; 59. A; 60. E; 61. C; 62. A; 63. B; 64. D; 65. A; 66. C; 67. B; 68. E; 69. D; 70. A; 71. E; 72. B; 73. D; 74. C; 75. E; 76. D; 77. C; 78. E; 79. E; 80. E; 81. B; 82. E; 83. D; 84. B; 85. B; 86. C; 87. C; 88. E; 89. A; 90. D; 91. E; 92. A; 93. C; 94. D; 95. C; 96. C; 97. B; 98. A; 99. A; 100. B; 101. B; 102. D; 103. A; 104. C; 105. C; 106. C; 107. E; 108. D; 109. C; 110. B; 111. A; 112. D; 113. B; 114. A; 115. B; 116. B; 117. A; 118. A; 119. B; 120. C; 121. A; 122. A; 123. C; 124. C; 125. A; 126. B; 127. B; 128. C; 129. C; 130. D; 131. C; 132. D; 133. A; 134. C; 135. A; 136. E; 137. C; 138. B; 139. A; 140. D; 141. B; 142. B; 143. A; 144. B; 145. A; 146. A; 147. D; 148. A; 149. B; 150. B; 151. B; 152. C; 153. A; 154. C; 155. B; 156. B; 157. A; 158. A; 159. D; 160. A; 161. D; 162. C; 163. A; 164. B; 165. B; 166. D; 167. A; 168. B; 169. B; 170. D; 171. D; 172. A; 173. B; 174. B; 175. C; 176. C; 177. D; 178. A; 179. B; 180. A; 181. E; 182. B; 183. A; 184. C; 185. D; 186. A; 187. B; 188. A; 189. C; Marquis reagent is formaldehyde-sulfuric acid which forms a purple complex with the opium alkaloids. 190. C; hashish is a concentrated form of marijuana. 191. A; Rauwolfia also belongs to this family. 192. D; The solubility of alkaloids and their salts is useful in pharmaceutical industry for the extraction and formulation of final pharmaceutical preparations. In general, the free bases of alkaliods are soluble in organic non-polar, immiscible solvents. The salts of most of alkaloids are soluble in water. In contrast, free base are insoluble in water and their salts are soluble in organic solvents. 193. E; it is a synthetic analog of morphine. 194. C; it is actually Mayer's reagent. 195. B; alkaloidal salts are freely soluble in water. 196. A; not used frequently because it produces emesis. 197. B; it is used only for research and testing purposes. 198. D; ephedrine is a sympathomimetic alkaloid. 199. E; Most alkaloids are weak bases ($pK_a^s > 7$) and form salts with acids (e.g., pilocarpine hydrochloride, morphine sulfate etc.). All alkaloids contain nitrogen (tertiary atom in their molecules. Stereoisomerism is common in alkaloidal structures and large differences in therapeutic activity can be expected among isomers. 200. A; By arresting mitosis at the metaphase and inhibits RNA synthesis. 201. A; Another product containing ipecac is quelidrine. 202. A; diacetylmorphine is commonly known as heroin or brown sugar. It is a Class I controlled substance; this means that it may be used only for experimental work by special permit. 203. A; Lanolin is hydrous wool fat containing 25 to 30% water and is a w/o emulsion into which more water can be incorporated if desired without much change in consistency. Wool fat is anhydrous lanolin and contains no water. 204. i-E; ii-A; iii-F; iv-B; v-G; vi-H; vii-C; viii-D; ix-K; x-L; xi-I. 205. i-G; ii-E; iii-A; iv-B; v-F; vi-C; vii-D. 206. i-D; ii-A; iii-E; iv-B. 207. i-A; ii-D; iii-B; iv-E. 208. i-E; ii-C; iii-A; iv-B. 209. i-C; ii-D; iii-E; iv-A. 210. i-D;

ii-B;iii-E; iv-C. 211. i-E; ii-C; iii-B; iv-D. 212. i-E; ii-C; iii-B; iv-D. 213. i-C; ii-B; iii-A; iv-D. 214. i-D; ii-B. 215. i-C; ii-D; iii-A. 216. i-C; ii-A; iii-E; iv-D. 217. i-C; ii-D; iii-A; iv-E. 218. i-E; ii-C; iii-D; iv-B. 219. i-C; ii-A; iii-B; iv-D. 220. i-B; ii-A; iii-C; iv-E. 221. i-A; ii-E; iii-B; iv-D. 222. i-D; ii-C; iii-E; iv-B. 223. i-A; ii-B; iii-E; iv-C. 224. i-A; ii-D; iii-B;iv-C. 225. i-D; ii-C; iii-B; iv-A. 226. i-D; ii-C; iii-E; iv-A. 227. i-C; ii-A; iii-B; iv-D. 228. i-B; ii-A; iii-E; iv-C. 229. i-D; ii-C; iii-B; iv-A. 230. i-C; ii-D; iii-A; iv-E. 231. i-C; ii-D; iii-A; iv-E 232. i-B; ii-; iii-C; iv-E. 233. i-B; ii-C. 234. i-B; ii-D. 235. i-D; ii-C. 236. i-A; ii-B. 237. i-D; ii-A. 238. i-A; ii-D. 239. i-B; ii-C (from these characteristics, cassia is distinguished from cinnamon). 240. i-E; ii-D; iii-C; iv-B; v-A. 241. i-D; ii-C; iii-B; iv-A. 242. i-H; ii-A; iii-D; iv-B; v-G; vi-C; vii-E. 243. i-D; ii-B; iii-C; iv-A. 244. i-B; ii-C; iii-A; iv-E. 245. Fill in the blanks : 1. 1. inactive 2. pinene 3. active 4. *Cinnamomum camphora* 5. water soluble category (ergometrine or ergonovine) 6. water insoluble category (ergotamine and ergotoxine) [levo form (-ine) is medicinally active whereas dextro form (-inine) is inactive] 7. amide (peptide linkage) 8. rhytidoma 9. 2% KOH 10. *Colchicum atumnale* and *C. luteum* Fam. Liliaceae 11. Keller-Kiliani test 12. proteolytic 13. potassium bismuth iodide solution 14. collection 15. drying 16. water 17. alcohol 18. disappears 19. reappears 20. hilum 21. striations 22. α-naphthol 23. deoxy 24. potassium mercuric iodide 25. alkaloids 26. trichome 27. arbutin 28. rose pink 29. blood red 30. ouabagenin 31. rhamnose 32. anthraquinone 33. scillaren - A 34. aloe emodin 35. p-hydroxybenzyl isothiocyanate 36. sinapin acid sulphate 37. glucose 38. *Coccus cacti* 39. phenanthrene 40. piperine 41. pipereltine 42. hyoscyamine 43. methanol, benzoic acid 44. ecgonine 45. thalleioquin 46. ergot 47. myrosin 48. *Myristica fragrans* 49. eugenol 50. (-) carvone 51. (+) limonene 52. bronyl chloride 53. p-cymene 54. Cocaine 55. Reserpine 56. methadone 57. euginol 58. tannins 59. coriander 60. mucilage 61. ricinoleic acid 62. opium (*Papaver somniferum*) 63. quinidine 64. Umbelliferae 65. amylose 66. amylopectin; 246. (i) False (ii) True.

Forensic Pharmacy /
Pharmaceutical Jurisprudence

CHAPTER 31

Forensic Pharmacy / Pharmaceutical Jurisprudence

1. The Pharmacy Act - 1948: The Act extends to the whole of India (except J & K State) and has been amended twice in 1959 and 1976 to cater to changed social needs. The Pharmacy Bill in 1945, which took full three years to take the shape of the **Pharmacy Act, 1948**. The first **Pharmacy Council of India (P.C.I.)** under this Act was constituted by the Central Government in 1949, with two main objects, namely - (i) to provide for uniform education and training for the "would-be", Pharmacists and (ii) to maintain a control over the persons entering the profession of Pharmacy, by providing for their registration in every state. The first Education Regulations have come in force under the P.C.I. in 1954. The latest E.R. is known as E.R. 1991. Before that they were in the year 1981.

The important functions of the Pharmacy Council of India include: **I.** Design of the Educational Pattern (Education Regulations). **II.** Approval of Institutions/withdrawal of approvals. **III.** Recognition of Foreign Qualifications. **IV.** Maintenance of Central Register of Pharmacists.

Important functions of the State Pharmacy Councils include: **I.** Maintenance of Registers. **II.** Entry & Removal of names. **III.** Printing of Registers. **IV.** Inspection by State Councils.

2. The Drugs and Cosmetics Act (1940) and Rules (1945): In 1940 came the Drugs Bill to regulate the import, manufacture, sale and distribution of drugs in British India. It was first published to elicit public opinion and then submitted to a select committee and was finally adopted as the **Drugs Act of 1940. The first Drugs Technical Advisory Board (D.T.A.B.) under this Act was constituted in 1941** by the Central Government to advise the Central Government and the State Governments on technical matters arising out of the administration of the **Drugs & Cosmetics Act**. The **Drugs Consultative Committee (DCC)** is also an advisory body, constituted by the Central Government for the purpose of advising the various governments and the DTAB, on any matter tending to secure uniformity in the administration of the Act throughout India. It consists of two representatives nominated by the Central Government and one nominee of each of the State Governments. The **Biochemical Standardization Laboratory** of **Calcutta** was reconstituted as the **Central Drugs Laboratory** for the purpose of the Act. It took another 5 years to frame the Drugs Rules under the Drugs Act 1940, which were published in **1945**. The Drugs Act has been amended several times (1955, 1960, 1962, 1964, 1972, 1982 & 1986) since its passage in 1940 and at the moment the provisions of Act cover Cosmetics, Ayurvedic, Unani and Homeopathic medicines in some respects.

Drugs and Cosmetics Rules have been divided into 18 parts each dealing with a particular subject. There are 2 schedules to the Act and 26 schedules to the Rules, which are as follows:

Schedules to the Act

First Schedule: Name of books under Ayurvedic and Sidha systems.

Second Schedule: Standard to be complied with by imported drugs and by drugs manufactured for sale, sold, stocked or exhibited for sale or distributed.

Schedules to the Rules

A - *List of forms that should be used under the Act for purpose of making applications for the licenses, issue of licenses, for sending memorandum etc.*

Form 1	Memorandum to the Central Drugs Laboratory.
Form 2	Certificate of test or analysis by the Central Drugs Laboratory.
Form 8	Application for licence to import biological and other special products specified in Schedule C and C1 to the Drugs and Cosmetics Rules, 1945.
Form 9	Form of undertaking to accompany an application for an import licence.
Form 10	Licence to import biological and other special products specified in Schedule C and C_1 to the Drugs and Cosmetics Rules, 1945.
Form 11	Licence to import drugs for the purposes of examination, test or analysis.
Form 12	Application for licence to import drugs for purpose of examination, test or analysis.
Form 12-A	Application for the issue of a permit to import small quantities of drugs for personal use.
Form 12-B	Permit for the import of small quantities of drugs for personal use.
Form 13	Certificate of test or analysis by Government Analyst under Section25(1) of the Drugs and cosmetics Act, 1940.
Form 14-A	Application from a purchaser for test or analysis of a drug under Section 26 of the Drugs and Cosmetics Act, 1940.
Form 14-B	Certificate of test or analysis by Government Analyst under Section 26 of the Drugs and Cosmetics Act, 1940.
Form 15	Order under Section 22(c) of the Drugs and Cosmetics Act, 1940, requiring a person not to dispose of stock in his possession.

Form 16	Receipt for stock of drugs seized under section 22(c) of the Drugs and Cosmetics Act, 1940.
Form 17	Intimation to person from whom sample is taken.
Form 18	Memorandum to Government Analyst.
Form 19	Application for grant or renewal of a licence to sell, stock or exhibit for sale, or distribute drugs.
Form 19-A	Application for the grant or renewal of a restricted licence to sell, stock or exhibit for sale, or distribute drugs by retail by itinerant vendors and other dealers who do not engage the services of a qualified person.
Form 19-B	Application for licence to sell, stock or exhibit for sale or distribute Homeopathic medicines.
Form 20	Licence to sell, stock or exhibit for sale or distribute drugs by retail other than those specified in Schedules C and C_1.
Form 20-A	Restricted licence to sell, stock or exhibit for sale or distribute drugs by retail other than those specified in Schedules C and C_1 for itinerant vendors and other dealers who do not engage the services of a qualified person.
Form 20-B	Licence to sell, stock or exhibit for sale, or distribute by wholesale, drugs other than those specified in Schedules C and C_1.
Form 20-C	Licence to sell, stock or exhibit for sale or distribute Homeopathic medicines by retail.
Form 20-D	Licence to sell, stock or exhibit for sale or distribute Homeopathic medicines by wholesale.
Form 21	Licence to sell, stock or exhibit for sale, or distribute by retail drugs specified in Schedules C and C_1.
Form 21-A	Restricted licence to sell, stock or exhibit for sale or distribute by retail drugs specified in Schedules C and C_1 for itinerant vendors and dealers who do not engage the services of a qualified person.
Form 21-B	Licence to sell, stock or exhibit or offer for sale or distribute by wholesale drugs specified in Schedules C and C_1.
Form 21-C	Certificate of renewal of licence to sell, stock or exhibit for sale or distribute drugs.
Form 22	General Warranty under Section 19(3) of the Drug and Cosmetics Act, 1940.
Form 23	Specific Warranty under Section 19(3) of the Drug and Cosmetics Act, 1940.
Form 24	Application for the grant of or renewal of a licence to manufacture.
Form 24-A	Application for grant or renewal of a loan licence to manufacture for sale drugs other than those specified in Schedules C and C_1.

Form 24-B	Application for grant or renewal of a licence to repack for sale or distribution of drugs, being drugs other than those specified in Schedules C and C_1.
Form 24-C	Application for grant or renewal of a licence to manufacture for sale of Homeopathic medicines.
Form 25	Licence of manufacture for sale drugs other than those specified in Schedules C and C_1.
Form 25-A	Loan Licence to manufacture for sale drugs other than those specified in Schedules C and C_1.
Form 25-B	Licence to repack for sale or distribution of drugs being drugs other than those specified in Schedules C and C_1.
Form 25-C	Licence to manufacture for sale Homeopathic medicines.
Form 26	Certificate of renewal of licence to manufacture for sale drugs.
Form 26-A	Certificate of renewal of loan licence to manufacture for sale drugs.
Form 26-B	Certificate of renewal of licence to repack for sale or distribution of drugs being drugs other than those specified in Schedules C and C_1.
Form 26-C	Certificate of renewal of licence to manufacture for sale of Homoeopathic medicines.
Form 27	Application for grant or renewal of a licence to manufacture for sale drugs specified in Schedule C and C_1.
Form 27-A	Application for grant or renewal of a loan licence to manufacture for sale drugs specified in Schedule C and C_1.
Form 28	Licence to manufacture for sale drugs specified in Schedule C and C_1.
Form 28-A	Licence to manufacture for sale drugs specified in Schedule C and C_1.
Form 29	Licence to manufacture drugs for purposes of examination, test or analysis.
Form 30	Application for licence to manufacture drugs for purposes of examination, test or analysis.
Form 31	Application for grant or renewal of a licence to manufacture cosmetics for sale.
Form 32	Licence to manufacture cosmetics for sale.
Form 33	Certificate of renewal of licence to manufacture cosmetics for sale.
Form 34	Certificate of test or analysis of the cosmetics by the Central Drugs Laboratory or the Government Analysis.

B - *Rates of fee for test or analysis by the Central Drugs Laboratory or the Government Analyst.*

C - *List of biological and other special products whose import, sale, distribution and manufacture are governed by special provisions:* 1. Sera, 2. Solutions of serum proteins intended for injection, 3. Vaccines for parenteral injections, 4. Toxins, 5. Antigens, 6. Antitoxins, 7 Neo-arsphenamine and analogous substances used for the specific treatment of infective diseases, 8. Insulin, 9. Pituitary (Posterior lobe) Extract, 10. Adrenaline and Solutions of Salts of Adrenaline, 11. Drugs and Preparations thereof in a form to be administered parenterally: Penicillin, Streptomycin, Chlortetracycline, Oxytetracycline, Chloramphenicol, Viomycin, Polymyxin B, Neomycin, Bacitracin, Tetracycline, Carbomycin, Erythromycin, Vancomycin, 12. Any other preparation which is meant for parenteral administration as such or after being made up with a suitable solvent or medium or any other sterile product which either requires to be stored in refrigerator or dose not require to be stored in a refrigerator, 13. Sterile ligature, 14. Bacteriophages.

C₁ - *List of other special products whose import, sale, distribution and manufacture are governed by special provision:* 1. Drugs belonging to the Digitalis group and the preparations containing drugs belonging to the Digitalis group not in a form to be administered parenterally, 2. Ergot and its preparations containing Ergot not in a form to be administered parenterally, 3. Adrenaline and preparations, 4. Fish Liver Oil and preparations containing Fish Liver Oil, 5. Vitamins and preparations containing any vitamin not in a form to be administered parenterally, 6. Liver extract and preparations containing liver extract not in a form to be administered parenterally, 7. Hormones and preparations containing hormones not in a form to be administered parenterally, 8. Vaccines not in a form to be administered parenterally, 9. Following drugs and preparations containing them not in a form to be administered parenterally: i. Penicillin, ii. Streptomycin, iii. Chlortetracycline, iv. Oxytetracycline, v. Chloramphenicol, vi. Viomycin, vii. Neomycin, viii. Bacitracin, ix. Tetracycline, x. Gramicidin, xi. Tyrothricin, xii. Carbomycin, xiii. Erythromycin, xiv. Vancomycin, xv. Polymyxin B, xvi. Framycetin, xvii. Griseofulvin, xviii. Novobiocin, xix. Nystatin, xx. Oleandomycin, xxi. Spiramycin.

D - *List of drugs exempted from the provisions of import of drugs.*

E₁ - *List of poisonous substances under the Ayurvedic (including Sidha) and Unani system of medicine.*

F & F₁ - *Provisions applicable to production, testing, storage, packing and labeling of Biological and other special products.*

FF - *Standards of ophthalmic preparations.*

F₂ - *Gives details of standards for surgical dressings.*

F₃ - *Standards for sterilized umbilical tapes.*

G - *List of substances that are required to be used only under medical supervision and which are to be labeled accordingly:* Aminopterin, L-Asparaginase, Bleomycin, Busulfan: its salts, Carbutamide, Chlorambucil: its salts, Chlorthiazide and other derivatives of 1,2,4-benzothiadiazine, Cisplatin, Chlorpropamide: its salts, Chlorthalidone and other derivatives of Chlorobenzene compound, Cyclophosphamide: its salts, Cytarabine, Daunorubicin, Disodium Stilboestrol Diphosphate, Doxorubicin hydrochloride, Ethacrynic acid: its salts, Ethosuximide, Glibenclamide, Hydantoin: its salts, Mercaptopurine: its salts, Methosuximide, Mustine: its salts, Paramethadione, Phenacemide, Phenformin: its salts, 5- Phenylhydantoin: its alkyl and aryl derivatives: its salts, Primidone, Procarbazine hydrochloride, Quinthazone, Sarcolysine, Testolactone, Thiotepa, Tolbutamide, Tretamine: its salts antihistaminic substances, their salts and derivatives: Antazoline,

Bromodiphenhydramine, Buclizine, Chlorcyclizine, Chlorpheniramine, Clemizole, Cyproheptadine, Diphenhydramine, Doxylamine Succinate, Isothipendyl, Mebhydroline napadisylate, Meclozine, Phenindamine, Pheniramine, Promethazine, Sarcolysine, Sodium-2-mercapto-ethanesulfonate, Tamoxifen citrate, Thenalidine, Triprolidine, tetra-N-substituted derivatives of Ethylene diamine or propylenediamine. (Note: Preparations containing the above substances excluding those intended for topical or external use are also covered by this schedule).

H - *List of prescription drugs (List of the drugs to be sold on the prescription of a Registered Medical Practitioner):* Adrenocorticotropic hormone (ACTH), Amyloride hydrochloride, Analgin, Androgenic, Anabolic, oestrogenic and progestational substances, the following: Benzestrol, derivatives of stibene, dibenzyl or naphthalene with oestrogenic or progestational activity, their esters, Allopurinol, Alphachymotrypsin, Amantadine hydrochloride, Amitriptyline: its salts, Ammidine, Ammodine, Antibiotics, Apil, Aprotinin, Arsenic, organic compounds for injection, Azathioprine, Barbituric acid: its salts,derivatives of barbituric acid their salts, compounds of barbituric acid, its salts, its derivatives, their salts with any other substance excluding those included in Schedule X, Beclomethasone dipropionate, Benactyzine: its salts, Betablistinem dihydrochloride, Betamethasone-17-benzoate, Bethanidine sulphate, Biperiden hydrochloride, Bioscanate bretylium tosylate, Bromhexine hydrochloride, Bumetidine, Bupivacaine hydrochloride, Carbanoxolone sodium, Carbidopa, Carisoprodol, Cephalethin sodium, Chloral hydrate, Chlordiazepoxide: its salts, Chlorisondamine chloride, Chlorpromazine: its salts, Chlorprothiaxene, Cimetidine, Citrated calcium carbimide, Clindamycin, Clidinium bromide, Clofibrate, Clonidine hydrochloride, Clopamide, Clotrimazole, Clorexolone, Corticosteroids: their esters, derivatives and esters, Dyclandelate, Danazole, Dapsone: its salts and derivatives, Deoxyribonuclease, Diazepam, Diazoxide, Dilazep hydrochloride, Dimethothiazine and mesylate, Diisopyramide, Dopamine hydrochloride, Dothiepin hydrochloride, Doxapram hydrochloride, Doxepiam hydrochloride, Drugs coming within the preview of the Narcotic Drugs and Psychotropic Substances Act, Econazole, Enfenamic acid, Epinephrine: its salts, Epsilon, Aminocaproic acid, Ergot, alkaloids of, whether hydrogenated or not, their homologues, any salt of any substance falling within this item, Estradiol succinate, Ethacridine lactate, Ethambutol hydrochloride, Ethinyloestradiol, Ethionamide, Fenfluramine hydrochloride, Flavoxate hydrochloride, Flufenamic acid: its salts, esters: their salts, Flupenthixol, Fluphenazine Enanthate and Decanoate, Flubiprofen, Galanthamine hydropromide, Galliamine: its salts, quaternary compound, Glucagon, Glycopytrolate, Glydiadinamide, guanethidine, Halofuginone, Halogenated hydroxyquinoline derivatives, Haloperidol, Heparin, Hyaluronidase, Hydroxyzine: its salts, Houprofen, Imipramine: its salts, Indapamide, Indomethacin: its salts, Intralipid intravenous fat emulsion, Iron preparations for parenteral use, Isocarboxazid, Isonicotinic acid hydrazide and other hydrazine derivatives of isonicotinic acid, their derivatives, their salts, Isosorbide dinitrate, Isoxsuprine, Ketamine hydrochloride, Ketoprofen, L-Dihydroxy phenylalanine, Levarterenol: its salts, Levodopa, Lidoflazine, Lithium carbonate, Loperamine, Lorazepam, Mebendazole, Mebevecrine hydrochloride, Medigoxin, Mefenamic acid: its salts, its esters: their salts, Megestrol acetate, Meglumine locarmate, Mephenesin: its esters, Mesterolone, Methicillin sodium, Methixene: its salts, Methocarbamol, Methossalen, Methylprenthyaol: its esters and other derivatives, 1-Methyl-1,3-phenylpiperidine-4-carboxylic acid esters of their salts, Metoclopramide, Metoprolol tartrate, Metrizamide, Metronidazole, Miconazole, Morphaninamide hydrochloride, Nalidixic acid, Naproxen, Natamycin, Nicofuranose, Niffumic acid, Nemorezole, Nitrazepam, Orphenadrine: its salts, Oxazepam, Oxethazaine hydrochloride, Oxolinic acid, Oxpremolol hydrochloride, Oxyfedrine, Oxymetozone, Oxytocin, Para-amino benzene sulfonamide: its salts, derivatives or para amino benzene sulfonamide having any of hydrogen atoms of the para amino group of the sulfonamide group substituted by another radical excluding carbutamide: their salts, Para amino salicylic acid: its salts, its derivatives, their salts, Pancuronium bromide, Pemidine: its salts, Penamecillin, D-penicillemine, Pentazocine, Pentoxyfylline, Phenelzine: its salts, Phenothiazine: derivatives of and salts of its derivatives not otherwise specified in the Schedule, Phenylbutazone: its salts, Phenylpropanolamine hydrochloride, Pimozide, Pindolol, Piracetam, Pituitary gland, the active principle of not otherwise specified in this Schedule and their salts, Prednisolone stearoglycolate, Promazine: its salts, Propanidid, Propranolol hydrochloride, Protrislyline hydrochloride, Pyrantel pamoate, Pyrazinamide, Pyridinium: its salts, Rauwolfia alkaloids: their salts, derivatives of the alkaloids of rauwolfia, their salts, Resoxacin, Salbutamol sulphate, Salicydazosulphayridine, Sisomicin sulphate, Sodium Chromoglycate, Sodium and Meglumine lethalamates, Sodium Valproate, Sotalol, Spironolactone, Sulfonal: alkyl sulfonals, Sulfadoxine, Sulphamethoxypyridazine, Sulphapenazole, Sulthiame, Terbutaline sulphate, Terizidone, Tetramisole hydrochloride, Thiabendazole, Thiacetazone, Thiethylperazine, Thiopropazate: its salts, Tretinoin, Tribromoethyl propanol, Trichloromethiazide, Trifluoperazine, Trifluoperidol hydrochloride, Trimeprazine: its salts, Trimetazidine dihydrochloride, Trimipramine, Tylosin tartrate, Urokinase, Vasopressin, Verapamil hydrochloride, Xipamid.

Note: 1. Preparations exempted under provision to para **2** of Note to Schedule X shall also be covered by this Schedule. **2.** Preparations containing the above substances excluding those intended for topical or external use are also covered by this Schedule. The inclusion of a substance in Schedule H does not imply or convey that the substances is exempted from the provisions of Rule 30A of the Drugs and Cosmetics Rules.

J - *Diseases or ailments which a drug may not purport to prevent or cure:* Appendicitis, Arteriosclerosis, Blindness, Blood poisoning, Brights' disease, Cancer, Cataract, Deafness, Diabetes, Diseases and disorders of the optical system, disorders of brain, diseases and disorders of uterus, disorders of prostatic glands, Dropsy, Epilepsy, Female diseases (in general), Fevers (in general), Fit's Gall stones, Kidney stones and bladder stones, Gangrene, Glaucoma, Goitre, Heart diseases, High or low blood pressure, Hydrocele, Infantile paralysis, Insanity, Leprosy, Leucoderma, Lock jaw, Locomotor ataxia, Lupus, Nervous debility, Obesity, Paralysis, Plague, Pleurisy, Pneumonia, Rheumatism, Sexual impotence, Small pox, Sterility in women, Trachoma, Tuberculosis, Tumors, Typhoid fevers, Ulcers of gastrointestinal tract, Venereal diseases, including Syphilis, Gonorrhoea, Soft chancre, Venereal granuloma, Lymphogranuloma.

K - *Drugs exempted from certain provisions relating to the manufacture of drugs.*

M - *Good Manufacturing Practices and Requirements of Pilot Equipment for Allopathic Drugs (The conditions and requirement should be conformed by the premises for manufacturing of drugs).*

M_1 - *Requirements of Factory Premises for the manufacture of Homeopathy Medicines.*

M_2 - *Requirements of Factory Premises for the manufacture of Cosmetics.*

M_3 - *Requirements of Factory Premises for the manufacture of Medical Devices.*

N - *List of minimum equipment for efficient running of a pharmacy.*

O - *Standards for disinfectant fluids.*

P - *Life periods of drugs.*

P$_1$ - *Pack sizes of drugs.*

Q - *List of coal tar colors permitted to be used in cosmetics.*

R - *Standards for mechanical contraceptives.*

R$_1$ - *Standards for medical devices.*

S - *Standards for cosmetics.*

T - *Requirements of factory premises and hygienic conditions for Ayurvedic (including Sidha) and Unani drugs.*

U - *Particulars to be shown in manufacturing, raw materials and analytical records of drugs.*

U$_1$ - *Particulars to be shown in manufacturing raw materials and analytical records of cosmetics.*

V - *Standards for patent or proprietary medicines.*

W - *List of drugs which are to be marketed under generic names only.*

X - *List of drugs whose import, manufacture and sale, labeling and packaging are governed by special provisions: Amobarbital, Amphetamine, Barbital, Cyclobarbital, Dexamphetamine, Ethchloronal, Glutethimide, Meprobamate, Methaqualone, Methylphenobarbital, Pentobarbital, Phencyclidine, Phenmetrazine, Phenobarbital, Secobarbital.*

Note: 1. Stereoisomeric forms, salts and preparations of the above substances are also deemed to be Schedule X drugs. **2.** Meprobamate or phenobarbital in combination with other drugs may be exempted if satisfactory evidence is produced that the same are not liable to misuse.

Y - *Requirements and guidelines on clinical trials for import and manufacture of new drugs.*

General Labelling Provisions for All Drugs

Containers of each and every drug should display the following particulars on their labels:

(i) Identity of the drug by disclosure of its official name, its manufacturer's name and licence No. Under which manufacture preceded by words Mfg Lic. No. or M.L. No. it's batch number preceded by words like Batch No., B.N., Lot no. etc. In case the drug has any trade name also its proper name should be more conspicuous than it's trade name. In case of Schedule W drugs and new drugs only generic names can be used. In addition the address of the premises of manufacture where the drugs has been manufactured should be given.

(ii) It's potency, standard, grade etc., as relevant. Quantities of active ingredients has to be expressed in oral liquid per 5 ml or multiples or per ml if dose is less than 5 ml.

For parenteral fluids quantities may be expressed per ml or as percentage by volume or for single dose containers quantities per dose. In solids quantities may be as unit's or weight per gram or per milligram. In tablets, capsules etc. quantities may be per unit or for other preparations as percentage by weight or volume or per gram or per milliliter as the case may be.

(iii) Net contents either by weight or by volume or as numbers in the case of unit dosage forms.

(iv) Date of manufacture and in case of drugs in Schedules P and C date of expiry.

(v) Precautions for handling, storage, sale, use etc.

(vi) Word "Physician's Sample not to be sold" on containers meant for distribution to physicians as samples.

Special additional provisions for special categories of drugs

Drugs	Particulars
Schedule G drugs	"Caution. It is dangerous to take this preparation except under medical supervision".
Schedule H drugs	(i) "Schedule H drug. Warning. To be sold on the prescription of a Registered Medical Practitioner only". (ii) Symbol Rx prominently on left hand top corner of the label. (iii) Symbol NR_x prominently on left hand top corner if drug is covered under Narcotic Drugs and Psychotrophic Substances Act.
Schedule X drugs	(i) "Schedule X drug. Warning: To be sold on prescription of RMPs only". (ii) Symbol XRx in red on left hand top corner.
Schedule C drugs	(i) Where a test for maximum toxicity is prescribed a statement that it has passed that test. (ii) Nature and percentage of antiseptic, if any.
Patent & Proprietary	(i) Names & quantities of active ingredients. (ii) If vitamins are present, the following words: "For therapeutic use" "For prophylactic use" "For paediatric use" and age of child/infant as the case may be.
Medicines for External use/Medicines containing Methylated spirit	"FOR EXTERNAL USE ONLY".
Alcoholic preparations	% of alcohol in terms of absolute alcohol.
Veterinary drugs	(i) Not for human use. For animal treatment only. (ii) Head of any domestic animal.
Colored preparations	Name and % of color.
Ophthalmic Solutions/ Suspensions	(i) Use within one month of opening. Not for injection. (ii) Name and concentration of preservative. (iii) Words: (a) If irritation persists or increases discontinue use and consult physician. Keep container tightly closed. (b) Do not touch the dropper tip/other dispensing tip to any surface since this may contaminate. "Before fixing dropper where there is possibility of touching it scrub hands with soap and rinse into water".

Ophthalmic Ointments	Warning: If irritation persists or increases discontinue use and consult physician.
Mechanical Contraceptives	Particulars specified in Schedule R.
Disinfectants	(i) Grade & phenol coefficient. (ii) Method of use.
Labelling of Dispensed Medicines	Medicines dispensed on prescription of RMPs are also exempt from the normal provisions. However, following particulars are to be included on their labels: (a) Name and address of the supplier. (b) Name of patient and quantity. (c) Serial No. in prescription record. (d) Dose, if it is for internal use and the words 'For External use only' if it is for external application.
Manner of Labelling	Labels of all drugs should bear conspicuous vertical red or orange or green lines running throughout the body of the label as per the following categorizations:
Red:	Narcotic analgesics, hypnotics, sedatives, tranquilizers, corticosteroids, hormones, hypoglycemics, antimicrobials, antiepileptics, antidepressants, anticoagulants, anticancer drugs, and all other drugs falling under Schedule 'G' and Schedule 'X'.
Orange:	All Schedule H drugs not covered under 'Red'.
Green:	All drugs other than those not covered under 'Red' and 'Orange' Further, when the drug is contained in an ampoule, it shall only be necessary to label the ampoule itself with (i) the name and quantity of the drug and (ii) the name of the manufacturer.

Other particulars may appear on the box or other device in which the ampoules are packed. The Letter I.P., B.P., B.P.C., etc., shall be entered on the label of a drug to indicate that the drug complies with the standards set out in these pharmacopoeias. Containers of Schedules H & G drugs, prior to manufacture in dosage forms, should be labelled in red letters against white background.

Colors

The following colors may be added to *medicines*, provided the common name and the percentage of the color are stated on the label of the container.

1. **Natural Colors:** Annatto, Carotene, Cochineal, Curcumin, Chlorophyll, Red oxide of Iron, Yellow oxide of Iron, Titanium dioxide.

2. **Artificial Colors:** Caramel.

3. **Coal Tar Colors:** *Green* - Quinazarine Green SS, Alizarin Cyanine Green F; Fast Green FCF, Green S; *Yellow* - Tartrazine, Sunset Yellow FCF; Quinoline Yellow WS; *Red* - Amaranth, Erythrosine, Eosine YS or Eosine G, Toney Red or Sudan III, Ponceau 4R, Carmoisine, Fast Red E; *Blue* - Indigo Carmine, Brilliant blue FCF; *Violet* - Alizurol purple; *Brown* - Resorcin Brown; *Black* - Naphthol Blue.

List of Colors Permitted to be Used in Soaps: Phthalocyanine Blue, Iragalite Rod CVPB paste or Pigment Orange 5, Citrus Red No. 2, Rhodamine B 500, Aqueous Green Paste, Pigment Yellow 3, Irgalite Carmine F. P. Powder or Pigments RED 5, Monolite Red 4R HV Paste or Pigment Red 7, Oil Red No. 1 or Solvent.

3. The Opium Act (1857, 1878).

4. The Dangerous Drugs Act 1930.

5. The Narcotic Drugs and Psychotropic Substances Act and Rules, 1985: The Dangerous Drugs Act 1930 which was enacted in accordance with the Geneva agreement of League of Nations of 1925 failed to curb the misuse of habit forming drugs like cocain, morphine, ganja (cannabis), etc. As such a more comprehensive Act namely Narcotic & Psychotropic Substances Act has been enacted by the Parliament in 1985 to protect Society from the dangers of addictive drugs, followed by another complementary Act namely **Prevention of Illicit Traffic in Psychotropic Substances Act 1988**. The Narcotic and Psychotropic Substances Act superseded the two Opium Acts of 1857 and 1878 and the Dangerous Drugs Act of 1930.

6. The Medicinal and Toilet Preparations (Excise Duties) Act (1955) and Rules (1956) ...came into force from 01.4.1957 ....In order to make a uniform law for the whole country.

Manufacture in Bond: *Preparations containing alcohol or other narcotic substances:* Preparations are deemed to be manufactured in bond when they are manufactured in a premise, licensed or approved for this purpose and on which duty is not paid until the finished products are removed from such licensed premises.

7. The Drugs and Magic Remedies (Objectionable Advertisements) Act, 1954: "Insulin no longer needed; it is better than insulin and reduces sugar in two weeks", "Sure remedy for helping expectant ladies to give birth to male children only" male off-spring guaranteed etc.

To counteract such nefarious advertisements the Drugs and Magic Remedies (Objectionable Advertisements) Act 1954 was passed and enforced.

8. The Poisons Act, 1904-1919: It was in 1904 that the first Act to control some operations over poisonous substances was passed in India known as Poisons Act, 1904. The U. P. Govt. in 1910, as well as in 1914, proposed some radical amendments in the Act to make it more effective.

The Poisons Act, 1919 was passed with a view to control the import, possession and sale of poisons. The provision of the Act are in addition to the rules, which have been made for the dispensing and sale of poisons under the Drugs and Cosmetics Act, 1940.

9. The Shops and Establishments Act: The Shops and Establishments Act are one of the numerous 'Social Acts' passed with a view to ensure fair deals by the employers to their employees.

10. The Prevention of Cruelty to Animals Act 1960: An Act aimed at preventing unnecessary pain and suffering to animals has been passed. This Act is known as the "Prevention of Cruelty to Animals Act" and is applicable to all parts of the country.

11. The Insecticides Act 1968: The Insecticides Act has been passed with a view to protect human beings and animals from the risks involved in the use of insecticides.

12. The Medical Termination of Pregnancy Act (1971) and Rules (1975): The first provision for termination of pregnancies was in the Indian Penal Code formulated in 1860 by the then British Rulers in accordance with the British Law on the subject. Under the provision abortion was deemed to be a crime for which the mother as well as person doing the abortion were culpable except when it was done to save the mother's life. This law was very strict but was breached to a very appreciable extent.

Hence, in view of the expansion in medical services throughout the country and to avoid the risks to the mother's health it was considered fit to liberalize the law regarding abortion specially keeping the following backgrounds in mind:

(a) *Humanitarian aspects:* like when a pregnancy arises due to sex crimes such as rape, intercourse with a lunatic woman, etc.

(b) *Health aspects:* when a pregnancy poses grave risk to the life or physical or mental health of a woman.

(c) *Eugenic aspects:* where the child to be born is likely to have deformities and/or serious defects.

13. The Indian Contract Act 1872.

14. The Standards of Weights and Measures Act 1976.

15. The Factories Act, 1948.

16. The Industries (Development and Regulations) Act, 1952.

17. The Patents and Designs Act, 1970.

18. The Trade and Merchandise Marks Acts, 1958.

19. The Prevention of Food Adulteration Act (1954) and Rules (1955).

Drug (Price Control) Order, 1995: This Order has been made under Sec. 3 of the Essential Commodities Act, 1955 with a view to exercise Governmental control over the prices of bulk drugs as well as drug formulations. It came in force repealing the Drug (Price Control) Order of 1987.

For calculation of retail price of any drug formulation the following formula has to be used:

$$R.P. = (M.C. + C.C. + P.M. + P.C.) \times (1 + MAPE)/100 + E.D.$$

where, 'R. P'. stands for retail price, 'M. C'. stands for material costs (inclusive of processing losses), 'C. C'. for conversion costs as per norms notified from time to time, 'P. M'. for packing material costs, 'P. C'. for packing charges, MAPE for maximum allowable post manufacturing expenses inclusive of trade margins and, 'E. D'. for Excise Duty.

Chemists and Druggists: Premises licensed for the sale of drugs which have a "qualified person" but wherein drugs are not compounded.

Drug Stores: Premises licensed for sale of drugs, which do not have a "qualified person".

Pharmacy: Premises licensed for the retail sale of drugs, which have a "qualified person" and indulge in the compounding of drug.

Opium: Coagulation juice of opium poppy (*Papaver somniferum*) or any other species of Papaverum from which opium or any phenanthrene alkaloid can be extracted and which may be declared to be opium poppy by notification by the Central Government or any mixture or opium poppy, with or without neutral materials, containing more than 0.2% morphine.

Registered Pharmacists: Persons registered as Pharmacists under the Pharmacy Act, 1948.

Vendors of Drugs: Persons who do not have fixed premises to sell drugs but are licensed to distribute them personally in specified areas.

Drugs Enquiry Committee and Aftermath: On 11th August, 1930, the Government of India, appointed a committee (the Drugs Enquiry Committee) under the Chairmanship of late Col. R. N. Chopra to explore and define the scope of the problem and to make recommendations as to the measures which should be taken, with some terms of reference.

In 1932, Prof. Mahadeva Lal Schroff initiated Pharmaceutical education at the University level in the Banaras Hindu University.

In 1948, a full fledged **Indian Pharmacopoeia Committee** was constituted under the chairmanship of late Dr. B. N. Ghosh of Calcutta and several sub-committees were set to work. The first edition of **The Indian Pharmacopoeia** was out in **1955**. Thereafter, the second edition of I.P. was published in the year **1966** and third edition of the same was published in two volumes in the year **1985**. Now the latest i.e., the fourth edition was published in the year **1996**.

MODEL QUESTIONS

1. License to sell drugs specified in Schedule C & C1 is given in form number
   A. 18   B. 19   C. 21   D. 24   E. 31.

2. For the registration of pharmacists in the various states, the Pharmacy Act provides for the constitution of
   A. Registration Tribunals
   B. Registrar of Co-operative Societies
   C. Registrar of State Pharmacy Council
   D. Registrar of Central Pharmacy Council
   E. None of the above.

3. In Drugs & Cosmetics Act & Rules thereunder, list of substances that should be sold by retail only on prescription of Registered Medical Practitioner is given in
   A. Schedule H   B. Schedule V   C. Schedule X
   D. Schedule Q   E. Schedule G.

4. The Pharmacy Council of India (Central Council) is constituted by the:
   A. Central Government   B. State Government   C. Parliament
   D. Legislative Assembly   E. Cabinet.

5. One of the following is an Ex- officio Member of the State Pharmacy Council:
   A. Chief Pharmacist of government hospital.

B. Chief administrative medical officer of the State.

C. Registered Pharmacist.

D. Assistant Drug Contoller.

E. Chief Minister of the State.

6. License for wholesale sales of drugs specified in Schedule C & C_1 are issued in form

   A. 20A   B. 20B   C. 21B   D. 22A   E. 31

7. The State Pharmacy Council is established by the

A. Central Pharmacy Council (P.C.I.)

B. Director of drugs control administration of the State

C. Central Government

D. State Government

E. Director of Health Services of the State.

8. Pharmacy Council of India is constituted as per the provision of

A. The Pharmacy Act, 1948

B. The Drugs & Cosmetics Acts, 1940

C. The Drugs & Cosmetics Rules, 1945

D. The Pharmacy (Amendment) Act, 1976

E. None of the above.

9. Importance of Drugs & Cosmetics (Amendment) Act, 1972 is

A. Act is extended to Jammu & Kashmir

B. Act has given higher powers to Inspector of Drugs

C. Toilets soaps are included

D. Ayurvedic & Unani medicines are brought under the Act

E. All of the Above.

10. Central Drugs Laboratory was established by

A. the private firms

B. Rajya Sabha

C. The Central Government

D. The State Government

E. Drugs Controller General of India.

11. Validity of drug manufacturing license is upto

   A. 30th March   B. 1st January

   C. 30th June   D. 30th April

E. 31st December of the year following the year in which it is granted or renewed unless sooner suspended or cancelled.

12. The label of the container of any preparation containing not less than "--------" percent of volume of alcohol shall include a statement of this effect

   A. 0.5   B. 1.0   C. 3.0   D. 5.0   E. 10.0

13. The factory premises shall comply with the conditions prescribed in which Schedule of the Drugs & Cosmetics Rules
    A. Schedule M   B. Schedule N
    C. Schedule P   D. Schedule O
    E. None of the above.

14. Importance of Drugs & Cosmetics (Amendment) Act, 1964 is/are
    I. To bring Ayurvedic & Unani drugs which were till then not covered
    II. To prohibit the import, manufacture sale etc., of adulterated, misbranded, spurious or sub-standard drugs
    III. To enlarge the definition of drug.
    A. I only   B. II only
    C. III only   D. I & II only
    E. I, II & III.

15. Importance of Drugs & Cosmetics (Amendment) Act, 1982 is/are
    A. The definition of the term drug has been enlarged - insect (including mosquitoes) repellants, formulation components (including empty gelatin capsule shell etc.) & diagnostic devices are included.
    B. Toilet soaps & cosmetics are required to be manufactured under licence.
    C. Misbranded & adulterated drugs have been redefined. Misbranded, Spurious, Adulterated, Ayurvedic, Siddha or Unani drug & cosmetic have been defined.
    D. Power to ban import & manufacture risky & therapeutically unsound drug.
    E. Drugs inspector can now stop & search any vehicle or vessel or any other Conveyance.
    F. All the above.

16. Importance of Drugs & Cosmetics (Amendment) Act, 1986 is/are
    A. This amendment empowers any person or a consumer association to take samples of drugs for test/analysis and they can also prosecute firms for manufacture/sale of sub-standered drugs.
    B. Punishment have been rationalized.
    C. Provision has been made for summary trial of offences under this Act.
    D. All the above.
    E. None of the above.

17. The name of pharmacist can be removed from the register if the Registrar is satisfied that:
    A. The name has been entered by error or on account of misrepresentation or suppression of material fact.
    B. The pharmacist has convicted of any offence or guilty of any infamous conduct.
    C. The pharmacist employed a person for the purpose of his business of a pharmacy who has been convicted of an offence or has been guilty of any infamous conduct.
    D. All of the above.
    E. None of the above.

18. Given below are drugs and their Schedules A to E. Match them correctly
    (i) B-Complex tablets   A. Schedule C_1
    (ii) Calcium gluconate injection B. Schedule F

(iii) Smallpox vaccine   C. Schedule H

(iv) Ampicillin capsules   D. Schedule L

                                 E. Schedule C

19. According to Drugs and Cosmetics Rules, a list of Schedules are given below. Match the appropriate statement A to E with them.

(i)   Schedule G   A. Drugs used under medical supervision

(ii)   Schedule P   B. Drugs marketed under generic name only

(iii) Schedule J   C. Minimum requirements needed for a retail pharmacy

(iv)   Schedule N   D. Diseases that a drug should not claim to cure

                     E. Life period of drugs

20. Match the following with the Schedules listed in A to E correctly.

(i)   Requirements of factory premises   A. Q

(ii)   Standard for disinfectant fluids   B. V

(iii) Coal tar colors used in cosmetics   C. S

(iv)   Standards for cosmetics   D. O

                                            E. M

21. The following forms under Schedule A of the Drugs & Cosmetics Rules are utilized for applying for licenses listed A to E. Match them

(i)   Form 8   A. Application to import drugs for personal use

(ii)   Form 12A   B. Application for grant of license to sell, stock or distribute the drugs

(iii) Form 19   C. Application to import biological products

(iv)   Form 24C   D. Application to manufacture homeopathic drugs

                  E. Application to import drugs for research purposes

22. Listed below are some Schedules i to iv and the Rules A to D. Match them correctly.

(i)   Schedule C   A. Biological and special products

(ii)   Schedule F   B. Provision applicable to Vaccines, Toxins, Antigens and Sera.

(iii) Schedule M   C. GMP requirements of factory premises, plant, equipments etc.

(iv)   Schedule FF   D. Standards for surgical dressings.

                     E. Standards for ophthalmic preparations.

23. The following drugs are included under the Schedules listed in A to E. Match them.

(i)   Meprobamate   A. Schedule E_1

(ii)   Poisonous drugs   B. Schedule C and C_1

(iii) Biological & special products C. Schedule X

                                    D. Schedule Q

24. A drug is deemed to be as indicated in 1 to 4 and the corresponding definitions are given in A to E. Match with the correct ones.

(i)   Misbranded drug   A. If it is marketed without prescription

(ii)	Adulterated drug	B.	If it is imported under a name which belongs to another drug
(iii)	Spurious drug	C.	If it is not labeled in the prescribed manner
(iv)	Drug of abuse	D.	If it contains any harmful or toxic substance
		E.	If it develops addiction

25. Listed below are some of the important drugs. Classify them as per the relevant Schedules of Drugs & Cosmetics Rules.

(i)	Chlorpropamide	A.	Schedule G
(ii)	Betamethasone benzoate	B.	Schedule M
(iii)	Amaranth	C.	Schedule H
(iv)	Dexamphetamine	D.	Schedule Q
		E.	Schedule X

26. Given below from A to D are the application forms for the specific purpose listed as per D & C Act. Match them.

(i)	Manufacture of cosmetics	A.	Form No. 31
(ii)	Retail sale of Schedule C and C_1 drugs	B.	Form No. 20C
		C.	Form No. 20
		D.	Form No. 21

27. Given below from A to E are the location of the following listed. Match them correctly.

(i)	Central Drugs Laboratory	A.	Lucknow
(ii)	Central Research Institute	B.	Kasauli
(iii)	Indian Veterinary Research Institute	C.	Calcutta
(iv)	Central Drugs Research Institute	D.	Izatnagar
		E.	New Delhi

ANSWERS

1 - C; 2 - A; 3 - A; 4 - A; 5 - B; 6 - C;

7 - D; State Pharmacy Councils & Joint State Pharmacy Councils are constituted under the Pharmacy Act, 1948 by the state governments;

8 - A; 9 - A; 10 - C; 11 - E; 12 - C; 13 - A; 14 - D; 15 - F; 16 - A; ["B" & "C" are included in Drugs & Cosmetics (Amendment) Act, 1982.];

17 - D; 18 - (i) A (ii) E (iii) E (iv) C; 19 - (i) A (ii) E (iii) D (iv) C; 20 - (i) E (ii) D (iii) A (iv) C; 21 - (i) C (ii) A (iii) B (iv) D; 22 - (i) A (ii) B (iii) C (iv) E; 23 - (i) C (ii) A (iii) B; 24 - (i) C (ii) D (iii) B (iv) E; 25 - (i) A (ii) C (iii) D (iv) E; 26 - (i)A (ii) D; 27 - (i) C (ii) B (iii) D (iv) A.